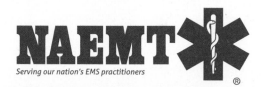

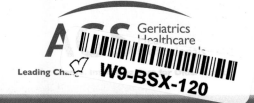

Geriatric Education

for Emergency Medical Services

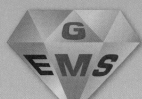

SECOND EDITION

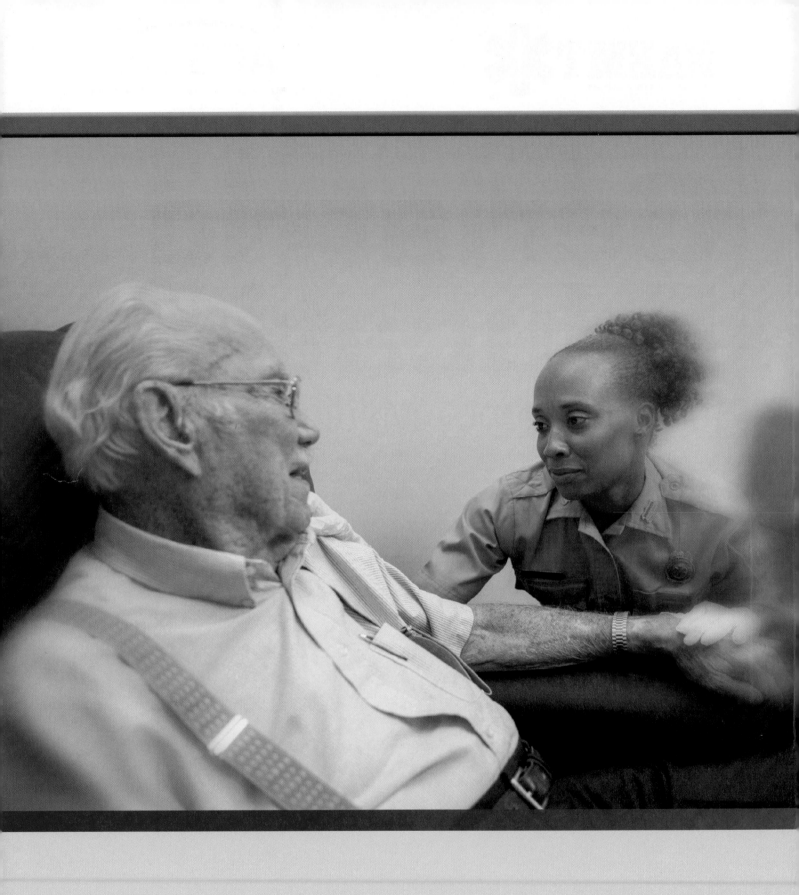

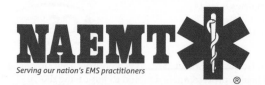

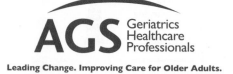

Geriatric
Education
for Emergency Medical Services

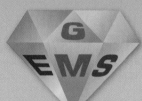

SECOND EDITION

David R. Snyder, MS, NRP
Editor

Manish N. Shah, MD, MPH
Medical Editor

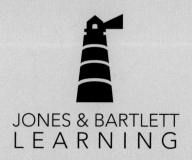

JONES & BARTLETT
LEARNING

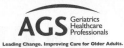

World Headquarters
Jones & Bartlett Learning
5 Wall Street
Burlington, MA 01803
978-443-5000
info@jblearning.com
www.jblearning.com

Jones & Bartlett Learning books and products are available through most bookstores and online booksellers. To contact Jones & Bartlett Learning directly, call 800-832-0034, fax 978-443-8000, or visit our website, www.jblearning.com.

American Geriatrics Society
40 Fulton Street
New York, NY 10038
212-308-1414

The American Geriatrics Society (AGS) is a not-for-profit organization of over 6,000 health professionals devoted to improving the health, independence and quality of life of all older people. The Society provides leadership to healthcare professionals, policy makers and the public by implementing and advocating for programs in patient care, research, professional and public education, and public policy.

Substantial discounts on bulk quantities of Jones & Bartlett Learning publications are available to corporations, professional associations, and other qualified organizations. For details and specific discount information, contact the special sales department at Jones & Bartlett Learning via the above contact information or send an email to specialsales@jblearning.com.

Production Credits

Chief Executive Officer: Ty Field
President: James Homer
Chief Product Officer: Eduardo Moura
VP, Executive Publisher: Kimberly Brophy
Executive Editor: Christine Emerton
Development Editor: Carly Lavoie
Production Editor: Cindie Bryan
VP, Sales: Public Safety Group: Matthew Maniscalco
Director of Sales: Public Safety Group: Patricia Einstein
VP, Marketing: Alisha Weisman

Art Development Editor: Joanna Lundeen
VP, Manufacturing and Inventory Control: Therese Connell
Composition: diacriTech
Cover Design: Scott Moden
Text Design: Kristin E. Parker
Manager of Photo Research, Rights & Permissions: Lauren Miller
Cover Image: © Jones & Bartlett Learning. Courtesy of MIEMSS
GEMS Diamond Logo Concept: Amy M. Snyder
Printing and Binding: Courier Companies
Cover Printing: Courier Companies

Library of Congress Cataloging-in-Publication Data
Geriatric education for emergency medical services : (GEMS) / American Geriatrics Society, National Association of Emergency Medical Technicians ; David Snyder, [editor]. —Second edition.
       p. ; cm.
Includes bibliographical references and index.
ISBN-13: 978-1-4496-4191-7 (pbk.)
ISBN-10: 1-4496-4191-1 (pbk.)
I. Snyder, David R., editor. II. American Geriatrics Society. III. National Association of Emergency Medical Technicians (U.S.)
[DNLM: 1. Emergencies—Programmed Instruction. 2. Aged. 3. Emergency Medical Technicians—education. 4. Emergency Treatment—Programmed Instruction. 5. Geriatrics—education. WB 18.2]
RC952.5
618.97—dc23
                           2014019227

6048

Printed in the United States of America
18 17 16 15 14   10 9 8 7 6 5 4 3 2 1

BRIEF CONTENTS

CHAPTER 1   Aging   1

CHAPTER 2   Changes with Age   15

CHAPTER 3   Communication   26

CHAPTER 4   Assessment of the Older Patient   38

CHAPTER 5   Psychosocial Aspects of Aging   65

CHAPTER 6   End-of-Life Care Issues   85

CHAPTER 7   Trauma   96

CHAPTER 8   Respiratory Emergencies   119

CHAPTER 9   Cardiovascular Emergencies   132

CHAPTER 10   Neurological Emergencies   147

CHAPTER 11   Other Medical Emergencies   169

CHAPTER 12   Pharmacology and Medication Toxicity   196

CHAPTER 13   Elder Abuse   211

CHAPTER 14   Mobile Integrated Healthcare   230

CHAPTER 15   Disasters and Older People   239

Procedures and Home Health Devices   *253*

Glossary   *285*

Index   *293*

CONTENTS

Acknowledgments xii

Preface xvii

CHAPTER 1   Aging 1

Older People and the EMS Provider 2
Historical View of Aging 2
The GEMS Diamond 3
Attitude and the EMS Provider 4
  Ageism 4
Sociology of Aging 5
  Influences in the Life Course 6
  End-of-Life Issues 6
Demographics of the
Older Population 7
  Life Expectancy 7
  Rate of Aging 7
  Geographic Distribution 7
  Living Arrangements 8
  Income and Poverty 8
  Overall Health 8
Older People and the Health Care System 9
  Use of Health Care Services 9

Types of Care Facilities for Older People 9
  Active Adult Communities 9
  Independent Living in Senior Apartments 10
  Independent Living in Congregate
  Housing 10
  Assisted Living 10
  Alzheimer's Care Facilities 10
  Nursing Homes 10
  Home Care 11
  Hospice Care 11
  Respite Care 11
Ethnogeriatrics 12
Summary 13
References 14
Additional Resources 14
Case Study 1 Summary 14
Case Study 2 Summary 14

CHAPTER 2   Changes with Age 15

Introduction 16
Nervous System 17
Sensory Changes 18
Psychological Changes 19
Respiratory System 19
Cardiovascular System 20
Integumentary System 21
Musculoskeletal System 22
Endocrine System 23

Gastrointestinal System 23
Immune System 24
Genitourinary System 24
Summary 24
References 25
Case Study 1 Summary 25
Case Study 2 Summary 25

CHAPTER 3   Communication 26

Communication and the Older Adult 27
Types of Communication Skills 27
  Verbal and Nonverbal Communication 27
  Listening 28
Age-Related Communication Challenges 28
  Vision 28
  Hearing 29
  Speech 31
Communication Disorders 32
  Aphasia 32

  Dementia 32
  Other Disorders Affecting
  Communication 34
Additional Communication Challenges 34
Communication Techniques 35
Summary 37
References 37
Additional Resources 37
Case Study 1 Summary 37
Case Study 2 Summary 37

CHAPTER 4   Assessment of the Older Patient 38

Introduction 39
Principles of Geriatric Assessment 40
Scene Size-Up 40
Initial Assessment 41
  Mental Status Assessment 41
  Circulatory Assessment 42
  Airway Assessment 43
  Breathing Assessment 44
  Patient Medications 44
Trauma Assessment 45
  Mechanism of injury 45
  Immobilization Concerns 47
  Physical Exam 48
  Putting It All Together 49
Assessing the Chief Complaint 50
  Identifying Priority Patients 50
  Detailed Physical Exam 51

Ongoing Assessment 51
Common Complaints of the Older
Patient 52
  Shortness of Breath 52
  Chest Pain 54
  Abdominal Pain 56
  Dizziness and Vertigo 58
  Fever 59
  Generalized Pain 60
  Nausea, Vomiting, and Diarrhea 61
Summary 62
References 62
Case Study 1 Summary 63
Case Study 2 Summary 63
Case Study 3 Summary 63

CHAPTER 5   Psychosocial Aspects of Aging 65

Introduction 66
Psychosocial Changes With Age 66
  Cognition 66
  Memory 66
  Personality 67
Depression 67
  Red Flags: Possible Depression 68
  Impact 68
  Screening for Depression 69
  Treatment 69
Suicide 70
  Etiology of Suicide 71
  Suicide among Older People in Long-Term
  Care Facilities 72

  Screening for Suicide Potential 72
  DOs and DON'Ts for Patients at Risk of
  Suicide 73
  Take Care of Yourself 74
Chemical Dependency and Substance
Abuse 74
  Epidemiology 74
  Medication Misuse and Abuse 75
  Risk Factors for Substance Abuse 75
  Pathophysiology of Substance Abuse in Older
  Adults 78
  Screening for Substance Abuse or Misuse 79
Approaching the Older Patient 79
  Assessment Goals 79

History 80
Environmental Observations 80
Medical Examination and Care 81
Social Setting 81
Management Considerations 82

Summary 83
References 83
Case Study 1 Summary 84
Case Study 2 Summary 84
Case Study 3 Summary 84

CHAPTER 6   End-of-Life Care Issues 85

Introduction 86
Definition of Death 86
Determination of Death 86
Pronouncement of Death 87
Certification of Death 87
Epidemiology 87
Palliative Care and Hospice 87
Good Death 88
Impending Death 88
Ethical and Legal Considerations 88
Autonomy and Consent 89
Advanced Health Care Directives 89
Surrogate Decision Maker 89
Implied Consent 90

Medical Orders for Life Sustaining Treatment
(MOLST) or Physician Orders for Life Sustaining
Treatment (POLST) 90
Do Not Resuscitate (DNR) and Do Not
Attempt Resuscitation (DNAR) Orders 90
**Communication With Families and
Companions of Deceased Patients 90**
Bereavement and Grief 92
Role of EMS on Scene 94
Critical Incident Stress Management 94
Summary 95
References 95
Case Study 1 Summary 95
Case Study 2 Summary 95

CHAPTER 7   Trauma 96

Introduction 97
**Epidemiology of Trauma in the Older
Population 97**
Falls 97
Motor Vehicle Collisions 98
Burns 99
**Physiological Changes Associated with Aging
That Impact Trauma 99**
Musculoskeletal Disorders 100
Specific Injuries in the Older Patient 101
Cervical and Spinal Injuries 101
Torso Trauma 102
Hip Fractures 102
Lower Extremity Injuries 103
Upper Extremity Injuries 103
Injuries Associated with Prosthetic
Joint Replacement 103
Assessment of Geriatric Trauma 104
Management of Geriatric Trauma 105

Immobilizing an Older Trauma Patient 106
**Preventing Falls and Injuries in Older
People 107**
Reducing Medications 108
Improving Sensory Function 108
Exercise and Balance Training 108
Use of Assistive Devices 113
Making the Home Safe 113
Proper Footwear 115
Hip Protectors 115
Personal Alarms 115
Teaching the Older Adult to Get Up Safely
After a Fall 116
Other Risk Reduction Tips 116
Summary 117
References 117
Case Study 1 Summary 117
Case Study 2 Summary 118
Case Study 3 Summary 118

CHAPTER 8   Respiratory Emergencies 119

Introduction 120
**Approach to the Older Patient with
Respiratory Signs and Symptoms 120**
Signs and Symptoms 120

Assessment 122
Specific Lung Conditions 123
Chronic Obstructive Pulmonary Disease 123
Influenza 125

Pneumonia   125
Pulmonary Embolism   125
Lung Cancer   126
Tuberculosis   127
Acute Respiratory Distress
Syndrome (ARDS)   127
Pulmonary Fibrosis   128

Congestive Heart Failure and Pulmonary
Edema   128
Patient Education   129
Summary   130
References   130
Case Study 1 Summary   131
Case Study 2 Summary   131

CHAPTER 9   Cardiovascular Emergencies 132

Introduction   133
Coronary Artery Disease   133
Acute Coronary Syndrome   134
Valvular Heart Disease   138
Arotic Value Disorders   138
Mitral Valve Disorders   139
Congestive Heart Failure   140
Assessment   140
Management   141
Electrical Disturbances   142
Assessment   142
Management   142

Hypertensive Emergencies   143
Assessment   144
Management   144
Syncope   144
Assessment   145
Management   145
Cardiac Arrest   145
Summary   145
References   145
Case Study 1 Summary   146
Case Study 2 Summary   146

CHAPTER 10 Neurological Emergencies 147

Introduction   148
Normal Age-Related Changes in the Nervous
System   148
Mental Function and Status   148
Cranial Nerve Function   148
Motor Function   149
Sensation and Reflexes   149
Posture and Gait   149
Neurological Examination of the Older
Patient   150
Complaints Related to the Nervous
System   152
Stroke and Cerebral Vascular Disease   152
Transient Ischemic Attack   155
Sudden Loss of Focal Neurological
Function   155
Generalized Weakness   156
Altered Mental Status   156
Delirium   157
Dementia   158
Delirium Versus Dementia   159

Alzheimer's Disease   159
Parkinson's Disease   160
Seizure Disorders   161
Lowered Level of Consciousness   162
Loss of Consciousness   163
Paraplegia and Quadriplegia   164
Head and Spine Trauma   165
Secondary Neurological Disorders   165
Behavioral Emergencies: Intervention,
Management, and Transport   166
Behavior That Is Potentially Threatening to
the Patient   166
Behavior That Is Potentially Threatening to
the Caregiver   167
Uncooperative Patients and Refusal of
Transport   167
Summary   168
References   168
Resources   168
Case Study 1 Summary   168
Case Study 2 Summary   168

CHAPTER 11 Other Medical Emergencies 169

Introduction 170
Infectious Diseases 170
  Age-Related Changes of Immune Function 170
  Infection in Community-Dwelling Versus Nursing Home Residents 170
  HIV 171
  Hepatitis 171
Sepsis 171
  Management 171
Urinary Tract Infections 172
  Management 172
Endocrine Emergencies 172
  Diabetes 172
  Thyroid Disorders 173
Integumentary System Emergencies 174
  Age-Related Changes in the Integumentary System 174
  Pressure Ulcers 176
  Infection in the Aging Skin 178
Gastrointestinal Emergencies 178
  Age-Related Changes in the Gastrointestinal System 178
  Gastroesophageal Reflux Disease (GERD) 179

  Gastrointestinal Bleeding 179
  Gallbladder Disease 182
  Colorectal Cancer 182
  Problems with Elimination: Constipation and Fecal Incontinence 182
Malnutrition and Dehydration 183
  Assessment 184
  Management 185
  Prevention 186
Environmental Emergencies 187
  Age-Related Changes in Temperature Regulation 187
  Hypothermia 187
  Hyperthermia 188
  Prevention 189
Burns 189
  Management 190
  Prevention 190
Cancer 191
Summary 193
References 193
Case Study 1 Summary 194
Case Study 2 Summary 195
Case Study 3 Summary 195

CHAPTER 12 Pharmacology and Medication Toxicity 196

Introduction 197
Medications and Age-Related Changes in the Geriatric Patient 197
  Passage of Medications Through the Body 197
Drug Interactions 199
  Drug–Drug Interactions 200
  Drug–Nutrient Interactions 200
  Drug–Disease Interactions 201
  Drug–Herb Interactions 202
Evidence-Based Research 203
Assessing Problems Related to Medication Toxicity or Adverse Effects 203
  History 204

  Medication Nonadherence 205
  Adverse Drug Events 206
  Drug Withdrawal Problems 207
Intervention, Management, and Transport 207
Prevention 208
Summary 209
References 209
Case Study 1 Summary 210
Case Study 2 Summary 210

CHAPTER 13 Elder Abuse 211

Introduction 212
Definitions 212
Incidence 213
Elder Abuse in Long-Term Care Facilities 213

  Characteristics of Elder Mistreatment in Long-Term Care Facilities 214
  The Nursing Home Reform Act 215
  Long-Term Care Ombudsman 217

Risk Factors   217
Theories of Abuse and Neglect   218
Observing for Clues to Elder Abuse   219
  Environmental Assessment   219
  Clinical Assessment   220
  Social Assessment   223
Sexual Assault in the Elderly   224
Interviewing the Patient   224
Interviewing Suspected Abusers   225
Putting It All Together   226

Documentation   226
Elder Abuse, Domestic Violence, and
Animal Cruelty   226
Summary   228
References   228
Additional Resources   228
Case Study 1 Summary   229
Case Study 2 Summary   229
Case Study 3 Summary   229

CHAPTER 14 Mobile Integrated Healthcare 230

Introduction   231
Mobile Integrated Healthcare
Defined   231
Health Care Reform and Mobile Integrated
Healthcare   231
MIH Program Development   232
  EMS Providers Versus MIH Providers   232
  *The Importance of Collaboration
  with Stakeholders   232*
Types of MIH Programs that Benefit Older
Persons   233
  Frequent Users of 911 Program   233
  Congestive Heart Failure Program   233
  *Observation Admission Avoidance
  Program   233*
  Other MIH Programs   233

The Role of the Primary Care Physician
in MIH   233
MIH and Quality of Life   234
  Emotional Health   234
  Physical Health: Nutrition and Hydration   234
  Social Connections   234
  Economic Security   235
  Safety   235
Resources   236
Summary   237
Case Study 1 Summary   237
Case Study 2 Summary   238

CHAPTER 15 Disasters and Older People. 239

Introduction   240
Emergency Management Phases   241
Preparedness Strategies for Older
People   241
  Personal   241
  Agency   242
  Community   242
Responsibilities of Assisted Living and Long-
Term Care Facilities During Disaster   244

Shelters   245
  *Determining Needs of Older Persons in
  Shelters   246*
Recommendations   246
Summary   250
References   251
Additional Resources   251
Case Study 1 Summary   252
Case Study 2 Summary   252

Procedures and Home Health Devices   253

Glossary   285

Index   293

ACKNOWLEDGMENTS

Editor

David R. Snyder, MS, NRP
Emergency Medical Services Lieutenant
Baltimore County Fire Department
Towson, Maryland

Medical Editor

Manish N. Shah, MD, MPH
Society for Academic Emergency Medicine
Rochester, New York

Contributors

Chapter 2: Changes with Age
Keith Widmeier, NREMT-P, CCEMT-P, EMS-I
University of Cincinnati
Cincinnati, Ohio

Chapter 4: Assessment of the Older Patient
Catherine Z. Curtis, RN, MSN, AGPCNP, CNL, CCRN
Director, The Caring Well Institute
D'Youville Life & Wellness Community
Lowell, Massachusetts

Chapter 5: Psychosocial Aspects of Aging
Laurie Weaver, RN, BSN, EMT-P
Massillon, Ohio

Chapter 6: End-of-life Care Issues
Andrew Bartkus, RN, MSN, JD, CEN, CCRN, CFRN,
   NREMT-P, FP-C
Emergency Department Director
Sandoval Regional Medical Center
Rio Rancho, New Mexico

Chapter 7: Trauma
Andrew N. Pollak, MD
The James Lawrence Kernan Professor and Chairman
Department of Orthopaedics, University of Maryland School
   of Medicine
Chief of Orthopaedics, University of Maryland Medical
   System
Medical Director, Baltimore County Fire Department
Special Deputy US Marshal
Baltimore, Maryland

Colleen Christmas, MD
Associate Professor of Medicine
Division of Geriatric Medicine, Johns Hopkins University
Baltimore, Maryland

Chapter 8: Respiratory Emergencies
Al Benney, CP, NREMTP
Hennepin Technical College
Brooklyn Park, Minnesota

Chapters 9: Cardiovascular Emergencies and Chapter 10:
   Neurological Emergencies
Alan Heckman, MSPAS, PA-C, NRP, NCEE
Assistant Professor
DeSales University
Physician Assistant Program
Center Valley, Pennsylvania

Chapter 12: Pharmacology and Medication Toxicity
Chris Coughlin, PhD, NRP
EMT Program Director
Glendale Community College
Phoenix, Arizona

Chapter 14: Mobile Integrated Healthcare
Nicholas J. Montelauro, NRP, NCEE
Terre Haute, Indiana

Matt Zavadsky, MS-HSA, EMT
Director of Public Affairs
MedStar Mobile Healthcare
Fort Worth, Texas

GEMS Steering Committee

Colleen Christmas, MD
American Geriatrics Society

Matt Zavadsky, MS-HSA, EMT
National Association of Emergency Medical Technicians

Zara Cooper, MD
American Association for the Surgery of Trauma

Howard Mell, MD, MPH, FACEP
American College of Emergency Physicians

Joan Somes, RNC, MSN, PhD, CEN, CPEN, FAEN, NREMT-P
Emergency Nurses Association

Keith Widmeier, NREMT-P, CCEMT-P, EMS-I
National Association of Emergency Medical Services Educators

COL Richard Hilburn, MD
National Association of State EMS Officials

Manish N. Shah, MD, MPH
Society for Academic Emergency Medicine

National Association of Emergency Medical Technicians 2014 Board of Directors

Officers
President: Don Lundy
President-Elect: C. T. Kearns
Secretary: James A. Judge, II
Treasurer: Dennis Rowe
Immediate Past-President: Connie Meyer

Directors
Rod Barrett
Aimee Binning

Chris Cebollero
Ben Chlapek
Bruce Evans
Paul Hinchey, MD
Scott Matin
Chad E. McIntyre
Cory Richter
James M. Slattery
Matt Zavadsky

National Association of Emergency Medical Technicians GEMS Committee

Chair: Daniel Talbert, MA EMT-P
University of Florida Health
Jacksonville, Florida

Lead Editor: Dave Tauber, BS NR-P, CCEMT-P, FP-C, NCEE
Yale New Haven Sponsor Hospital Program
New Haven, Connecticut

Medical Director: Manish Shah, MD, MPH
University of Rochester School of Medicine and
    Dentistry
Rochester, New York

Committee Members
Gregory Adams, BS, NREMT-P
Turlock, California

Linda Bell, MSN, ARNP, EMT-P
Consultant Services
Middleburg, Florida

Lance Villers, PhD, LP
Department of Emergency Health Sciences, University of Texas
    Health Science Center
San Antonio, Texas

Connie Meyer, RN, EMT-P
Anderson County, Kansas

Reviewers

Linda M. Abrahamson, BA, ECRN, EMT-P, NCEE
Advocate Christ Medical Center—EMS Academy
Oak Lawn, Illinois

Dennis Baier BSN, RN, EMT-P
Ozarks Technical Community College
Springfield, Missouri

Terri Bailey, EMT, Educator, Training Officer
Hart County EMS/State Fire Commission Area #4
Kentucky Technical College
Munfordville, Kentucky

Michael W. Baker, Paramedic
U.S. Army Department of Combat Medic Training
Converse, Texas

Stanley Baldwin, EMT, MA
Foothill College
Los Altos Hills, California

Stephen J. Barney, NR EMT-P, EMS Coordinator
Vance Granville Community College
Wise, North Carolina

Bruce Barry, RN, BSN, CEN, NRP, CIC
Peak Paramedicine, LLC
Wilmington, New York

Ryan Batenhorst, BA, NRP, EMSI
Southeast Community College
Lincoln, Nebraska

Alan Batt, NQEMT-P, CCP, Clinical Educator
National Ambulance LLC
Abu Dhabi, UAE

Andrew Binder, MS, NRP, CCEMT-P, I/C
Spearfish Ambulance
Spearfish, South Dakota

Christopher Black, M.A.Ed, BA, CEP, NCEE
Estrella Mountain Community College
Avondale, Arizona

Leo Bosner
Director of Training, Education, and Research
International Institute of Global Resilience
Bethesda, Maryland

Patt Cope, MEd, NRP
Arkansas State University—Beebe
Beebe, Arkansas

Chris Coughlin, PhD, NRP
Public Safety Sciences
Glendale, Arizona

Amanda T. Creel, RN, BS, NRP
University of South Alabama
Mobile, Alabama

Sean Davis, CICNRP, EMS-I
Auburn Career Center
Concord, Ohio

Mark Deavers, Paramedic
SUNY Canton
Gouverneur, New York

Stephanie Dornsife, MS, RN, NRP, CCEMT-P, EMS-IC
Wentworth Douglass Hospital
Dover, New Hampshire

Michael J. Dunaway, Assistant Professor, BHS, NRP, CCP, NCEE
Greenville Technical College
Greenville, South Carolina

Jeffrey L. Foster, NRP, I/C, CCEMT-P, EMD
Delta Ambulance, Education Coordinator
Waterville, Maine

Victoria Gallaher, CCP, FP-C
Nauvoo Fire Protection District
Nauvoo, Illinois

Scott A. Gano, BS, NRP, FP-C, CCEMT-P
Columbus State Community College
Columbus, Ohio

Jason A. Grafft, M.Ac, NREMT
Laerdal Medical Corp., Metropolitan State University
Saint Paul, Minnesota

Kevin M. Gurney, BS, CCEMT-P, I/C
Delta Ambulance
Waterville, Maine

Randy Hardick, NREMT-P, BA, Department Chair, Program Director
Saddleback College EMS Programs—EMT and Paramedic
Mission Viejo, California

Rick Hilinski, BA, EMT-P
Community College of Allegheny County Public Safety Institute
Pittsburgh, Pennsylvania

Paul J. Honeywell, CEP, NRP
Flagstaff Medical Center
Flagstaff, Arizona

Justin Hunter, BAS, NRP, FP-C
Oklahoma State University—Oklahoma City
Oklahoma City, Oklahoma

Rianne Kemphorst, Manager of Training and Education
RAV Gooi en Vechtstreek
The Netherlands

Randall Kirby, BS/EMTP, CCP, I/C
Macon County EMS
Lafayette, Tennessee

Ashley Knights, Registered Nurse & Paramedic
School of Health, The University of Northampton
United Kingdom

Daniel W. Lewis, MBA, NREMT-P
Indianapolis EMS
Indianapolis, Indiana

Michael E. Lisa, BS, NJ EMT Instructor
TRINITAS Medical Center
Elizabeth, New Jersey

Christy Little, RN, AAS, CCEMT-P
Utica, Mississippi

Jeanette S. Mann RN, BSN, NRP
Director of Emergency Medical Services Program
Dabney S. Lancaster Community College
Clifton Forge, Virginia

Amy Marsh, BA, NRP
Sioux Falls Fire Rescue
Sioux Falls, South Dakota

Scott A. Matin, MBA, NREMT-P
MONOC Mobile Health Services
Wall, New Jersey

Mitchell A. Matlow, MICP
San Jose Fire Department EMS Division
San Jose, California

Donna McHenry, MS, NREMT-P
Los Alamos Fire Department
Los Alamos, New Mexico

Janis J. McManus, MS, NREMT-P
Virtua Emergency Medical Services
Mt. Laurel, New Jersey

Melisa McNeil, EMT-P, MHS
Western Carolina University
Cullowhee, North Carolina

Howard K. Mell, MD, MPH, CPE, FACEP
Department of Surgery, University of Illinois at Urbana, College
    of Medicine
South Russell, Ohio

Fred Mueller, NRP, FPC
Temple University Health System
Holland, Pennsylvania

Richard L. Naumann, BS, AAS, SEI, AEMT
Waitsburg EMS
Waitsburg, Washington

Keith Noble, MS, LP, NREMT-P, Commander
Austin–Travis County EMS
Austin, Texas

Amiel B. Oliva, BSN, RN, REMT-A
EMR Healthcare and Safety Institute
National Ambulance (Abu Dhabi, UAE)
Quezon City, Philippines

**Chris Ottolini, EMT-P, Paramedic Supervisor, Adjunct
    Instructor, NASM-CPT**
Coast Life Support District
Gualala, California
Santa Rosa Junior College Public Safety Training Center
Windsor, California

Sean F. Peck, M.Ed, EMT-P
WestMed College
Chula Vista, California

Stephen Post, NREMT-P, CIC, RF
New York Methodist Hospital Center for Allied Health
    Education
Brooklyn, New York

John Reed, MPH, BSN, RN, NRP
Birmingham Regional EMS System
Birmingham, Alabama

Mike Reilley, NREMT-P
MONOC
Toms River, New Jersey

Timothy J. Reitz, BS, NREMT-P, NCEE
Conemaugh Memorial Medical Ctr. Conemaugh School of EMS
Johnstown, Pennsylvania

Nicholas Russell, AAS, FI-2, EMS-I, NRP
Edgewood Fire/EMS
Edgewood, Kentucky

Karen Scheuch, RN, NRP
Eastern Panhandle EMS Education System
Inwood, West Virginia

Shadrach Smith, BS Bio, NRP, LP
CME Associates, Paramedic Advantage
Anaheim, California

Joan Somes, RNC, MSN, PhD, CEN, CPEN, FAEN, NREMT-P
Regions Hospital EMS
St. Paul, Minnesota

Daniel A. Svenson, BA, NR-Paramedic
Portland Fire Department
Portland, Maine

Michael E. Tanner, FP-C, NRP, MCCP
Air Evac Lifeteam, RESA-V
Parkersburg, West Virginia

**Annmary Thomas, M.Ed., NREMT-P, EMS Program
  Director**
STAR Career Academy
Philadelphia, Pennsylvania

Justin G. Tilghman, MS, CEM, EMTP
Lenoir Community College
Kinston, North Carolina

John C. Tomlinson, Sergeant, EMT-P, EMSI
City of Cleveland, Division of EMS
Cleveland, Ohio

William F. Toon, Ed.D, NREMT-P
Battalion Chief–Training (ret.)
Johnson County MED-ACT
Lenexa, Kansas

Rebecca Valentine, BS, Paramedic, I/C, NCEE
Wellesley College EMS
Wellesley, Massachusetts

Sara VanDusseldorp, CCTP, NREMT-P, NCEE
North Lake County EMS
Waukegan, Illinois

David A. Vitberg, MD
Director, Division of Medical & Surgical Critical Care, Greater
  Baltimore Medical Center
Associate Medical Director, Baltimore County Fire
  Department
Baltimore, Maryland

David Watson, NREMT-P, CCEMT-P
Pickens County EMS
Pickens, South Carolina

Jackilyn E. Williams, RN, MSN, NRP
Portland Community College Paramedic Program
Portland, Oregon

Evelyn Wilson, MHS, NCEE, NRP
Western Carolina University
Cullowhee, North Carolina

Robert Wise, MD
Johns Hopkins University School of Medicine
Baltimore, Maryland

Andrew Wood, MS, NREMT-P
Emergency Medical Training Professionals, LLC
Lexington, Kentucky

The American Geriatrics Society and the National Association of Emergency Medical Technicians are pleased to present the second edition of *Geriatric Education for Emergency Medical Services (GEMS)*. Since the program's inception 10 years ago, over 4,000 Course Coordinators have taught GEMS in the United States and a dozen other countries throughout the world. This is a testimonial to the number of prehospital providers who have sought the knowledge to improve the care delivered to older patients.

In an affirmation of the significance of the GEMS program, the *Journal of the American Geriatrics Society* published the results of a study that concluded that the majority of EMS providers, EMS leaders, and physicians perceive a deficit in EMS education aimed at the care of older patients and desire more continuing education opportunities for EMS providers, particularly in the areas of communication and psychosocial issues (JAGS, March 2009, Vol. 57, No. 3, pp. 530–535). Another study published by the journal evaluated the effect of the GEMS course on a rural community of EMS providers. The study concluded that provision of the GEMS course resulted in an increase in the providers' comfort level in caring for older patients (JAGS, June 2008, Vol. 56, No. 6, pp. 1134–1139). Additional course feedback received from EMS providers who care for older patients every day has been centered on gaining the knowledge necessary to provide better outcomes and an improved quality of life for their geriatric patients.

As with the first edition, the development of the second edition of GEMS was achieved through a collaboration of physicians, nurses, gerontologists, EMS educators, and providers. This edition is built upon the advances in geriatric care and the lessons learned by EMS providers caring for older patients. For example, we now know that geriatric trauma patients are often undertriaged to trauma centers. The second edition's revised trauma chapter discusses the challenges of geriatric trauma care so that these patients can be correctly triaged and transported to the appropriate level of care. Additionally, the second edition includes a new chapter that addresses the needs of older people in times of disaster and introduces the reader to the concept of mobile integrated healthcare as it relates to older people.

Geriatric patients account for some of the most complex and challenging cases that the EMS provider will encounter; however, this group of patients can also be some of the most interesting and rewarding. The GEMS course has been revised and updated to include improved educational strategies and delivery methods to better prepare EMS providers to respond to the needs of older people.

David R. Snyder, MS, NRP
Editor, GEMS

CHAPTER 1

Aging

LEARNING OBJECTIVES

1. Discuss aging in society today, including demographic trends.

2. Discuss gerontology, geriatrics, and the historical view of aging.

3. Discuss the social aspects of aging, including ageism, retirement, lifestyles, family, social roles, and the financial status of older people.

4. Demonstrate sensitivity to the negative stereotyping of older people and be able to educate others about stereotyping.

5. Describe the living arrangements of older people.

6. Describe cultural differences in older people (ethnogeriatrics), particularly as they relate to the provision of medical care.

Older People and the EMS Provider

Aging is a part of the life cycle. As an EMS provider, you encounter older people in the community every day. Have you ever wondered what older people think about themselves? About their health? As a prehospital care professional, your views about aging most likely affect your perceptions about the older patients you serve.

Attitude Tip

It is an honor to be involved in the life of an older person in any way.

One of the major issues for those who study or work with older people is defining what constitutes "old" or "old age." Depending upon what discipline one is working in or what text one is reading, old or old age can be defined as 55, 60, or 65 years. This particular text defines older people as age 65 or older. In 2011, 41.4 million people in the United States were 65 years or older, representing 13% of the U.S. population, or over one in every eight Americans.[1] This number is expected to increase dramatically during the 2010–2030 period, as the "Baby Boomers" (those born between 1946 and 1964) turn 65.[2]

With such an expected increase in the older population, it is important for the EMS provider to understand the differences that exist between patients of different age. For example, variability increases dramatically with age. Whereas most 50-year-old adults are quite similar to most other 50-year-old adults, an 85-year-old adult is quite different from another 85-year-old adult. In fact, the over-65 population is the most heterogeneous of all **cohorts**.

As a result of the aging process, many older people suffer from one or more medical conditions. They often take multiple medications to treat these conditions and are more easily affected by poor nutrition and changes in temperature. Older people may suffer from a temporary failing in memory or from Alzheimer's disease. They may experience grief and loss from the death of loved ones, struggle with feelings of isolation, suffer a loss of independence, or experience depression. The differences older people face will complicate the way in which you deliver emergency medical care to them. For example, for an older patient who experiences trauma, you must consider whether the trauma was precipitated by a medical event. If an older person

calls 911 but appears to have no real medical emergency, what could this mean? Would you know what questions to ask to discover the underlying problem? Providing appropriate and compassionate care to older patients can often have a positive impact on the quality of their lives.

Attitude Tip

The EMS provider should value and respect the older patient and his or her unique concerns and fears, regardless of whether the older patient is clear minded and independent, frail and dependent, or suffering from dementia and living in a nursing home.

Historical View of Aging

The history of aging has its origins in the archaic period, the beginning of recorded history. For the ancient civilizations of China, India, and Asia Minor, aging personified achievement. In first century A.D. the Greek physician Galen used the term "gerocomy" to describe the medical care provided to older people. Still, it was not until the advent of science in the 1600s that researchers and scientists began to undertake a systematic study of the processes of aging.

In 1903, the term **gerontology** was coined at the Pasteur Institute in Paris to describe the study of aging; in 1909, Dr. Ignatius L. Nascher used the term **geriatrics** to describe the branch of medicine concerned with the health of older people. By the 1930s, the groundwork was laid for many of the developments in gerontology. One of the concepts that came from this period is that aging is best studied in an interdisciplinary context—that is to say, aging is a *process* involving both physical and psychological changes.

In the decade between 1950 and 1960, the generated amount of literature on aging was equivalent to the total amount that had been produced in the preceding 115 years. This increased interest in the aging process may be the reason that, while the average **life expectancy** in 1900 was 49 years, a child born in 2011 can expect to live for about 79 years. That is a gain of approximately 30 years in just one century—a gain that is unparalleled in the history of mankind.[3]

What does the history of aging mean for EMS? The organized approach to EMS began with the passage of the Emergency Medical Services Systems Act of 1973. The original intent

CASE STUDY 1

You are called to a senior citizen complex for an "unknown medical emergency." You do not know how old the patient will be or exactly what condition they are in.

■ What assumptions can be made about the patient you will encounter at this facility?
■ What do you need to determine and do once you encounter the patient?

of the system was to combat the growing number of highway traffic fatalities and out-of-hospital cardiac arrests. As EMS providers became proficient in providing emergency medical care, the scope of care and the number of patients served by the system increased. EMS providers are now increasingly called upon to care for the variety of needs of older people.

The GEMS Diamond

In caring for older patients, it is important to remember certain key concepts. The **GEMS Diamond** was created to help you remember what is different about the older patient (**Table 1-1**). The GEMS Diamond is not intended to be a format for the

Table 1-1 The GEMS Diamond
G Geriatric Patients
■ Present atypically ■ Deserve respect ■ Experience normal changes with age
E Environmental Assessment
■ What is the physical condition of the home? Is the interior or exterior of the home in need of repair? Is the home secure? ■ Are hazardous conditions present (e.g., poor wiring, rotten floors, unventilated gas heaters, broken window glass, clutter that prevents adequate egress)? ■ Are smoke detectors present and working? ■ Is the home too hot or too cold? ■ Is there a fecal or urine odor in the home? ■ Are pets well cared for? ■ Is food present in the home? Is it adequate and unspoiled? ■ Are liquor bottles present (lying empty)? ■ Is bedding soiled or urine-soaked? ■ Are there burn patterns on the walls, cabinets, or floors? ■ If the patient has a disability, are appropriate assistive devices (such as a wheelchair or walker) present and in adequate condition? ■ Does the patient have access to a telephone? ■ Are medications prescribed to someone else, out of date, unmarked, or from many physicians? ■ If the patient is living with others, is he or she confined to one part of the home? ■ If the patient is residing in a nursing facility, does the care appear to be adequate to meet the patient's needs?
M Medical Assessment
■ Older patients tend to have a variety of medical problems, making assessment more complex. Keep this in mind in all cases—that is, both trauma and medical. A trauma patient may have an underlying medical condition related to the traumatic event. ■ Obtaining a medical history is very important in older patients—no matter what the primary complaint is. ■ Initial assessment ■ Ongoing assessment
S Social Assessment

■ Assess ADLs:
  ▪ Eating
  ▪ Dressing
  ▪ Bathing
  ▪ Toileting
■ Are these activities being provided for the patient? If so, by whom?
■ Are there delays in obtaining food, medication, or toileting? The patient may complain of this, or the environment may be suggestive of this.
■ Does the patient have regular visits from family members, live with family members, or live with a spouse?
■ If in an institutional setting, is the patient able to feed himself or herself? If not, is food still sitting on the food tray? Has the patient been lying in his or her own urine or feces for prolonged periods of time?
■ Does the patient have a social network? Does the patient have ways to interact socially with others on a daily basis?

approach to the older patient; instead, it serves as an acronym for the issues to be considered when assessing an older patient. The GEMS Diamond will appear throughout the text whenever one of the four aspects of the diamond is being discussed.

"G" stands for Geriatric. In other words, the first thing you should think of when you respond to an emergency involving an older patient is that older patients are different and may present atypically. You will need to remember the changes that occur with age. Just as important, remember that an older person is as human as a child or younger adult. Treat him or her with respect and dignity.

"E" stands for Environmental assessment. The environment may contain clues to the cause of the emergency. For example, older people are more sensitive to temperature. Is the home too hot or too cold? Is the home well-kept and secure? Are there hazardous conditions (poor lighting, throw rugs, faulty wiring, broken windows, etc.)? These conditions could be clues to elder abuse, neglect, depression, inability of the person to care for self, or a number of other problems.

"M" stands for Medical assessment. Older patients tend to have a variety of medical problems and may be on numerous prescription, over-the-counter, and/or herbal medications. Obtaining a thorough medical history is very important.

"S" stands for Social assessment. Older people may have less of a social network, due to the death of a spouse, family member, or friend. This can lead to depression. Additionally, the older person may need help with **activities of daily living (ADLs)**—such as dressing and eating—and not have anyone to help. You will need to find out if the patient has sufficient social support to care for both their physical and emotional needs. Last, but not least, a social assessment—like an environmental assessment—can help you uncover signs of elder abuse and neglect.

Attitude and the EMS Provider

As noted, older people have unique needs and problems that must be managed with skill and compassion. In order to properly manage these needs, you must educate yourself about the older patients you serve and have the appropriate attitude when managing their needs (**Figure 1-1**).

It is an honor to be involved in the life of an older person. Your attitude as an EMS provider must reflect this. Just as it is your responsibility to care for the medical needs of the older patient, you must manage the social, psychological, and environmental needs of the older patient as well. No other age group served by prehospital professionals presents such unique

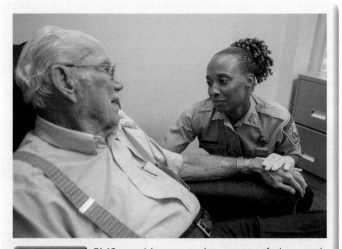

Figure 1-1 EMS providers must be aware of the needs and concerns of older people.
© Jones & Bartlett Learning. Courtesy of MIEMSS.

challenges. With proper training and an attitude of caring and compassion, you can have a profound positive impact on the lives of older patients.

Ageism

The term **ageism** was coined in 1969 by Dr. Robert Butler. Dr. Butler defined ageism as systematic stereotyping of, and discrimination against, people who are old: "Old people are categorized as senile, rigid in thought and manner, old fashioned in morality and skills…Ageism allows the younger generation to see older people as different from themselves; thus they subtly cease to identify with their elder as human beings."[4] Referring to an older person as "honey," "dear," or "pops," or calling the older person by his or her first name without permission, is a subtle form of ageism. It is never appropriate to refer to the older person using these or similar terms, even if you think the older person cannot hear or understand you.

One of the myths of aging is that when a person reaches retirement age, they become nonproductive. The reality is that the majority of older people are healthy and active, and continue to be engaged in society long after retirement (**Figure 1-2**). **Table 1-2** lists notable accomplishments made by people aged 65 years or older.

Using derogatory terms, speaking in a condescending tone, or having a negative attitude toward older patients undermines the care you provide and will erode the trust that you are trying

Attitude Tip

With an attitude of compassion and caring, you can have a profound positive impact on the lives of older patients.

Attitude Tip

"Age is an issue of mind over matter. If you don't mind, it doesn't matter." –Mark Twain

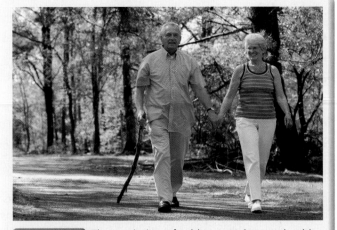

Figure 1-2 The majority of older people are healthy, active, and continue to be engaged in society long after retirement.
© Simone van den Berg/ShutterStock, Inc.

to establish. There may be instances where you are disgusted or disturbed by what you see on a scene. This is no excuse for a negative attitude. It unjustly punishes the person simply for being old—something over which they have no control.

As human beings, we must understand and accept aging as part of the life cycle and, as a society, we must reverse the attitude that aging is an affliction. As professionals, we must understand the physiology and psychology of the aging process, know how to manage the acute care needs of older patients, and educate older people about prevention techniques that promote and enhance their quality of life. EMS providers should not treat older patients with disdain and disgust, but rather with an understanding of their situations and needs and with the respect they have earned.

Keep this in mind: a person who is 90 years old has experienced the Depression, two World Wars, the Korean and Vietnam conflicts, the Cold War, the civil rights movement, the peace movement, the space age, and terrorism on our own soil. Older people are unique individuals with a lifetime of experiences. Take time to get to know some of the older patients

you serve—your life will be more enriched. By exemplifying a caring and compassionate attitude toward older people, the EMS community can begin to win the battle against ageism.

Sociology of Aging

How individuals perceive life as they grow older has a large effect on their aging process. People who have a healthy attitude may be running marathons when they are 90 years old. Conversely, people who fear growing older may feel useless and depressed. Throughout the stages of life, people have emotional reactions to the aging process, especially during major life events. For example, parents who build their lives around their children may have difficulty when their children grow older. The difficulties they have in dealing with their new lifestyle as the children grow can lead to

Table 1-2   Notable Accomplishments of Older People
■ At 65, Harlan David Sanders—better known as Colonel Sanders—started the Kentucky Fried Chicken franchise.
■ At 69, Ronald Reagan became President of the United States.
■ At 70, Benjamin Franklin signed the Declaration of Independence.
■ At 72, Oscar Swahn won a silver medal at the 1920 Olympics, holding the record as the oldest medalist.
■ At 73, Peter Mark Roget published Roget's Thesaurus. His book has never been out of print since it was first published in 1852.
■ At 74, Nelson Mandela became the oldest elected president in South Africa.
■ At 77, John Glenn became the oldest person to venture into space.
■ At 80, George Burns won an Academy Award for his performance in *The Sunshine Boys*.
■ At 81, Johann Wolfgang von Goethe finished writing *Faust*.
■ At 82, Leo Tolstoy wrote *I Cannot Be Silent*.
■ At 84, Thomas Edison produced the telephone.

(Continued)

Table 1-2 Notable Accomplishments of Older People (*Continued*)

- At 85, Claude Monet painted his famous Water Lily series.
- At 88, Michelangelo was still designing churches.
- At 89, Albert Schweitzer headed a hospital in Africa.
- At 90, Pablo Picasso was producing drawings and engravings.
- At 93, George Bernard Shaw wrote the play *Farfetched Fables*.
- At 100, Tesichi Igarishi climbed the 12,395-foot summit of Mount Fuji.

uncertainty and depression, adversely affecting the aging process. On the other hand, if parents have a healthy attitude and enjoy watching their children grow into adulthood, they will most likely view their role as evolving in their children's lives, not ending.

Later in life, women undergo **menopause**, and men undergo the lesser-known "male menopause," or **andropause**—a time of lessening of testosterone and sexual hormone activity. Just as every individual is unique, these changes affect each individual differently. In some instances, individuals alter their lifestyle, which in turn alters their aging process. Having a positive outlook on major life events can make the aging process smoother.

Views about retirement also have an effect on aging. People retire at different ages for different reasons. For some, the decision may be influenced by economic reasons. Once people stop working, they may feel the need to find another purpose in life. Those with hobbies and interests are often better able to enjoy their retirements, while those who feel they have lost their purpose age more rapidly and with greater difficulty. Coping with life's changes can be difficult, especially as one ages. The personality of the individual determines how well he or she will react to the process. Additionally, expectations regarding how the aging process will occur will directly influence the individual's own aging process.

Attitude Tip

When errors are detected regarding the attitudes or approach of others toward older people, correct them with adequate information and your positive example.

Influences in the Life Course

A variety of societal factors influence the process of aging. The following sections give an overview of some of these factors.

Social Class and Environment

The social class and environment in which a person lives directly influence how that person deals with the aging process. Social institutions and their policies often dictate how issues of modesty, dignity, self-esteem, and independence are to be accepted.

Race and Ethnicity

Our society is diverse in its ethnic culture. A person's race, ethnicity, and culture will influence how they deal with issues of aging. In some cultures, the aging process is viewed differently depending on the gender of the individual.

Independence and Decision Making

As they age, individuals will most likely want to maintain their independence as long as they possibly can. It is important to take the older person's wishes into consideration when faced with situations that could negatively impact their independence.

However, for those afflicted by certain ailments such as dementia, the ability to make sane and rational decisions decreases as their mental capacity diminishes. Bad decision making can lead to financial and health problems. Consideration of decision-making ability with regard to health care issues is vital in the prehospital setting.

Family

The family needs to consider the responsibility they have to their aging members. Specifically, physical distance between members should be taken into consideration. The nuclear family is often extended miles apart, and younger family members may not be in close proximity to their aging members (**Figure 1-3**).

Crime

Although older persons have the lowest crime victimization rates, there is disagreement among researchers about the specific fears and perceptions older people have regarding crime. Some research suggests that older people fear crime less and are more confident in the ability of law enforcement than any other age group; other studies report a general fear of crime among both urban and rural older people. There is also research that suggests that older people are aware of crime and alter their lifestyles to avoid becoming victims.

End-of-Life Issues

There are several controversial issues with regard to ending one's life to honor the individual's modesty, dignity, self-esteem, and

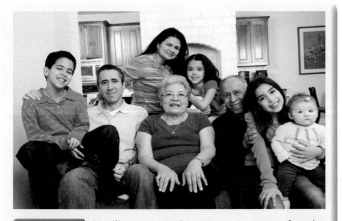

Figure 1-3 Families are an important resource for the older person.
© Jack Hollingsworth/Photodisc/Thinkstock

independence. Many feel they should have the right to determine how and when they will die. Late-life suicide often results from the loss of a spouse or the lack of wanting to continue to live with a terminal illness. Euthanasia has been legalized in a few states, but continues to be controversial. The right-to-die movement has focused on a variety of issues and circumstances; however, not all are accepted.

Most states have prehospital **do not resuscitate (DNR) orders** that emergency medical technicians and paramedics are bound to honor by state law. Most DNR orders give specific direction for the EMS provider to follow. To simplify, DNR orders specify the type of care that the EMS provider is able to render (based on the patient's or the patient's physician's request). Care may range from palliative measures to advanced life support procedures up until cessation of breathing and/or pulselessness occurs. A complete discussion of end-of-life care issues can be found in the *End-of-Life Care Issues* chapter.

Demographics of the Older Population

To understand the older population better, the EMS provider needs to understand the demographics of the older population as a whole. This section provides a brief overview of the older population in the United States.

Life Expectancy

People are living longer than ever before, increasing the number of older patients who will be served by the EMS system. As previously noted, overall life expectancy for someone born in 2011 is about 79 years.[5]

> **Attitude Tip**
>
> Always attempt to serve as an advocate for older people. Be a positive role model and a force for positive changes in the attitudes of others and in the quality of services provided to older people.

Rate of Aging

The number of people older than age 65 years has dramatically increased over the last century (**Table 1-3**). The older population began to grow rapidly in 2011, when members of the Baby Boomer generation began to turn 65. This growth is expected to continue through 2030. As a result, the population of people age 65 years and older is projected to rise from 40 million in 2010 to 55 million by 2020. By 2030, the population of that age group will be more than 72 million. In addition, the population of those age 85 years and older is expected to jump from 5.8 million to 6.6 million between 2010 and 2020. Since the trend in growth of the older population will continue, EMS providers must be knowledgeable and skilled in caring for these diverse older populations (**Figure 1-4**).

Geographic Distribution

Currently, 13% of the U.S. population is 65 years of age and older. In twenty-three states, the percentage of the population aged 65 years and older is higher than the national average. The states with the largest populations of people over the age of 65 are shown in **Figure 1-5**. The top five states with the highest percentage of resident population aged 65 or older are:[6]

1. Florida—17.3%
2. West Virginia—16.0%
3. Maine—15.9%
4. Pennsylvania—15.4%
5. Iowa—14.9%

Table 1-3 Number of Older Adults in the United States in 2011		
Age	**Number of People**	**Increase Since 1900**
65–74 years	21.4 million	10 times more
75–84 years	12.8 million	16 times more
85 years and older	5.0 million	40 times more
Source: Data from *A Profile of Older Americans 2012.* Administration on Aging, U.S. Department of Health and Human Services.		

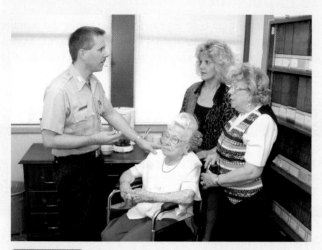

Figure 1-4 Life expectancy in the United States has increased significantly. EMS providers must know how to care for older patients.
© Jones & Bartlett Learning. Courtesy of MIEMSS

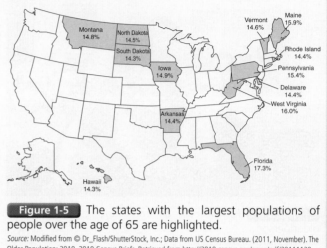

Figure 1-5 The states with the largest populations of people over the age of 65 are highlighted.
Source: Modified from © Dr_Flash/ShutterStock, Inc.; Data from US Census Bureau. (2011, November). The Older Population: 2010. 2010 Census Briefs. Retrieved from http://2010.census.gov/news/pdf/20111130_slides.pdf

People age 65 and older are less likely to live in metropolitan areas. It is estimated that 50% of older people live in suburbs, 27% live in cities, and 23% live outside of a metropolitan area.[7]

Living Arrangements

Older people live in a variety of settings—for example, with family, alone, or in institutions. For some, living arrangements are linked to income, health status, and the availability of caregivers. In 2012, among older, non-institutionalized adults in the United States, 72% of men lived with a spouse, compared with only 45% of women. This discrepancy is even sharper among women age 75 and older, only 32% of whom lived with a spouse in 2012. Some older adults also take on new family responsibilities during this period of their lives. In 2011, about 2 million older adults had one or more grandchildren living with them.

In contrast, about 28% of the older, non-institutionalized adult population lived alone in 2012, with 36% of older women living alone, compared with 19% of older men. The percentage is even higher among women age 75 and older, with nearly half living alone. These women are more likely than other women in their age group to use paid caregivers rather than rely on family to help with the activities of daily living.[8] Out of all persons 65 years of age or older, only 3.6% live in an institutional setting, with the rate of institutionalization increasing with age (**Table 1-4**).

Income and Poverty

Inadequate income can affect older adults' eating habits, the upkeep of their homes, and their access to health care. In 2011, older adults had a median income of $21,534.50, with men earning $27,707 and women earning $15,362. That same year, six million older adults were classified as living either below the poverty level or at a "near-poor" level. Older women fared worse

Table 1-4 Percentage of Older People Living in Institutions

Age in Years	Percentage Living in Institutions
65-74	1%
75-84	3%
85 and over	11%

Source: Data from *A Profile of Older Americans 2012*. Administration on Aging, U.S. Department of Health and Human Services.

than their male counterparts, with 10.7% of the former living in poverty, compared with 6.2% of the latter. Older people who lived with families were better off than those who lived alone, with 5% of those in family settings likely to be poor, compared with 16.5% of those living by themselves.[9]

Overall Health

In 2012, 44% of non-institutionalized older adults rated their health as being excellent or very good. This figure is 20% lower than that cited by adults age 18 to 64. By definition, declining health is a part of aging, and chronic conditions are common. A look at the 2-year period from 2009 to 2011 gives us a clear snapshot of the most prevalent conditions among older adults. During that time frame, just over half of all older people had arthritis, about one third suffered from heart disease, and nearly one quarter had been diagnosed with cancer. In addition to those chronic conditions, studies show that about 35% of men and 38% of women age 65 years and older report problems with hearing, vision, cognition, mobility, self-care, or other activities that allow them to continue living independently.[10]

Older People and the Health Care System

Older people are the largest single consumer of health care resources. People over the age of 65 years account for 13% of the U.S. population, but they consume more than 30% of all prescription medications and outpatient resources, including EMS, and account for almost 30% of all emergency department visits.

The emergency department is an important means of access to health care by older people. Studies have concluded that the types of illnesses for which older people use the emergency department are distinct from those of younger adults. Younger adults are typically seen for surgical problems—mostly minor trauma—whereas older patients are seen in the emergency department for medical illnesses, many of which are serious or life threatening and require admission to the hospital. Studies have also shown that younger adults tend to use the emergency department after working hours, whereas older people tend to utilize the emergency department fairly consistently around the clock. Additionally, older patients, upon presentation to the emergency department, are more likely to be acutely ill and have several coexisting conditions at the time of admission.

The emergency department serves older patients in one of three ways: for treatment of emergency conditions, as a provider of primary care, and as an entry point into the long-term-care system. Social and physical isolation often influence the older person's decision to utilize the emergency department. People who are single, widowed, or divorced are more likely to visit the emergency department, as these individuals live alone and have no immediate sources of help. Older people living in rural areas use the emergency department less frequently than their urban counterparts, but tend to require ambulance transport more frequently.

The frequency of emergency department use by older patients has a direct impact on EMS. The EMS provider is the only health care worker outside of the emergency department immediately available to assist the older person in crisis 24 hours a day, 7 days a week. The older a person is, the more likely they are to arrive to the emergency department by ambulance.

Use of Health Care Services

Tracking the number of hospital discharges, the average length of stay, and the number of visits to health care providers helps researchers analyze these trends in older adults' use of health care services. In 2010, three times as many people age 65 years and older were discharged from the hospital compared with all other age groups. The average length of stay for older adults was nearly a day longer than the average for all other age groups. Not surprisingly, older people also visit the doctor more often than their younger counterparts. In 2010, 21% of adults age 75 years and older had visited a doctor or other provider at least 10 times during the preceding year, compared with 14% of adults ages 45 to 64.

Another measure of older adults' use of health care services is their access to primary care. In 2012, nearly 96% of older adults reported that they visited a regular provider. Lack of financial resources prevented 2.4% of older adults from accessing such routine care. Researchers also pay attention to trends in older adults' spending on health care, which rose 46% between 2000 and 2011. This rapid increase considerably outpaced the rate at which health care spending rose in the adult population overall.

In 2011, 93% of non-institutionalized older adults relied on Medicare to cover a portion of their acute care services, 58% received at least some benefits from a private health insurer, and more than 9% had health insurance related to veteran's benefits. Another 9% of non-institutionalized older adults were covered by Medicaid, which also covered the cost of care for about 50% of institutionalized older adults. Fewer than 2% lacked health benefits of any kind.[11]

The **old-age dependency ratio** depicts the dependency individuals place on society as they age. It is defined as the number of older people for every 100 adults between the ages of 18 and 64 (potential caregivers). In 2010, there were 22 older people for every 100 "caregivers." By the year 2030, it is projected that there will be 35 older people for every 100 caregivers.[12] The supply of caregivers is not keeping pace with the growth of the older population. The need for caregivers is going to increase, and society will most likely have difficulty keeping up with the demand for services as the population continues to age.

Attitude Tip

"The diseases of the aged are worthy of the most careful study. Let us not dismiss his ailments with the facile diagnosis: 'you are old'." –I.L. Nascher

Types of Care Facilities for Older People

There are a variety of living facilities for older people that provide a range of care. Some facilities are more prevalent in certain geographical locations, depending on the number of older people residing in the area, to meet the community's needs. The following sections describe the different types of care facilities for older people.

Active Adult Communities

Active adult communities have become very prevalent in the United States. Also known as active adult living and active retirement communities, these communities offer age-restricted housing specifically created for seniors who enjoy participating in physical and social activities. The communities boast resort-type amenities, such as golf courses, tennis courts, pools, education classes, bike paths, and restaurants. Some of the larger communities provide their own EMS (including transport), or have first responder services available. Fees are paid by private funds only.

Independent Living in Senior Apartments

There are a number of rental developments that contain multiple units restricted to lease to those over the age of 55 years. Individuals who reside in these facilities may want additional physical or emotional security or prefer to live with other seniors. These complexes often have restricted access and may have someone on duty, such as a desk clerk, to monitor access 24 hours a day. Many are mid-rise or high-rise buildings.

Independent Living in Congregate Housing

Congregate housing contains convenience services for residents of community. Provisions may include meals, housekeeping services, transportation, or social events. Residents may have minor health concerns and need the added security of having staff and other residents located nearby. This type of housing is typically paid for on a monthly basis by private funds. Independent living is unlicensed and may vary greatly.

Assisted Living

Assisted living is also known as residential care, board and care, and boarding house. Residents residing in these facilities require assistance with one or more ADLs and/or 24-hour supervision to maintain safety. Residents tend to need assistance with medication administration, but not more significant daily medical care. They enjoy the security of 24-hour staffing. Some facilities specialize in the care of Alzheimer's patients or those with other dementias. Fees may be paid for with private funds, supplemental security incomes (SSI), long-term care insurance, or Medicaid. These facilities are typically licensed by state, and licensing varies by each state. Assisted-living facilities may be built as such, or may be contained in regular neighborhood homes (**Figure 1-6**). Assisted-living facilities also offer a variety of activities for their residents in a home-like atmosphere (**Figure 1-7**).

Alzheimer's Care Facilities

Alzheimer's care facilities are specialized care facilities for those with signs of Alzheimer's disease or other dementias. The residents of these facilities typically exhibit signs of impaired cognitive ability, forgetfulness, and/or wandering. The facility is designed to prevent residents from wandering off and to maintain safe activities, and may include features such as alarm systems on all doors and hallways that allow residents to wander in a continuous path without obstacles. Private funds, Medicaid, and long-term care insurance typically pay the fees associated with Alzheimer's care facilities.

Nursing Homes

Nursing homes are also known as skilled nursing facilities, convalescent homes, or long-term care facilities. Residents cannot perform ADLs without assistance and require 24-hour nursing care. In most cases, they are unable to ambulate without the assistance of a walker, wheelchair, or another person. A resident may need therapeutic or rehabilitative services including speech therapy, physical therapy, occupational therapy, respiratory therapy, or wound care.

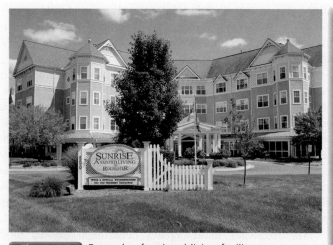

Figure 1-6   Example of assisted-living facility.
© RiverNorthPhotography/iStockphoto.com

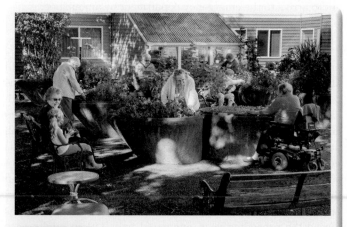

Figure 1-7   Assisted-living facilities offer a variety of activities for older people.
© Jamie Hooper/Shutterstock, Inc

These facilities are regulated by both federal and state governments to ensure quality of care. Private funds, long-term care insurance, Medicare, and Medicaid pay for the fees associated with long-term care. In 2009, there were approximately 15,700 nursing homes in the United States, comprising some 1,707,808 nursing home beds.

Home Care

Home care allows the older person to remain in his or her own home and receive assistance from family, home care nurses, and other professionals. This type of care is also known as home health care, personal care, and in-home care. Many of the patients receiving this type of care are homebound (unable to leave the home to seek routine health care) and only see a hospital physician when emergency situations arise.

With the increase in insurance regulations and restrictions in payment, home health care has become an economical alternative to facility living. Services offered include assistance with bathing, feeding, and exercising; administration of medication therapy; IV therapy; and chores (**Figure 1-8**). Private funds, long-term care insurance, private health insurance, Medicare, and Medicaid may pay for the fees.

Hospice Care

Hospice care is provided for those with terminal illnesses, either in the patient's own home or in a hospice facility (**Figure 1-9**). It allows for peace, comfort, and dignity. In 2012, an estimated 1.5 million patients received services from about 5,500 hospice programs. Of those patients, 83.4% were 65 years of age or older. The majority of hospice care is provided in the patient's place of residence, whether that be a private residence, a nursing home, or a residential facility; however, it may also be provided in a hospice inpatient facility or an acute care hospital.[13]

Hospice care focuses on **palliative care**, or relieving pain and controlling symptoms, as opposed to a primary focus on curative care. **Table 1-5** summarizes the primary diagnosis of hospice enrollees for 2012. Hospice services include supportive medical, social, and spiritual services to the terminally ill, as well as support for the patient's family. Health insurance, Medicare, or Medicaid typically covers payment for hospice services.

Respite Care

Respite care provides temporary relief for caregivers, ranging from hours to days. This care can be provided in the patient's own home or in a nursing home, assisted-living facility, or adult day

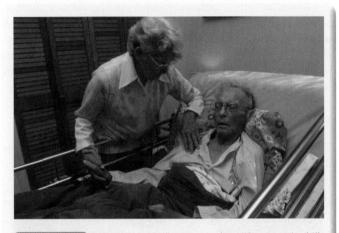

Figure 1-9 Hospice care allows people with a terminal illness to receive palliative care in their own homes or an inpatient hospice facility.
© Joel Gordon Photography

Table 1-5	Primary Diagnosis of Hospice Patients in 2012	
Cancer	**36.9%**
Noncancer diagnosis	**63.1%**
Debility unspecified	14.2%
Dementia	12.8%
Heart disease	11.2%
Lung disease	8.2%
Other	5.2%
Stroke or coma	4.3%
Kidney disease (ESRD)	2.7%
Liver disease	2.1%
Non-ALS motor neuron	1.6%
Amyotrophic lateral sclerosis (ALS)	0.4%
HIV/AIDS	0.2%

Source: Data from National Hospice and Palliative Care Organization. *NHPCO Facts and Figures: Hospice care in America.* Alexandria VA, Author, October 2013.

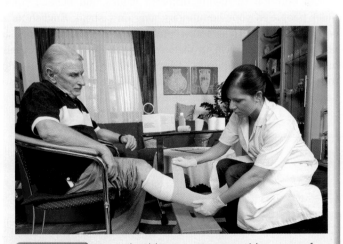

Figure 1-8 Home health care covers a wide range of activities, and can be occasional or around-the-clock.
© Lisa S./ShutterStock, Inc

care center. The care ranges from assistance with ADLs to skilled nursing care, depending on the level of care needed by the patient. In most cases, payment for respite care comes from private funds.

Ethnogeriatrics

EMS providers are encouraged to learn about the ethnic older people within the community they serve. **Ethnogeriatrics** is defined as health care for older people from diverse ethnic populations. It is important for EMS providers to study ethnogeriatrics, as demographic projections indicate that the number of ethnic older people in the United States is rapidly increasing and will continue to do so in the future.

Racial and ethnic influences impact the prevalence, morbidity, and mortality of diseases and access to hospital and community services (**Figure 1-10**). Studies indicate that on average, older persons from most ethnic minority populations use formal health care services less than their white counterparts—with the exception of emergency services and acute care.

Providing Care to Ethnic Groups

EMS providers must have an understanding of the wide degree of variation among traditional minority groups in the United

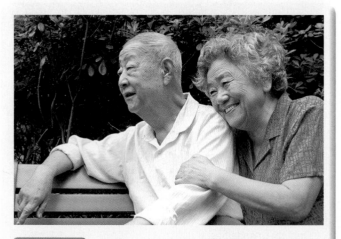

Figure 1-10 Racial and ethnic influences impact the prevalence, morbidity, and mortality of diseases and access to hospital and community services.
© Jack.Q/ShutterStock, Inc.

States, as well as the differences between older adults born in the United States and those born abroad. Providers who do not have experience working with older patients of other ethnicities may have a tendency to prejudge them based on hearsay and emotions. In order to overcome this tendency, EMS providers should:

- Examine the community's cultural values and the values that could affect their interactions with patients.
- Have adequate knowledge of the ethnic groups in their communities.
- Develop the appropriate skills necessary to manage the needs of older people of different ethnicities, such as by learning the appropriate ways of showing respect and acknowledging the older person's health beliefs.

Getting to know the cultures you serve will allow you to understand how the older population perceives and utilizes health care, as well as help you to provide professional and compassionate care. One way to do this is to interview an older person of a different ethnicity in the community who is willing to share his or her cultural values and beliefs. Another way is to invite a community leader from another ethnic group to become part of the training process. Taking the time to learn about the ethnic groups you serve will allow community cultural values to be incorporated into educational programs.

Communication Tip

Get to know the various cultures you serve in order to understand how the older population perceives and utilizes health care.

In addition to having different values and beliefs, some older people in your community may only speak English as a second language. These individuals may be able to read English perfectly but still wish to discuss complicated issues in their native language with family. Allow the older person time to do this, as others in the family may not speak English. It may also have a calming effect on the family.

CASE STUDY 2

© 123dartist/Thinkstock

You are called to the home of an older female. When you arrive at the residence you are greeted by the patient's family member who briefly speaks with you about the patient's condition before leading you to a bedroom where the patient is lying in bed.

The patient is moaning and crying out in distress. She appears to be of ethnic origin, and the family member who is present begins communicating with her in a foreign language.

- Can you assess the patient?
- What should be your first step in caring for this patient?

There also may be times when the older patient does not speak English and you must rely on a family member or interpreter to help with communication. The following are general guidelines to be employed when working with an interpreter:

- Ask short questions.
- Avoid technical terminology, abbreviations, and jargon.
- Avoid colloquialisms, abstractions, idiomatic expressions, slang, similes, and metaphors.
- Encourage the interpreter to translate the patient's own words as much as possible. This will allow for a better grasp of the patient's understanding and emotional state.
- During the interaction, look and speak directly to the patient.
- Listen to the patient, even though you do not understand. Be alert for nonverbal clues. Obvious or subtle body language is present in all cultures. If you observe particular body language cues that appear significant, take note, and attempt to learn their significance.

Communication Tip

Allow an older patient the time to discuss complicated issues in his or her native language with family if the patient desires to do so.

There are many differences in the explanations of disease and treatment that are based on a person's culture. Some patients may rely on beliefs such as nature, balance, and spiritual interventions to explain physical states. All of these beliefs have an impact on how the patient defines wellness, illness, and decision making regarding health care.

The following are general points that should be considered when conducting a physical examination on an older person of another ethnicity:

- Cross-gender examinations (a male provider examining a female patient, or vice versa) are unacceptable in

many cultures; however, do not delay care in these circumstances. The preservation of life is most important.
- Ask the patient for preference of the presence of family during the physical examination. Again, the severity of the situation will determine if time allows for this.
- Symptom recognition, meaning, and reporting will vary culturally. For example, "air heavy" or "air not right" may mean dyspnea for some Native American older people. "Heavy heart" may indicate depression among Chinese Americans.
- Dementia and depression are considered mental illnesses in some cultures and are, therefore, highly stigmatized. In other cultures, dementia is seen as part of aging and is defined as a minimal problem.
- Talking about death is considered inappropriate in some cultures, such as Chinese and Navajo.

Take the time to learn about the ethnic groups you serve. Not only do intergenerational differences exist, but cultural differences exist as well. Being a health care professional means being a student as well as a provider.

Attitude Tip

An informed mind and a positive attitude toward the older population will result in a higher interest level, improved communication and assessment, and more effective care and management of older patients.

Attitude Tip

"'One hallmark of a civilized society,' it was said, 'is its willingness to care for its poor, ill, elderly...and handicapped.'" –*Saturday Review*, May 1970

Summary

The premise of geriatric EMS is clear: care for every older patient in every sense of the word. By taking the time to study geriatrics, you are extending your knowledge beyond that of initial certification and licensure and preparing yourself to properly manage the diverse needs of the older patient. Most importantly, however, you embrace the older population you are caring for. Remember, aging is a process, and older patients are people.

One day, you and your parents, siblings, friends, and extended family will be part of the older population, perhaps living in a facility and in need of emergency care. The measures you take to improve the emergency care of the older population today will shape the emergency care you receive tomorrow.

References

1. U.S. Department of Health and Human Services. Administration on Aging (AoA), *A Profile of Older Americans: 2012* Washington, DC, Author, 2012.
2. Federal Interagency Forum on Aging-Related Statistics. *Older Americans 2012: Key Indicators of Well-Being.* Federal Interagency Forum on Aging-Related Statistics. Washington, DC, U.S. Government Printing Office, June 2012.
3. Ibid.
4. Enright, R. B. Jr. *Perspectives in social gerontology.* Needham Heights, MA, Allyn and Bacon, 1994, p 3.
5. *A Profile of Older Americans 2012.*
6. *Older Americans 2012: Key Indicators of Well-Being.*
7. U. S. Census Bureau. *The Older Population: 2010.* 2010 Census Briefs.
8. *A Profile of Older Americans 2012.*
9. Ibid.
10. Ibid.
11. Ibid.
12. *The Older Population: 2010.*
13. National Hospice and Palliative Care Organization. *NHPCO Facts and Figures: Hospice care in America.* Alexandria VA, Author, October 2013.

Additional Resources

Administration on Aging (www.aoa.gov)
American Geriatrics Society (www.americangeriatrics.org)
Assisted Living Federation of American (www.alfa.org)
Gerontological Society of America (www.geron.org)
Indian Health Service (www.ihs.gov)
National Asian Pacific Center on Aging (www.napca.org)
National Association of Area Agencies on Aging (www.n4a.org)
National Caucus and Center on Black Aged (www.ncba-aged.org)
National Center on Elder Abuse (www.elderabusecenter.org)
National Hispanic Council on Aging (www.nhcoa.org)
National Indian Council on Aging (www.nicoa.org)
National Institute on Aging (www.nih.gov/nia)
National Pacific/Asian Resource Center on Aging (www.napca.org)
U.S. Bureau of the Census (www.census.gov)

CASE STUDY SUMMARIES

Case Study 1 Summary

No other age group served by prehospital professionals presents such unique challenges as the older population. Some 60 year olds are bed bound, while some 90+ year olds are still living independently at home. The age and condition of patients in senior citizen complexes vary widely. Not all patients are bedridden or sitting in a wheel chair; many are up and about, engaging in activities that involve the mind and body. This patient may only be in the care center for a short time period while receiving post-op care following recent surgery. Additionally, the patient may not even be a resident at the center; he or she may only be visiting a loved one or friend, or attending a community activity sponsored by the center.

As you approach the patient, consider speaking more loudly and clearly, and positioning yourself in such a way that the patient can see your lips when you speak. You may need to give the patient a little more time to organize answers and have patience as the patient relates his or her history and medications to you. Additionally, you will need to compare the patient's "normal" vital signs and usual findings to your current findings. For example, the patient may have been suddenly stricken with chest pain or weakness while attending a community activity, or he or she may have been bedridden and is now worsening. Regardless of the patient's condition, remember to stay calm, patient, and gentle as you provide care to the older adult.

Case Study 2 Summary

Just because the patient does not appear to speak English does not mean she cannot. Elicit help from the family member who is able to communicate with the patient, but do not assume the patient is unable to understand and/or speak English. She may be fearful, in too much distress, or unwilling to attempt to show how much, or how little, English she knows. Additionally, if the patient appears to be unable to understand what you are saying, reasoning may include hearing loss or even stroke. You must do your best to assess the patient and gather the patient's history regardless of your assumption.

Ask simple questions and give simple explanations; if necessary, this can be accomplished via the family member. Ask permission to perform an exam, keeping in mind that the physical exam should include the same steps, whether the patient speaks English or not. You must also remember that disrobing the older adult can lead to modesty issues and also may have cultural implications. In addition, different cultures have different approaches to aging, so it is a good idea to identify and learn about the different cultures in your area and use this information during patient assessment. Ask about symptoms such as vomiting, bleeding, or pain. Have the patient point to where it hurts. If you put in the time and effort, much information can be obtained through the family member who is translating for you; however, never assume the patient cannot share the information with you.

CHAPTER 2

Changes with Age

LEARNING OBJECTIVES

1. Define the factors that cause older people to be at risk for increased medical care.

2. List the major diseases and disorders common to older people.

3. Define normal psychological changes affecting older people.

4. Identify the general decline in organ systems in older people.

5. Explain why the special needs of older people and the changes that the aging process brings about in physical structure, body composition, and organ function provide a fundamental knowledge base for maintenance of life support functions.

Introduction

The human body has the ability to age for about 115 years. However, in the everyday process of replacing dead cells with new ones, the body's ability to regenerate cells is surpassed by the amount of cell death, which ultimately leads to tissue death, organ death, and, finally, death of the body. The top causes of death in older patients include heart disease, cancer, and cerebrovascular accident (CVA) (**Table 2-1**).[1] Aging of body systems makes the older person more prone to the effects of these disease states.

With advancing age, everyday activities take on new requirements. Activities of daily living (ADLs) include basic everyday functions needed to sustain life, such as feeding oneself, walking, dressing, and getting up from a chair. **Instrumental activities of daily living (IADLs)** include basic tasks that require a higher level of function, such as going shopping, making a meal, cleaning up, or using the telephone. As a person ages, ADLs and IADLs may take more planning or may require additional help that the person did not need in his or her younger years (**Figure 2-1**). For instance, a decrease in muscle mass can mean that the individual can carry only lighter loads of groceries from the store, making additional or more frequent trips necessary. Additionally, deterioration in eyesight, hearing, and peripheral nervous system response can make driving more difficult. Older drivers may compensate for these deficiencies by taking commonly traveled routes or making three right turns in order to avoid one left turn. They may also develop medical complaints upon overexertion.

Seemingly minor ailments can be excessively burdensome to an already compromised older person. For example, an upper respiratory infection can make the patient weaker, keeping him or her from getting up and having meals or drinking the appropriate amount of liquids. This could then lead to dehydration,

Table 2-1	Top Ten Causes of Death in 2010 for Persons Age 65 and Older in the United States
Cause	**Number of Deaths**
1. Diseases of the heart	477,338
2. Cancer	396,670
3. Chronic lower respiratory diseases	118,031
4. Cerebrovascular diseases	109,990
5. Alzheimer's disease	82,616
6. Diabetes	49,191
7. Influenza and pneumonia	42,846
8. Nephritis, nephrotic syndrome, and nephrosis	41,994
9. Accidents	41,300
10. Septicemia	26,310

Data from: National Vital Statistics Reports, December 20, 2013; 62 (6).

CASE STUDY 1

You are at the local senior citizens center performing educational outreach. A resident named Lisa comes up to your booth and requests a blood pressure check. After taking her blood pressure, you note that she is hypertensive with a blood pressure of 154/96. You inquire further and she reveals that she has a history of hypertension but is out of her Lopressor medication. She tells you a friend from the senior center offered her Capoten—the hypertension medication of the friend's deceased husband—and she asks if it would be okay to take it even though it is a different medication than what she was prescribed.

- Is it okay for her to take the medication?
- What should your response be?

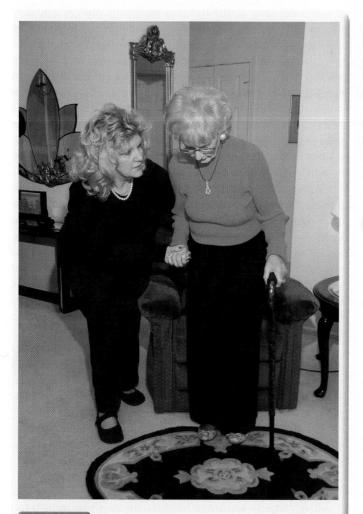

Figure 2-1 For older adults, activities of daily living may require help or additional planning.

Courtesy of John Valentini, Jr.

Attitude Tip

Realize that while changes in anatomy and physiology occur as people get older, growing old does not naturally or normally include confusion, dementia, delirium, depression, falls, weakness, syncope, or other conditions related to disease processes. Establish a baseline for your patient based off of a history provided by the patient or the patient's caretaker.

Nervous System

Nervous system changes can result in the most debilitating of age-related ailments. The central and peripheral nervous systems significantly change during a person's lifetime. The brain weight will shrink 10% to 20% by age 80. There is a selective loss of 5% to 50% of **neurons**—the cells that make up nerve tissue and receive and transmit impulses—and the remaining neurons shrink in size. The frontal lobe will lose up to 20% of its **synapses**, the junctions between neurons. Motor and sensory neural networks become slower and less responsive. Despite all of these changes, the metabolic rate in the older brain does not change, and oxygen consumption remains constant throughout a person's lifetime.

Sandwiched between the meninges and protected by cerebrospinal fluid (CSF), the brain takes up almost all of the space provided for it in the skull. Age-related shrinkage (**atrophy**) of the brain produces a void between the brain and the outermost layer of the meninges—the dura mater. Atrophy of brain tissue can result in an estimated 25% loss of deep sleep as well as a 55% loss of short-term memory. Brain shrinkage also provides room for the brain to move when stressed and stretches the bridging veins that return blood from inside the brain to the dura mater. If trauma moves the brain forcibly, the bridging veins can tear and bleed (**Figure 2-2**). Bleeding can empty into the void, resulting in a **subdural hematoma**, and go unnoticed for some time. Due to brain atrophy, the typical signs of increased intracranial pressure (ICP) will take longer to develop in the older patient. Intracranial pressure will not rise until the void space has been filled and pressurized, although there may be other signs that a head injury has occurred, such as abrasions, lacerations, and facial bruising.

Considering the breakdown of the various components of the neurological system, the older patient may experience a variety of issues that are baseline. For example, because of changes in sodium levels and plasma osmolality, the patient may experience excessive thirst. Changes in electrolytes may also affect the compensatory mechanisms and feedback loops utilized in thermoregulation.

Peripheral nerve function slows with aging, and peripheral neuropathies may develop, causing peripheral sensations to become diminished and misinterpreted. Patients may also develop optic neuropathies, which can cause dimmed vision and a decreased field of vision. This makes for slow reflexes,

making the patient's respiratory symptoms even worse. Because the older person does not have the reserves that a younger person might have, he or she may have a harder time compensating for illness and often will be forced to seek medical care. The same holds true for patients who have an acute exacerbation of a chronic condition, such as chronic obstructive pulmonary disease (COPD).

Multiple health conditions combine to make assessing and caring for the older person difficult. Conditions affecting one system can produce problems that affect another; for example, the patient who has both congestive heart failure (CHF) and COPD will have a build-up of fluid from the CHF that can worsen the COPD, making assessment and management more difficult.

Changes in anatomy and physiology can also lead to an increase in patient complaints. The older patient may become short of breath more easily due to decreases in normal lung function, or may trip more often because of a reduction in the muscle mass needed to move around. Utilizing a systems approach, this chapter looks at some of the body changes that occur in older patients.

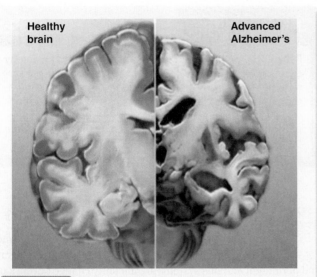

Figure 2-2 Brain atrophy with age can make tearing of the bridging veins more likely with trauma, as well as create a space into which bleeding can occur without producing immediate signs of increased intracranial pressure.

a contributing cause of trauma. As nerve endings deteriorate, the ability of the skin to sense the surroundings becomes hindered. Hot, cold, sharp, and wet items can all become dangerous because the body cannot sense them quickly enough. In addition, pain from an injured area may not be felt in the affected tissue, but rather in the surrounding areas. This can alter the classic presentation of disease states. Pain from a cardiac event, such as angina, may present only as neck or jaw pain in the older person; and chest pain or pressure, which is normally associated with cardiac problems, may be absent or lessened. As providers, we rely on the sensation of pain to treat a patient's illness or injury; however, some older patients may not experience any pain at all despite having a cardiac problem.

Sensory Changes

Pupillary reaction and ocular movements become more restricted with age. The pupils are generally smaller in older patients, and opacity of the eye's lens lowers visual acuity and makes the pupils sluggish in responding to light. Visual distortions are also common in older people. Cloudiness of the lens, known as cataracts, as well as thickening of the lens makes it harder for the eye to focus, especially at close range. Approximately 30% to 40% of patients who suffer retinal detachment have had previous cataract surgery.[2] Retinal detachment is a disorder in which the retina separates from the retinal pigment epithelium, causing loss of vision. In addition, the amount of light on the cornea that reaches the photoreceptors in the retina decreases dramatically with age, ultimately affecting the patient's color vision. Night adaptation, commonly referred to as night vision, diminishes because of decreased rods, smaller pupils, lens alterations, and vitamin A deficits. Presbyopia is a condition in which the eyes' ability to focus on nearby objects gradually decreases. In contrast, myopia is a condition in which objects far away appear blurry but the ability to see nearer is unaltered.

A variety of eye diseases may develop throughout the aging process. The most notable of these is glaucoma, a disorder in which the intraocular pressure increases and causes optic nerve atrophy. Glaucoma takes on a variety of forms that can cause a range of symptoms, from cloudy vision to blindness. Macular degeneration causes a portion of the patient's retina to break down over time. Patients with macular degeneration may require more light to see, have blurry vision, or see spots.

During eye exams in the field, upward gaze may be limited in many normal older patients because of degenerative changes in the elevator muscles. Additionally, tear production may be diminished as a potential side effect from a variety of medications. Peripheral fields of vision become narrower and there is a greater sensitivity to glare, which leads to a constricted visual field. These patients may become disoriented and anxious when they cannot adjust to the surroundings. Make every effort to allow the patient to wear eyeglasses and adjust the light to reduce this stress (**Figure 2-3**).

Beyond disorders that originate in the eye, some disorders originate in other areas but affect the eyes. For example, patients who have chronic hypertension may experience visual disturbances due to an increase in intraocular pressure. These symptoms are usually temporary and resolve when the blood pressure is controlled. Diabetes can cause several issues, including glaucoma, cataracts, and damage to the retinal vasculature known as retinopathy. Visual disturbances can also be caused by many neurological disorders such as strokes and brain tumors.

Hearing loss is about four times more common than loss of vision. Older people often have the greatest loss at high frequencies. With age, changes in several structures of the ear produce loss of high-frequency hearing, or even deafness. If an older

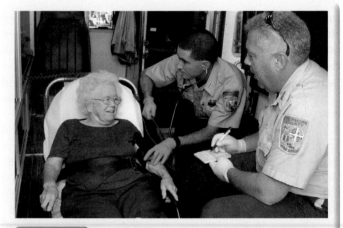

Figure 2-3 Ensuring that an older patient who has eyeglasses (or a hearing aid) is using it may reduce the patient's disorientation and stress, and will likely improve your communication with the patient during assessment.

patient uses a hearing aid for everyday activity, it is best to keep it in place to provide for better communication both during your assessment and for transport to the hospital, where there will be further medical evaluation.

Some patients may develop neuropathies (diminished or loss of sensation). The most common neuropathy encountered in the field is diabetic neuropathy, which generally affects the lower extremities. Some patients lose sensation to the point that they cannot feel when swelling and constriction of the foot is causing circulation loss to the extremity. Neuropathies can also cause patients to have difficulty differentiating temperatures, which can lead to accidental trauma. Beyond diabetic neuropathy, some patients may have neuropathies from a variety of medical disorders that cause vascular compromise as well as nerve damage.

Attitude Tip

Avoid assumptions or thoughts like "They're just old—what do you expect?" or "He's supposed to be confused/demented/delirious—look at his age!" Always rule out medical problems (head trauma, infection, metabolic problems, depression) before concluding that an older patient is demented.

Psychological Changes

Older adults often find themselves dealing with medical illness, physical limitation, and social loss all at the same time. Psychological problems of this age group include depression, anxiety, and adjustment disorders. These conditions are quite common, but they are by no means a normal part of the changes that occur with aging. (The *Psychosocial Aspects of Aging* chapter discusses these subjects in more detail.) Depression and anxiety can be associated with medical conditions such as heart disease or diabetes, and with medication use. These factors may contribute to excessive demanding and controlling behavior on the part of the older adult, and may cause family members or caregivers to be resistant, frustrated, or angry, making the situation more difficult to handle.

Respiratory System

The respiratory system changes many times throughout a person's lifetime. All parts of the system are affected by aging, and age-related changes in the respiratory system result in a predisposition to respiratory illness. A minor respiratory infection may propel the older patient into a life-endangering episode, and even normal activity can produce shortness of breath that necessitates resting.

Musculature of the upper airway weakens with age. This weakness may allow the tongue and soft tissue of the oropharynx to close in easily, narrowing the airway when the patient becomes overtaxed or less responsive. In addition, changes to bones and teeth can alter the shape of the face and mouth, making an airway harder to maintain when attempting to ventilate these patients.

Many older patients require dentures or dental appliances to eat. Improperly fitted or loose plates can result in an airway obstruction. Dentures are also associated with food-related obstructions due to the loss of sensation of the hard palate (roof of the mouth). A denture made for the upper jaw has a plastic connection that covers the hard palate, an area that provides sensory information required for determination of food particle size. When the denture blocks this sensation, the patient may attempt to swallow a larger piece of food than is tolerable. (You may be familiar with the same risk caused by alcohol intoxication.)

The loss of mechanisms that protect the upper airway is a concern in older adults. These can include a decreased ability to clear secretions, as well as decreased cough and gag reflexes. The cilia that line the airways lessen as we age, hindering the body's ability to move mucus out of the respiratory system, and the innervation of the structures in the airway provides less sensation. Without the ability to maintain the upper airway, aspiration and obstruction are more likely.

The smooth muscle of the lower airway also weakens with age. When a younger patient inhales, the airway maintains its shape, allowing air to enter (**Figure 2-4A**). As these muscles weaken with age, strong inhalation can make the walls of the airway collapse inward and cause inspiratory wheezing, just as strong exhalation can cause expiratory wheezing (**Figure 2-4B**). The collapsing airways result in low flow rates because less air can move through the smaller airways, and air trapping may occur because air does not completely exit the alveoli

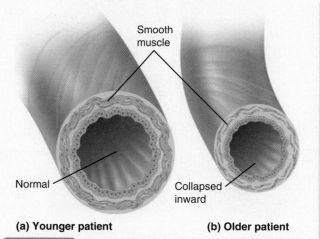

(a) Younger patient   **(b) Older patient**

Figure 2-4 A. Healthy muscle in the younger patient's airway helps maintain the open airway during the pressures of inhalation. B. Muscle weakening with age can lead to airway collapse that may produce wheezes.

(incomplete expiration). Gas exchange becomes even more problematic as the alveoli lose their shape and the sacs become baggy.

By age 75, the **vital capacity** (volume of air moved during the deepest inspiration and expiration) can drop to 50% of what it was in young adulthood.[3] This occurs because of the loss in respiratory muscle mass, increases in the stiffness of the thoracic cage, and decreases in the available surface area for the exchange of air. The total lung capacity—a combination of vital capacity and **residual volume** (the amount of air left in the lungs after the maximum possible amount of air has been expired)—increases significantly as well. As the total lung capacity increases, patients may develop the physical appearance of a large front-to-back diameter of the chest, commonly referred to as "barrel chest." The result is stagnant air resting in the alveoli and the hampering of good gas exchange, which can produce a relative **hypercarbia** (increased carbon dioxide in the bloodstream) and related acidosis, even at rest.

Aging adversely affects ventilatory function. The spine, ribs, breastbone, and muscles work together to pump air in and out of the lungs (**ventilation**). With age, the muscles of the chest wall and the diaphragm weaken. **Kyphosis**, or exaggeration of the curvature of the upper spine, can further reduce the body's ability to compensate during respiratory distress.

The brain's processing of sensory input from the nervous system is the most overlooked aspect of the respiratory system affected by age. **Chemoreceptors** located in the aortic arch sense carbon dioxide and oxygen concentrations in the blood and signal the brainstem to trigger each breath (**Figure 2-5**). With age, the sensitivity of these receptors decreases. Nerve impulse transmission from the brainstem through the phrenic nerve (which controls the diaphragm) and intercostal nerves slows, which can lead to a sluggish response to signals from the chemoreceptors. This sluggish response will lead to a lowered arterial oxygen concentration of approximately 1 mm Hg/year from age 65 to 80. A pulse oximetry reading of 93% to 95% may be normal because of these changes.

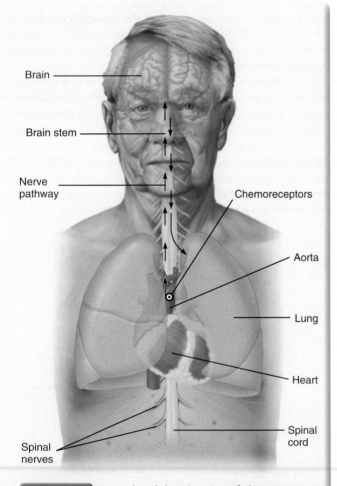

Brain

Brain stem

Nerve pathway

Chemoreceptors

Aorta

Lung

Heart

Spinal cord

Spinal nerves

Figure 2-5 Age-related deterioration of chemoreceptor sensitivity in the aortic arch and nerve signal transmission can slow signals to and from the brainstem that control ventilation.

Cardiovascular System

Cardiac function declines with age consequent to anatomic and physiologic changes that are largely related to the high incidence of coronary disease caused by **atherosclerosis**. In this disorder, cholesterol and calcium build up inside the walls of the blood vessels, forming plaque. The accumulation of plaque eventually leads to partial or complete blockage of blood flow. Age-related changes typically include a decrease in heart rate, a fall in **cardiac output** (the amount of blood pumped out of the heart in one minute) secondary to lowered **stroke volume** (the amount of blood pumped out of the heart in one beat), and the inability to elevate cardiac output to match the demands of the body.

Arrhythmias, or irregular or abnormal heart rhythms, also become common as aging alters the heart's electrical system. By age 75, the number of cells in the sinoatrial (SA) node decrease by 90%. Because the SA node is the origin of the normal heart beat, the loss of cells in this area hinders the heart's ability to produce a normal sinus rhythm. The SA and atrioventricular (AV) nodes both see a decline in pacemaker cells. Fibrosis and fatty deposits along the electrical pathway add to the risk of aberrancy. There is also a progressive loss of bundle branch fibers, leading to aberrant conduction syndromes. Common cardiac arrhythmias such as atrial fibrillation and junctional rhythms result in an uncoordinated filling of the ventricles by the atria, or the loss of "atrial kick," which accounts for 30% of the total stroke volume. As the atria fibrillate, they pool small amounts of blood, which can clot. If these clots flow into the system (embolize), they can plug up small vessels and cause ischemia to the tissues supplied by those vessels. Thus, atrial fibrillation increases the risk of **pulmonary embolus** (a blood clot that breaks off from a large vein and travels to the blood vessels of the lung, causing obstruction of blood flow), myocardial infarction, infarction of the extremities, and strokes.

With age, the vascular system becomes stiff, resulting in increases in the systolic blood pressure. As the pressure of systole increases, the left ventricle works harder and becomes thicker, similar to what happens to a muscle when it is trained. The ventricular muscle also loses its elasticity in this process. The thickening and stiffening of this muscle decreases filling of the ventricle, thus decreasing the cardiac output. This stiffening also occurs with the heart valves, which may impede normal blood flow into and out of the heart. As the blood passes through these stiffened valves, a heart murmur may be heard, even in the absence of disease.

Older patients are prone to a 20 mm Hg drop in systolic blood pressure when moving from a sitting to a standing position. This drop in blood pressure is known as **orthostatic hypotension** or postural hypotension, and occurs because the **baroreceptors** in the aortic arch and carotid sinus become less sensitive to changes in blood volume. These receptors sense the change in blood pressure and send a signal to the adrenal glands to secrete hormones, such as epinephrine and norepinephrine, to alter the blood pressure. However, the heart's response to epinephrine and norepinephrine decreases with age (**Figure 2-6**). The aging heart takes longer to speed up and then return to normal when the adrenal glands secrete these hormones, and so the body is less able to compensate quickly for low perfusion states or rapid postural changes.

Blood vessels become stiff with age because of decreased elastin and collagen in the vessel walls, and the peripheral vessels' elasticity reduces by as much as 70%.[4] Compensation for blood pressure changes will be hampered by the lessened distensibility and contractibility of the peripheral vessels.

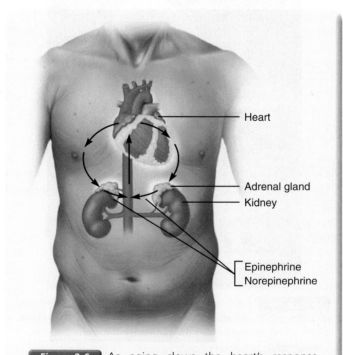

Heart

Adrenal gland
Kidney

Epinephrine
Norepinephrine

Figure 2-6 As aging slows the heart's response to epinephrine and norepinephrine from the adrenal glands, it takes longer for the heart to speed up and then slow again in response to the demands of the body.

Atherosclerotic disease affects more than 60% of people older than 65 years.[5] The process begins in the early teens and progresses throughout life. The coronary vessels are most commonly associated with this disease. Atherosclerosis, however, presents problems throughout the circulatory system. With this condition, the blood vessels narrow, making them unable to increase the supply of blood when there is an increased demand. Further, atherosclerosis can contribute to the development of an **aneurysm**, or the weakening and bulging of the blood vessel wall, with risk of rupture if subjected to high stretching forces.

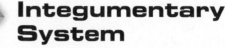

Integumentary System

Wrinkling and loss of resiliency of the skin (the integumentary system) are the most visible signs of aging. Wrinkling occurs because of atrophy of the epidermis, which causes the skin to become thinner, drier, less elastic, and more fragile. Accurately assessing skin turgor in the older patient may be difficult because tenting of the skin may exist without the associated dehydration. Subcutaneous fat becomes thinner, making a loosened outer cover for the body and inhibiting thermoregulation.

Elastin, the substance that makes the skin pliable, and **collagen**, the substance that makes the skin strong, both decrease with age. Skin tears or injuries from what is considered light contact or bumps occur frequently. For example, skin tears may occur while transferring patients, assisting patients, or performing standard procedures. In addition, attempts to establish an intravenous (IV) line can be more difficult because the thinner skin may tear during insertion of the catheter, or while holding the patient still when making the attempt. As the provider, you may choose to alter your equipment, such as exchanging various adhesive tapes for transparent dressings, in order to limit the possibility for skin tears.

The tightened skin of youth allows subcutaneous injuries to easily **tamponade**, or close and stop bleeding; however, with aging skin, bleeding may go unnoticed or uncontrolled, producing large hematomas underneath the skin (**Figure 2-7**). Injuries to the skin are slow to heal because of diminished capillary blood flow. Pressure ulcers, also called decubitus ulcers or pressure sores, may occur when an older patient remains stationary and the weight of the body compresses the already thinned skin. With little blood flow to regenerate the cells damaged by the pressure, tissue dies and a sore results.

Additionally, sebaceous glands produce less oil, making skin drier. With the lack of oil and moisture, the patient's fingernails and toenails may become brittle and crack. Sweat gland activity also decreases, hindering the body's ability to sweat and help regulate heat. Hair follicles atrophy, become brittle, and produce less **melanin**, a pigment that provides color to the skin and hair. The lowered production of melanin results in less color in the hair; without color, the hair is gray.

A hair strand has a life expectancy of 4 to 5 years. Hair follicles will produce thinner, smaller hair during the aging process, and many follicles will even stop producing hair as they age (more common in men).

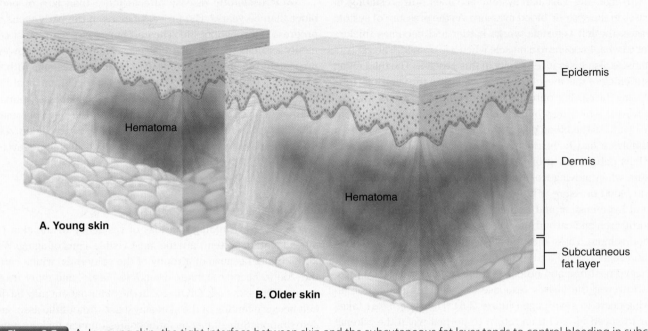

Figure 2-7 A. In young skin, the tight interface between skin and the subcutaneous fat layer tends to control bleeding in subcutaneous injuries. B. The looser connection between skin and fat in older skin exerts less control on bleeding and may result in larger hematomas.

Musculoskeletal System

While most older people maintain the ability to carry out daily activities, changes in physical abilities can affect the older adult's confidence in their mobility. The muscle system atrophies and weakens with age. Muscle fibers become smaller and fewer, motor neurons decline in number, and strength declines. The ligaments, tendons, and cartilage of the joints lose their elasticity. Cartilage and synovial fluid also go through degenerative changes with aging, contributing to arthritis.

Muscle atrophies and decreases in mass over time, and is replaced by fat. With the decreased muscle, increased fat, and decreased activity levels, patients may experience a decrease in physical strength. The increase in fat also alters the body's capacity to use some drugs. Diazepam, for instance, is distributed in the patient's fat. The more fat, the greater the spread of the drug, the lower the concentration, and the longer it is stored in the body. Alcohol, on the other hand, is distributed in lean tissue. Because older adults have less lean tissue, their blood alcohol level rises more quickly.

The stooped posture of older people comes from atrophy of the supporting structures of the body. Two out of three older patients will show some degree of kyphosis, a condition commonly known as "humpback," "hunchback," or "Potts curvature" (**Figure 2-8**). Lost height in older adults generally results from compression in the spinal column—first in the disks and then from the process of **osteoporosis** in the vertebral bodies. This change in shape affects how older patients are positioned for opening airways and spinal immobilization.

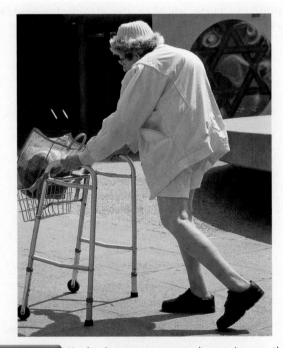

Figure 2-8 Kyphosis, seen to some degree in two-thirds of older adults, affects how you should position the patient when you open the airway or immobilize the spine.
© Bill Aron/PhotoEdit

Osteoporosis, which is the generalized loss of bone mass caused when bone reabsorption exceeds new bone production, occurs as the skeleton ages. Postmenopausal osteoporosis is by far the most common form. Clinically significant postmenopausal osteoporosis, present in one-third of older women, is the basic cause of vertebral body collapse, hip fractures, and forearm fractures in this group.[6]

Endocrine System

Older patients are prone to a variety of endocrine disorders. Women, in particular, are at risk for hypothyroidism and hyperthyroidism, as well as hyperparathyroidism. Women may also suffer from a decrease in estrogen production, increasing the likelihood of osteoporosis. With these endocrine changes, many patients experience an increase in antidiuretic hormone production, causing issues with fluid balance. These issues are often diagnosed with routine lab work performed at the patient's primary care physician's office.

The most common chronic disease seen throughout the older population is diabetes, specifically noninsulin-dependent diabetes mellitus. About 26% of the older population has diabetes and approximately half of those patients have some degree of hypertension.[7] Diabetes and hypertension place patients at an increased risk for myocardial infarctions, cerebrovascular accidents, and renal failure.

Gastrointestinal System

The gastrointestinal (GI) system goes through a variety of changes with age. The mastication process becomes more complex due to dental issues. Patients may have dentures, which can present issues during ventilation if not seated appropriately. Salivation also decreases, which reduces the initial release of digestive enzymes. Diminished muscle of the esophageal sphincter causes an increase in heartburn and acid reflux, causing damage to the esophageal lining. Diminished muscle control of the rectal sphincter causes fecal incontinence, which can cause psychosocial issues. Older patients may also experience hypochlorhydria, a decrease in the availability of hydrochloric acid in the stomach. Older patients tend to have less intake and poor absorption of nutrients and electrolytes. Peristalsis slows down with aging, causing constipation when combined with a poor diet.

Hepatic metabolism, the liver's use of enzymes to break drugs down into more water-soluble compounds, diminishes with age for two reasons: hepatic blood flow decreases, and the production and function of metabolic enzymes decline. In addition, environmental stresses—such as tobacco smoke, alcohol, and drugs—hinder the liver's ability to produce metabolizing enzymes. The body uses these enzymes to metabolize drugs into more water-soluble compounds, making it possible to use and dispose of these drugs (**Figure 2-9**). Impaired liver enzyme activity or impaired blood flow to the liver results in accumulation of the drug at higher, possibly toxic, levels.

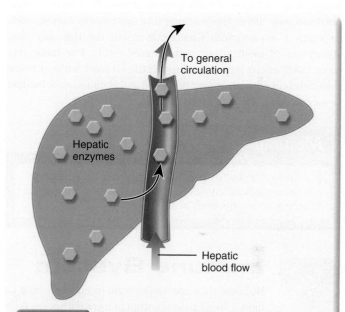

Figure 2-9 The ability of the liver to break some medications down into forms the body can use and dispose of depends on hepatic blood flow and the production and function of metabolizing enzymes. Both diminish with age.

CASE STUDY 2

You are dispatched for a lift assist. A 68-year-old male patient, Tom, has fallen and needs assistance getting up. This is the fourth time this week that this has occurred. Tom says that his arthritis has been getting worse and it hurts to move around. His doctor has prescribed some medication and Tom has been compliant, but it does not seem to help.

- Will every older person experience the effects of arthritis?
- Can these aches and pains be a sign of something more serious?

Changes in gastric and intestinal function may inhibit nutritional intake and utilization. Taste bud sensitivity to salty and sweet sensation decreases. Saliva secretion also decreases, lowering the body's ability to process complex carbohydrates. Gastric motility slows with age because of the loss of intestinal tract neurons, which can lead many patients to feel constipated or not hungry. There is a decrease in the gastric acid secretion. Blood flow in the **mesenteries**, the membranes that connect organs to the abdominal wall, may drop by as much as 50%, decreasing the ability to extract nutrients from the intestines.[8] Gallstones are increasingly common with age, and anal sphincter changes reduce elasticity and can produce fecal incontinence.

The condition of the oral cavity has important implications for eating. Loose-fitting dentures can cause pain when chewing, and when combined with gastrointestinal changes, the patient may experience poor oral intake and loss of appetite, leading to weight loss and loss of body protein stores. This form of malnutrition may affect medications that are protein bound, such as warfarin or phenytoin. Changes in gastric function may alter absorption of medications administered orally. For these reasons, medications may pass through the GI tract without being completely absorbed, or may be stored and accumulated, leading to increased medication levels and actions.

Medication Tip

Malnutrition and renal, hepatic, and gastrointestinal changes can cause medications either not to be absorbed properly, or to accumulate in the body at abnormally high levels.

Immune System

Because they are more prone to and less able to fight it, older patients often present with some type of infection. Systemic and cellular immune responses become less effective. Pneumonia and urinary tract infections (UTIs) are common in bed-bound patients. There is also an increase in abnormal immune system substances in the aging body, which has been correlated with an increased incidence of infection.

In general, due to the decreased muscle mass, increased fat, and the existence of other thermoregulatory issues, many older patients get cold easily. The warm temperatures that older patients find comfortable are ideal for the transmission of a variety of bacteria and viruses that can cause respiratory and integumentary infections. Integumentary infections, particularly decubitus ulcers, take longer to heal in hot environments.

It is imperative that clinicians take appropriate body substance isolation (BSI) and personal protective equipment (PPE) precautions—not only for the safety of the provider but also for the patient with the weakened immune system. Older patients are at increased risk for hospital-acquired infections due to a decrease in the amount of antibodies and the presence of autoimmune disorders.

Genitourinary System

In the kidneys, both structural and functional changes occur with age. For example, kidney mass decreases by 20% and, between the ages of 30 and 80, there is a loss of **nephrons**, the basic filtering units in the kidneys. Aging kidneys respond less efficiently to stress because of decreased bloodflow and degeneration of the tubules, causing **hemodynamic** stress along with fluid and electrolyte imbalances. In addition, kidney filtration function falls an average of 50% between the ages of 20 and 90.[9] Because many drugs are eliminated by renal excretion—including some drugs used to treat common cardiac conditions (digoxin, procainamide, disopyramide) and psychiatric disorders (lithium), as well as most antibiotics—the cause of many drug interaction problems in older patients is underlying renal dysfunction.

Patients may also experience changes in urinary output. Older men may experience prostate hypertrophy, which will cause an increase in the urge to urinate; however, the urinary output will be minimal. A decline in urinary sphincter control may cause incontinence and nocturnal voiding. Bladder capacities diminish with age, which also contributes to the urine output issues. It is imperative that providers protect patient modesty and are understanding of the situations at hand.

Summary

From birth to old age, the body undergoes many changes. As we get older, these changes alter the ways that the body can compensate for the stress of illness or injury. It is important to understand the physiology of normal aging in order to anticipate an older person's response to changing conditions. Activities that were done easily as a younger person may become more difficult or impossible, requiring additional help or changes in the task.

Physical changes take place in every system of the body. Different communication methods must often be used to compensate for sensory deterioration. Physical and psychological changes require the EMS provider to be able to assess and differentiate complicated medical conditions. Treatment choices may require changes to match the aging body's decreased responses.

References

1. Centers for Disease Control and Prevention. *National Vital Statistics Reports.* December 20, 2013: 62 (6).
2. Brinton, DA, Wilkinson, CP. *Retinal Detachment: Principles and Practice, Third Edition.* (2009). New York, NY: Oxford University Press.
3. American Academy of Orthopaedic Surgeons. *Nancy Caroline's Emergency Care in the Streets, Seventh Edition.* (2013) Burlington, MA: Jones & Bartlett Learning.
4. Ibid.
5. Ibid.
6. Reginster, JY, Burlet N. Osteoporosis: A still increasing prevalence. *Bone* 2006; 38: S4–S9.
7. Centers for Disease Control and Prevention. *National Diabetes Statistics Report: Estimates of Diabetes and Its Burden in the United States, 2014.* (2014). Atlanta, GA: U.S. Department of Health and Human Services.
8. American Academy of Orthopaedic Surgeons.
9. Ibid.

CASE STUDY SUMMARIES

Case Study 1 Summary

An increased blood pressure is normal with age. However, there are many factors involved in evaluating blood pressure. Your answer should be based on your system's programmed response (which may be to just give the numbers and not to advise, or to have the patient follow up with her personal physician). Because blood pressure is made from a combination of cardiac output and systemic vascular resistance, issues related to hypertension can affect multiple areas within the body. Common organs affected by hypertension include the heart, lungs, kidneys, brain, and the vessels throughout the body.

It is important to evaluate the cause of the poor medication compliance. If it is a financial issue, see what resources are available in your community to provide sliding scale or low-cost medications. While the patient's friend was just trying to be helpful, she does not have a thorough understanding of pharmacodynamics and could ultimately cause harm to the patient.

Case Study 2 Summary

Not every person will experience the pain of arthritis. During the aging process, pain in the joints can be a sign of arthritis, muscle fatigue, swelling from any number of causes, or referred pain from something more serious. Often, older people do not feel chest pain from cardiac muscle ischemia or infarction. The first clue may be an ache in the neck, back, or arm. Older patients often misinterpret these signs for something much less serious.

CHAPTER 3

Communication

LEARNING OBJECTIVES

1. Understand the process of communication.

2. Discuss and recognize communication challenges in the older person, including visual, hearing, speech, and disease processes that affect communication.

3. Describe the principles that should be employed when communicating with the older person.

Communication and the Older Adult

Every day, as an EMS provider, you communicate with many people, including your partner, the dispatcher, and the public. This **communication** is often hurried and, at times, wrought with emotion. It is important to take the time to think about how communication takes place, and what makes it effective. For example, how do we interact with the public? More specifically, how do we interact with the older people we come in contact with? Do we, as EMS providers, know how to communicate effectively with the senior citizens in the community?

Communication is the basic life experience. It allows us to receive information that keeps us alive and healthy. For older people, the ability to communicate is crucial to life maintenance and personal satisfaction. For the healthy older person, communication may be the crucial skill in negotiating the right to remain independent. For the older person with a disability, it is important to maintain communication throughout rehabilitation in order to prevent further deterioration, isolation, and dependence.[1] Older people have a greater need for good human relations than younger adults do—in order to counterbalance the forces of aging, older people need ties to reality, and to their family and friends. Enhancing communication with older people helps to maintain their integrity, preserve their wisdom, and enhance personal relations.[2]

Communication does not just involve talking; it also involves listening. Your first communication sets the tone with the patient—what you say and how you say it can mean success or failure in the communication process. It is important from the very beginning that, as an EMS provider, you present yourself as competent, confident, and concerned (**Figure 3-1**). Good communication skills will help you gain the information necessary to aid in your management of the situation. When your patients trust you, it is easier for them to explain their problem and to answer your questions. No matter how difficult the situation may be, EMS professionals can find effective ways to enhance communication with older people, and thus make the experience a positive one.

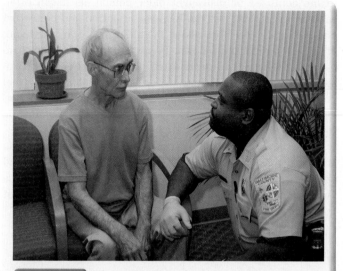

Figure 3-1 It is important to present yourself as competent, confident, and concerned.
© Jones & Bartlett Learning. Courtesy of MIEMSS.

Communication Tip

Communication includes both talking and listening.

Types of Communication Skills
Verbal and Nonverbal Communication

There are two types of communication—verbal and nonverbal—and the nonverbal type of communication is just as important as the verbal type. **Verbal communication** includes words and the volume, pitch, inflection, and tone of the voice. **Nonverbal communication** includes eye contact, hand gestures, body position, facial expressions, and touch. Touch can be important

CASE STUDY 1

You are dispatched to a local shopping mall for a patient who has fallen. Upon your arrival, you discover a few people standing around an older woman who is lying on the sidewalk at the bottom of a staircase. You learn from the bystanders that they heard the woman scream as she fell down several steps. Your first observation is that the woman looks very upset. You also note that her right leg is rotated laterally. As you lean over the woman, you begin your interview by attempting to obtain the woman's name and age, and what occurred. The older woman repeatedly says, "I don't know…I'm so upset, I can't think."

■ What are your next steps?

to the confused or distraught older person, as it can often calm and reassure, and can increase attention and nonverbal understanding. Consider taking the older patient by the hand, or touching them on the arm. Be aware, however, that some patients prefer not to be touched. Cultural beliefs may prohibit touching as well. Some older female patients may feel uncomfortable when touched by a male EMS provider. Whatever the reason, you should respect a patient's wish not to be touched.

It is important that verbal and nonverbal communication is congruent. Be sure that your words, facial expressions, and body language are consistent with each other. Patients can sense inconsistencies and insincerity, which will undermine the trust you are trying to establish.

Listening

Listening is a vital communication skill. Older people may need time to process the questions that are being asked of them. Unless the need to treat is urgent, take the time to listen patiently for the answers to your questions (**Figure 3-2**). Additionally, listen to the way patients say their words. Their tone may convey fear or confusion. Effective listening may allow you the opportunity to comfort and calm the person.

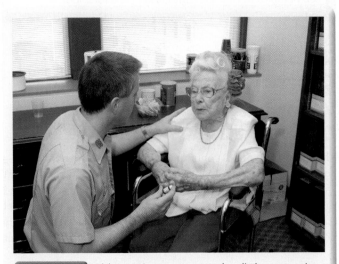

Figure 3-2 Older patients may need a little more time to process your questions, and may speak slowly when responding.
© Jones & Bartlett Learning. Courtesy of MIEMSS.

Attitude Tip

Be patient when interviewing older people. Take the time to recognize any physical, intellectual, or psychosocial barriers that slow or interfere with effective communication.

Age-Related Communication Challenges

Communication disorders constitute the nation's number one handicapping disability. Studies indicate that more people suffer from hearing, speech, and language impairment than from heart disease, venereal disease, paralysis, epilepsy, blindness, cerebral palsy, tuberculosis, muscular dystrophy, and multiple sclerosis combined. Conditions such as stroke, cancer, degenerative neurological diseases, and trauma can affect the older person's ability to communicate.[3] The aging process brings about changes in vision, hearing, taste, smell, and touch; in addition, changes in communication abilities may accompany aging, dementia, and other diseases. Advanced age can make a person's voice tremulous, weak, hoarse, and higher or lower pitched than it was in middle age. Older people may say, "My voice tires." These symptoms may be bothersome, but they are considered a normal consequence of aging (in the absence of any medical conditions that may be causing them).

The sections that follow discuss those changes that primarily affect the interaction between the older patient and the EMS provider.

Vision

Diseases of the eye, such as cataracts, glaucoma, **macular degeneration**, and visual problems secondary to stroke or diabetes, are more common in the older population. Fifteen percent of all adults older than the age of 65 have serious visual impairments. Any time you are called to the scene where an older person is not wearing eye glasses, ask if he or she has eye glasses and would like to put them on. If the patient says yes, ask where the eye glasses are kept and if you can get them. Carefully help the person put the eye glasses on. If the patient is blind, tell him or her everything you are going to do. For example, you may need to put the patient's hand on the equipment you are using (**Figure 3-3**). Do not assume that a patient who is blind is also deaf.

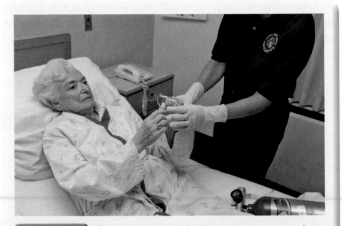

Figure 3-3 If your patient is blind, you may want to have him or her touch the equipment you are using.
© Jones & Bartlett Learning. Courtesy of MIEMSS.

Be aware of visual changes when assessing and transferring patients, making sure to support patients to prevent them from falling.

Hearing

Hearing loss is the most common communication disorder in the older population, and is the third most prevalent chronic condition in this group. Approximately 36 million adults in the United States report some degree of hearing loss. Of those adults, 18% are 45 to 64 years of age, 30% are 65 to 74 years of age, and 47% are over 75 years of age.[4]

There are three basic types of hearing loss: conductive, sensorineural, and central auditory processing disorders. Conductive hearing loss occurs when sound is not conducted efficiently through the outer and middle ears. It may be caused by absence or malformation of the pina, ear canal, or ossicles (the tiny bones of the middle ear); impacted cerumen; fluid in the ear associated with colds, allergies, or ear infections; or poorly functioning eustachian tubes. Conductive hearing loss usually involves a reduction in sound level or the ability to hear faint sounds, and can often be corrected with medicine or surgery.

Sensorineural hearing loss occurs when there is damage to the inner ear (cochlea) or to the nerve pathways from the inner ear to the brain. This type of hearing loss not only involves a reduction in sound level or the ability to hear faint sounds, it also affects speech understanding or the ability to hear clearly. Causes include disease, birth injury, medications that are toxic to the auditory system, genetic syndromes, noise exposure, viruses, head trauma, tumors, and aging. Sensorineural hearing loss is permanent and affects about 17 million people in the United States. Sensorineural hearing loss can occur in combination with conductive hearing loss.

A central auditory processing disorder occurs when auditory centers of the brain are affected by injury, disease, tumor, or heredity. These disorders do not necessarily involve hearing loss. Instead, central auditory processing involves sound localization and lateralization, auditory discrimination, auditory pattern recognition, the temporal aspects of sound, and the ability to deal with degraded and competing acoustic signals. A deficiency in any of these processes may constitute a central auditory processing disorder.

There are many causes of hearing loss in adults, including **otosclerosis**, **Meniere's disease**, **ototoxic** medications, exposure to harmful levels of noise, acoustic neuroma, and trauma. Hearing loss as a result of aging is called **presbycusis**. Presbycusis is progressive in nature, with high-frequency sounds being affected first. Although the process begins after age 20, it is often between ages 55 and 65 that high-frequency sounds are affected. Thus, a lower-pitched voice may be easier to hear than a higher-pitched voice. **Table 3-1** offers more tips for communicating with a hard-of-hearing patient.

If the patient does not have a hearing aid, try using the "reverse stethoscope" technique: Put the ear pieces of your stethoscope in the patient's ears and speak softly into the diaphragm of the stethoscope (**Figure 3-4**). This will amplify your voice.

Table 3-1	Communicating with Hard of Hearing Older Patients
1.	Ask the patient if he or she has a hearing aid and would like to use it.
2.	Stand approximately 18 inches in front of the patient.
3.	Reduce background noise, such as from a television or radio.
4.	Arrange to have light on your face, not behind you, if possible.
5.	Position yourself within the visual level of the listener.
6.	Speak at a natural rate, unless you see signs of incomprehension.
7.	Speak *slightly* louder than normal, but do not shout.
8.	Always face the hearing impaired patient, and let your facial expression reflect your meaning.
9.	Never speak from another room or out of the sight of a hearing-impaired patient.
10.	Use short sentences.
11.	Rephrase misunderstood sentences.
12.	Remember that the hearing-impaired person will not hear and understand as well when tired or sick.

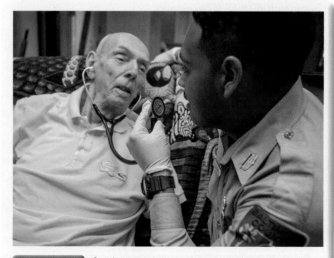

Figure 3-4 If a hearing-impaired patient does not have a hearing aid, you can amplify your voice with the "reverse stethoscope" technique.
© Jones & Bartlett Learning. Courtesy of MIEMSS.

Hearing Aids

A hearing aid is essentially a device that makes sound louder. Just as eye glasses cannot cure vision problems, hearing aids cannot restore hearing to normal. Instead, hearing aids improve a person's hearing and listening ability, ultimately improving the quality of life.

Although there are different types of hearing aids, four basic components remain the same: the microphone, amplifier, receiver, and power supply. The microphone collects sound energy and converts that energy into a weak electronic signal. The amplifier receives the electronic signal and increases the amplitude. The receiver acts like a miniature speaker, converting the amplified electrical signal into sound energy similar to that initially received by the microphone. It is this amplified signal which is then directed into the ear. The battery (power supply) provides power to the amplifier.

When sound leaves the receiver, it must have a means of being directed into the ear canal. This is accomplished through the use of a custom-fitted ear mold. An impression is taken of the outer ear and sent to a laboratory that will make the mold. Squealing that is often heard from a hearing aid is the result of feedback—sound escaping from the ear canal that is picked up by the microphone and further amplified.

Ask the patient if he or she has a hearing aid. Use hand gestures to signify putting a hearing aid in your ear. If the patient says yes, ask where the hearing aid is, retrieve it, and assist him or her in putting it in, if necessary.

Types of Hearing Aids

The different types of hearing aids are (**Figure 3-5**):

- *In-the-canal and completely-in-the-canal.* These hearing aids are contained in a tiny case that fits partly or completely into the ear canal.
- *In-the-ear.* This type of hearing aid is generally larger than the canal-type hearing aid. All of the components are contained in a shell that fits in the outer part of the ear.
- *Behind-the-ear.* All parts of this hearing aid are contained in a small plastic case that rests behind the ear. The case is connected to an ear mold by a piece of clear tubing.
- *Conventional body.* This type of hearing aid is an older style that is usually worn by people with profound hearing loss. It is generally worn on the chest, either in a shirt or coat pocket or in a harness. The microphone, amplifier, and battery are contained within the case

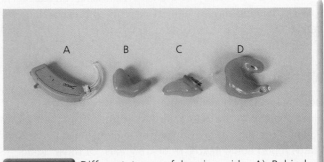

Figure 3-5 Different types of hearing aids. A) Behind-the-ear type. B) Conventional body type. C) In-the-canal type. D) In-the-ear type.
© Jones & Bartlett Learning. Courtesy of MIEMSS.

of the hearing aid. A cord carries the electrical signal to the receiver that is attached to the ear mold placed in the external ear.

Many hearing aids have optional features that can be built in to assist in different communication situations. Two of the more common options are directional microphones and telephone switches. A directional microphone responds to sound coming from a specific direction, as occurs in face-to-face conversation. A hearing aid with this feature will have a switch that, when activated, can change from the normal setting, which picks up sound almost equally from any direction, to focus on a sound coming from the front of the person and reduce the sound coming from behind the person.

With the telephone switch option, a change can be made from the normal microphone "on" setting to the "T" setting, which allows the user to hear better on the telephone. Hearing aids with the telephone switch feature contain an induction coil. In the "T" setting, environmental sounds are eliminated, and the person can only pick up sounds from the telephone.

First Aid for Hearing Aids

Occasionally, you may be asked to assist an older patient with his or her hearing aid. Hearing aid users often disconnect the batteries when the aids are not in use to prolong the life of the batteries (hearing aid batteries generally need to be changed every 5 to 7 days). If the back of the hearing aid is open and the battery is inside, simply close the battery door. If the battery is not inside the hearing aid, you will have to insert it. Some hearing aids have a preset volume; others will need to be turned on and the volume set. If the volume needs to be set, set it in the mid-range. It can always be adjusted later, but this will prevent a sudden loud burst of noise that may scare the patient. The hearing aid with the red dot always goes in the right ear; remember, red equals right.

When inserting the hearing aid, follow the natural shape of the ear. If a whistling sound occurs, the hearing aid may not be far enough in the ear to create a seal, or the volume may be up too loud. Try repositioning it, or remove it and turn the volume down. If, after two tries, the hearing aid still will not go in properly, do not try any further.

Communication Tip

The hearing aid with the red dot always goes in the right ear. Remember, red equals right.

You should not attempt to do anything you are not familiar with; however, there are a few basic things that can be done to solve hearing aid problems. If necessary, assist the patient with contacting their audiologist.

If the hearing aid will not work at all:

- Be sure the hearing aid is turned on.
- Try a fresh battery.
- Check the tubing to make sure it is not twisted or bent.
- Check the switch to make sure it is on M (microphone), not T (telephone).
- Try a spare cord (for a body aid). The old cord may be broken or shorted.
- Check the ear mold to make sure it is not plugged with wax.

If sound from the hearing aid is weaker than usual:

- Try a fresh battery.
- Check the tubing for bends and the ear mold for wax or dirt.
- If the hearing aid has been exposed to extreme cold, it may not work until it is at room temperature.
- There may be excessive wax in the ear. The patient should consult their physician.

If the hearing aid goes on and off or sounds scratchy:

- Work the switches and dials back and forth, as lint or dust will interfere with electrical contacts.
- On body hearing aids, try changing cords.

If the hearing aid whistles continuously:

- A new ear mold or new tubing may be needed. The patient should see his or her audiologist.

Additional things that can be done include the following:

- If excessive dirt or wax collects on the mold, it can be washed in warm water using mild soap. The mold must be removed from the hearing aid prior to washing. Wipe excess water from the mold, blow to clear any moisture from the tube, and allow the hearing aid to dry overnight.
- Discard any batteries that appear to be leaking. Clean the battery case.

Hearing aids must be handled with care, and some things should never be done with hearing aids. For example:

- Never attempt to remove wax from any opening of an in-the-ear hearing aid.
- Never expose a hearing aid to excessive heat.
- Never allow a hearing aid to become wet. Should a hearing aid become wet:
  - Immediately remove the batteries.
  - Wipe the exterior of the case with a dry absorbent cloth.
  - Place the hearing aid in a warm place. The low-heat setting of a hair dryer can be used for drying.
- Never take a hearing aid apart to examine the insides. This may void warranties.
- Do not wash the ear mold in alcohol, acetone, cleaning fluid, or extremely hot water. The use of chemicals may dissolve the plastic material of the ear mold. Hot water may soften the plastic and allow the ear mold to change shape.

If the older person will be transported to the hospital, ensure that the person's hearing aid is transported with the person.

Speech

For many older people, it is difficult to produce speech that is loud enough, clear enough, and well-spaced enough. Normal speech requires a delicate balance of energy and relaxation. Energy is required in skeletal muscles to support posture; in abdominal and breathing muscles to support loudness; and in the tongue, jaw, lips, and palate to support intelligibility. Relaxation is required in skeletal muscles to support pitch, in throat muscles to support a clear tone, and in vocal tract muscles to support resonance. Weakness, paralysis, poor hearing, or brain damage can destroy this balance.[5]

Dentures

Although dentures may not be thought of as a communication concern, they do help the person who wears them to communicate. Without dentures, a patient's speech may be slurred or mumbled, and he or she may be embarrassed to try to talk. Ask if your patient wears dentures. If the answer is yes, offer to get them. Dentures kept in a soaking solution need to be rinsed before inserting.

Ask the patient if he or she can put the dentures in. If the patient can insert the dentures, hand him or her the top plate first, the way it would fit in the mouth (**Figure 3-6**). After the top plate is inserted, hand the patient the bottom denture in the same manner. If the patient cannot insert the dentures and wants you to, insert the top plate first, holding it securely with your thumb, then lay the bottom denture along the bottom ridge. Ask the patient if the dentures are comfortable.

Never allow the older person with dentures to lie on their back unmonitored. Dentures can come loose and create an airway obstruction.

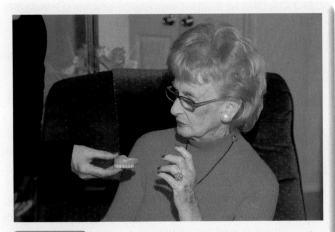

Figure 3-6 Hand dentures to a patient the way the dentures would fit in the mouth, with the top plate first.

Courtesy of John Valentini, Jr.

Communication Disorders

Aphasia

Aphasia is an impairment of language that affects the production or understanding of speech and the ability to read or write. Aphasia is caused by injury to the brain, most commonly from a stroke. Aphasia can range from very mild to so severe as to make communication with the patient almost impossible. Aphasia may mainly affect a single aspect of language use, such as the ability to recall the names of objects, to put words into sentences, or to read; or it may affect multiple aspects of communication. Approximately one million people in the United States are affected by aphasia.

There are several varieties of aphasia. These include:

- *Global aphasia.* The most severe form of aphasia may be seen after a person has suffered a stroke, and may improve rapidly if the damage has not been too extensive. The patient with global aphasia is the most difficult to communicate with, because they can produce few recognizable words, understand little or no spoken language, and can neither read nor write.
- *Broca's aphasia.* Often referred to as nonfluent or expressive aphasia, this form of aphasia is characterized by a severely reduced speech output, limited mainly to short utterances of less than four words. The patient may be able to read and understand speech, but vocabulary is limited and the formation of sounds is often laborious and clumsy for the patient.
- *Mixed nonfluent aphasia.* This type of aphasia is applied to persons who have sparse and effortful speech, resembling a severe form of Broca's aphasia. However, unlike with Broca's aphasia, comprehension of speech is limited and the patient will not read or write beyond an elementary level.

- *Wernicke's aphasia.* This type of aphasia is often referred to as fluent or receptive aphasia, as speech production is not affected. However, comprehension deficit is affected and patients tend to produce sentences that do not hang together and are intruded by irrelevant words. Reading and writing are also often severely impaired.
- *Anomic aphasia.* This type of aphasia applies to patients who have a persistent inability to find specific words in their vocabularies. However, patients with anomic aphasia understand speech well and, in most cases, read adequately.

There are additional forms of aphasia that do not fit into the above categories. While most family members or caretakers will be able to identify that the patient suffers from aphasia, they may not be able to identify the type. **Table 3-2** offers tips to help make communication easier and less frustrating for those with aphasia.

Dementia

Dementia, covered in detail in the *Neurological Emergencies* chapter, is a medical condition that affects the patient's ability to communicate. Language difficulties common in dementia patients affect the patients' ability to name things or say what they want to say. In fact, this is an early indication of the disease. Patients with dementia are often aware of their inability to perform as they once did, especially in the early stages of the disease. Other characteristics of patients with dementia include an appearance of frustration, withdrawal, suspiciousness, irritability, and restlessness—all of which affect the communication process. Paranoia, delusions, or hallucinations may also accompany dementia.

Dementia patients may no longer be able to recognize close friends, family members, or themselves. They may forget that you are an EMS provider. They may become very concrete or literal, no longer able to think in abstractions. There is also a delayed reaction time in conversation. Dementia patients may forget what was just said to them or what they were in the middle of saying. As the disease progresses, language difficulties become more severe. In addition, symptoms may worsen in the evening, a condition known as sun-downing.

Patients with dementia may have difficulty understanding language, though at times they may understand. You may be tempted to talk about the severely demented patient as though he or she were not there, but it is best to assume that the patient can understand. **Table 3-3** offers some tips that may prove helpful when communicating with dementia patients. If the patient cannot understand spoken language, written communication may be helpful; however, toward the middle stages of the disease, patients may be able to read words but not understand their meaning. Try a bit harder to communicate with the dementia patient. The result will be an increase in the quality of the person's life, if only for a short time.

Table 3-2 Communicating with the Aphasic Patient

1. Ask the family member or caretaker if the patient has difficulty with listening or talking. If the difficulty is with listening, use an environmental "show me" approach—in other words, show the patient what you want them to do. If the difficulty is with talking, use multiple-choice questions.

2. Talk to the person with aphasia as an adult and not as a child. Avoid talking down to the person.

3. Avoid open-ended questions. Use focused questions instead.

4. During conversation, minimize background noise.

5. Make sure you have the person's attention before communicating.

6. Praise all attempts to speak. Encourage the use of all modes of communication.

7. Give the person time to talk and permit a reasonable amount of time to respond. If the person takes too long to answer, ask the person to repeat the question to see if he or she comprehended it. Accept all communication attempts (speech, writing, gesture) rather than demanding verbal communication. Avoid insisting that each word be produced perfectly.

8. Keep your own communication simple, but adult-like. Simplify sentence structure and reduce your own rate of speech. Keep your voice at a normal volume and emphasize key words.

9. Augment speech with gesture and visual aids whenever possible. Repeat a statement when necessary.

10. Be patient; aphasia patients may experience poor language comprehension when they feel rushed or embarrassed. Give the patient time to grope for words and ideas, and listen without negative reactions. Expect telegraphic messages from the expressive aphasic.

Table 3-3 Communicating with Patients with Dementia

1. Use clear, concrete, familiar language.

2. Convey only one idea at a time, speaking simply and not too fast.

3. Do not use medical jargon.

4. Use short sentences. If the patient does not understand, repeat exactly what was just said. This allows time for the person's brain to process the information. If words are varied, greater effort is required by the patient. If the patient still cannot understand, repeat using different words.

5. Accompany your words with gestures.

6. If the patient tries to answer, but loses his or her train of thought, repeat back the last few words the person said as a reminder.

7. Do not give lengthy explanations as to why something is being done; the patient may not understand.

8. Use nouns instead of pronouns. The patient may lose track of who the pronouns are referring to. Don't say, "Your husband is here, may I ask *him* some questions about you?" Instead, say, "Your husband is here, may I ask your *husband* some questions about you?" Even better, refer to the husband by name. "Your husband John is here, may I ask *John* some questions about you?"

9. Avoid using the word *don't*. Patients with dementia sometimes cannot understand this commonly used contraction.

Other Disorders Affecting Communication

Apraxia

Apraxia is an impairment in carrying out purposeful movements. Commonly, patients with apraxia will show you something in their wallet, or lead you to show you something, but this is the extent of their nonverbal communication. These patients are unable to perform common expressive gestures on request (such as waving good-bye); this is referred to as limb apraxia. Apraxia may also primarily affect oral, non-speech movements, such as pretending to blow out a candle; this is referred to as facial apraxia. Apraxia can also manifest as a speech impairment, with the inability to voluntarily produce the correct rhythm and timing. The speech of a person with apraxia is characterized by highly inconsistent errors.

People with severe apraxia are usually limited in explaining themselves by pantomime or gesture, except for expressions of emotion. This disorder may even extend to the ability to manipulate real objects.

Dysarthria

Dysarthria refers to a group of speech disorders resulting from weakness, slowness, or incoordination of the speech mechanism due to damage to the nervous system. Dysarthria is a disorder of speech production, not language. It may affect some or all of the basic speech processes: respiration, phonation, resonance, articulation, or prosody. Unlike apraxia of speech, the speech errors that occur with dysarthria are highly consistent from one occasion to the next.

Patience is important when communicating with dysarthric patients because they cannot form the sounds that go into a ready answer. Expect poor articulation. Read gestures and nonverbal clues, and listen for the slow motion core of intelligibility.

Parkinson's Disease

Parkinson's disease is a chronic nervous disease characterized by a fine, slowly spreading tremor; muscle weakness and rigidity; and a peculiar gait. **Table 3-4** offers some tips to enhance communication with patients who have Parkinson's disease.

Additional Communication Challenges

In addition to the communication challenges related to vision, hearing, and speech, the patient may have concerns that lead to decreased communication. Being aware of common fears of the older person will help you communicate in a caring and compassionate manner. For example, it is natural for older people to want

Table 3-4 Communicating with Patients with Parkinson's Disease
1. Choose an environment with reduced noise.
2. Allow (and encourage) the patient to speak slowly.
3. Communicate face to face with the patient. Look at the patient as they are speaking. A well-lit room also enhances communication.
4. Encourage the patient to use short phrases. Have the patient say one or two words or syllables per breath.
5. Have the patient choose a comfortable posture and position that provides support during long and stressful conversations.
6. Fatigue significantly affects a person's speaking ability. Plan for periods of vocal rest before conversations.
7. If the patient has difficulty being understood and is able to write without difficulty, have the patient write what he or she is trying to say.

Attitude Tip

Though the older person's fears and anxieties may not seem important to you, they are very real and important to the older person. By acknowledging concerns and making it clear—with your words and your actions—that you understand their importance, you will do much to calm and reassure.

to stay in their own homes or in a home-type situation for as long as possible. Some older people may stay home longer than is safe for them because they do not want to give up their independence, cannot afford other care, or do not realize that their condition has deteriorated beyond the point where they can safely care for themselves. It is important that EMS providers be respectful to older patients' need for independence and the emotional attachment they may have to their homes. Older people may fear that when they leave their home to go in an ambulance, they will be moved to a nursing home or, even worse, never leave the hospital.

With this in mind, there are a few steps that you can take to make the patient more comfortable. If the patient seems fearful, ask what he or she is specifically nervous about; simply vocalizing these concerns may help the patient establish a sense of trust in your care. Remember, it may be helpful to touch an older person who is anxious or confused (**Figure 3-7**).

Your patient could also be concerned about a longtime companion; **separation anxiety** is common in older people. If possible, transport the patient's loved one in the front of the ambulance, or suggest that a friend or neighbor drive the companion to the medical facility. Pets can also be a source of anxiety for

Communication Techniques

In general, when interviewing the older patient, the following techniques should be employed:

- Identify yourself. Do not assume the older person knows who you are.
- Be aware of how you present yourself. Frustration and impatience can be portrayed through body language.
- Explain what you are going to do before you do it. Avoid using medical jargon or slang. Avoid complex grammar. For patients who are visually impaired, detailed explanation is especially important. If assisting a visually impaired patient with transfer, keep one hand on the patient and tell him or her what you want them to do and in which direction to turn.
- Show the older patient respect. Never use the patient's first name without his or her permission. Refer to the patient as Mr., Mrs., or Miss.
- Do not talk about the patient in front of him or her; to do so gives the impression that the patient has no say in any decision making. This is easy to forget when the patient is cognitively impaired or has difficulty communicating. If a caretaker or someone else is involved in the patient's decision-making process, continue to talk to the patient as well as to the patient's caretaker or decision maker.
- Maintain a relaxed, friendly, and calm manner when working with an older patient who is in distress or acutely ill.
- Be a good listener. EMS providers must listen empathetically. Patients who are nonverbal may refuse to display their disabilities to someone they perceive as cold and uncaring.
- For the laryngectomee, expect low-pitched monotone. Listen for shortened phrases that lack melody, and look for lip reading cues.

The National Victim Center has also identified useful techniques for communicating with older adults in stressful situations (**Table 3-5**).

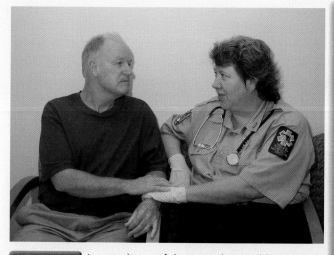

Figure 3-7 It may be useful to touch an older patient who is anxious or confused.

the patient. A patient who lives alone may not want to go to the hospital and abandon a pet. If there is no family present, ask a neighbor or friend to watch the pet.

Money can also be a concern. Health care is expensive, and many older people are on budgets. Be aware that your patient could be deeply concerned that hospitalization could cause the loss of their savings or even their home. Listen to your patient's fears with compassion, and acknowledge their importance.

There may be other considerations that make it difficult for an older person to tell you about his or her condition. The patient may take several medications, some of which may mask symptoms. He or she may have been in pain for a prolonged time and not notice a gradual worsening of symptoms, or could have dementia, delirium, stroke, a psychiatric disorder, or another disorder that affects the ability to communicate thoughts. In these circumstances, it is very useful to not only collect information from the patient, but to also confirm this information with another source such as a caregiver, family member, or bystander. Finally, the patient who comes from an ethnic or cultural background different from yours may communicate differently.

CASE STUDY 2

© 123dartist/Thinkstock

At 11:00 a.m. you receive an "unknown ambulance call" from the manager of a continuing care retirement community. The manager states other residents informed him that Ms. Telman, an 85-year-old resident who resides alone, was not seen at breakfast that morning. Additionally, there was no answer at Ms. Telman's door. The manager informs you that Ms. Telman has no immediate family and rarely leaves the complex. She is very socially active and never misses breakfast. The manager states that he has a master key and can gain access to Ms. Telman's apartment.

Once at Ms. Telman's apartment, you knock repeatedly on the door but do not get an answer. With the master key, you enter the apartment and observe Ms. Telman lying on the living room sofa. You call her name, but she does not answer. You gently touch her arm, at which time she awakes. You identify yourself as an Emergency Medical Technician. Ms. Telman looks at you confused and does not answer. You repeat what you have just said. Ms. Telman shakes her head as if she does not understand, at which point you notice her trying to adjust a hearing aid in her right ear.

- What are your observations?
- What is your course of action?

Table 3-5   Techniques for Communicating with Older Patients in Stressful Situations

- Do not assume that an older adult has a sensory or cognitive impairment. Be sensitive to the individual's particular needs.
- If circumstances permit, choose an environment that is conducive to communication. Eliminate factors that interfere with effective listening, such as the television or radio, and minimize distractions. This may involve moving the person to a quiet environment where one-on-one communication can take place. One-on-one communication is especially important if the older person has been victimized and must recount or give details of the event (**Figure 3-8**).

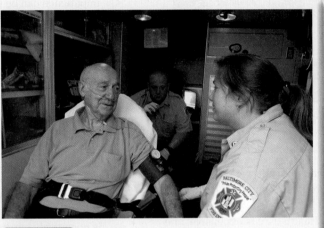

Figure 3-8 Try to find a quiet environment that encourages communication.
© Jones & Bartlett Learning. Courtesy of MIEMSS.

- If the patient's story appears rehearsed, be aware that the patient could be experiencing abuse.
- If the patient appears fearful while relaying facts, be sure to listen carefully. There could be a number of different reasons for their fears. Additionally, the older patient in crisis may not readily volunteer information.
- Try to position the older patient so that the light is not shining in their eyes.
- Sit or stand facing the older person at eye level, so that your eyes and mouth are clearly visible. Be sure to have the patient's attention before speaking.
- Keep interactions short and simple.
- If multiple providers are on the scene, have one provider conduct the interview, rather than multiple providers asking different questions.
- Keep your voice and mannerisms calm.
- Do not shout. If necessary, speak slightly louder without shouting or yelling.
- Show a willingness to listen through effective nonverbal communication. Be attentive.
- Ask questions to clarify confusion, but ask only one question at a time. Wait for a response to one question before asking another.
- Allow time for hearing and comprehending.
- Be especially sensitive to the older patient who is tired and not feeling well. Tired or ill people are less able to understand or remember what is asked or said.
- Observe nonverbal clues that the patient has understood what you have said. For example, are you receiving a blank stare?
- Be patient. Expect to repeat what you say often. If the older patient does not understand, rephrase the question, rather than repeating the same words.
- Never interrupt. It discourages free speaking, and the interruption may cause the patient to forget what he or she was going to say.

Data from Focus on the Future: A Systems Approach to Prosecution and Victim Assistance by the National Center for Victims of Crime.

Summary

Good communication is essential to successful assessment and treatment of older patients. There are many things that make communicating with older patients challenging. Keep in mind the age-related changes in the older person, disease processes that may affect communication, and differing cultural values. Be aware of not only what you say, but also how you say it.

Communication consists of both gathering and providing information. Listen and observe. You can learn a lot about your patient by being aware of potential vision impairments, hearing impairments, and underlying fears. A few minutes spent enhancing communication with your older patient is time well spent. Our oldest and most vulnerable patients deserve nothing but the kindest and most sensitive care.

References

1. Wilder CN & Weinstein BE (eds.): *Aging and Communication.* New York, NY, The Haworth Press, 1984, p 51.
2. Dreher BB: *Communication Skills for Working With Elders.* New York, NY, Springer, 1987, p xi.
3. Ibid., p 49.
4. National Institute on Deafness and Other Communication Disorders: *Quick Statistics*. National Institutes of Health, 2010, June 16. Available from: http://www.nidcd.hih.gov/health/statistics/Pages/quick.aspx.
5. Dreher, p 28.

Additional Resources

American Speech-Language-Hearing Association (ASHA): http://www.asha.org

National Aphasia Association: http://www.aphasia.org

National Institute of Health—National Institute on Deafness and Other Communication Disorders: http://www.nidcd.nih.gov

CASE STUDY SUMMARIES

Case Study 1 Summary

Your first priority, of course, is to treat life-threatening injuries. You notice that the patient's right leg is laterally rotated, indicating a possible hip fracture. Further assessment of the patient reveals minor abrasions to her hands and face. You learn that the woman is 85 years old; her name is Mrs. McDonald and she lives in a senior apartment complex across the street. You are not able to gather any additional information from Mrs. McDonald.

Having learned about communicating with older people, particularly older people in crisis, you know that a more productive interview can be accomplished in an environment that is more conducive and beneficial for the patient. In most cases, this type of environment can be found inside the ambulance: it is out of the elements (be it hot or cold weather) and there is less external stimulus. The communication process will be enhanced, as the patient will be more calm and able to focus on the interview.

As you conduct the interview, use all of the applicable techniques learned in the chapter. Remember, the patient has just suffered a traumatic injury (a possible hip fracture); this situation is as emotionally difficult as it is physically difficult. A calm, reassuring manner and good communication is just as important as the treatment you provide.

Case Study 2 Summary

You encounter an 85-year-old female who appears confused. Your first priority should be to ensure that there is no life-threatening emergency. The person appears to be displaying purposeful movements by attempting to adjust her hearing aid. You attempt to assist her. Taking a piece of paper, you write the word "batteries." The person reaches in the end table and takes out an envelope containing hearing aid batteries. The person then removes her hearing aid. You replace the batteries and hand the person back her hearing aid, at which time she places the hearing aid in her ear.

Once again, you identify yourself and explain why you are there. The person intelligibly states that she fell asleep last evening on the sofa and apparently did not hear anyone knocking at the door or realize what time it was.

No further intervention is necessary. What you do learn is that in most senior housing complexes there is a vast communication network among the residents, which includes checking on each other frequently.

CHAPTER 4

Assessment of the Older Patient

LEARNING OBJECTIVES

1. Compare the assessment of the older patient with that of a younger adult patient.

2. Describe normal and abnormal findings in the assessment of older patients.

3. Recognize common emotional and psychological reactions to aging.

4. Recognize normal and disease states in older patients.

5. Describe common complaints of the older patient, including shortness of breath; chest pain; abdominal pain; dizziness or weakness; fever; generalized pain; and nausea, vomiting, and diarrhea.

Introduction

As an EMS provider, it is important to give special consideration to the complexity of the older patient. The **Occam's razor** approach to assessment, diagnosis, and treatment is based on the assumption that the simplest diagnosis is the most likely diagnosis and, therefore, does not take into account a comprehensive evaluation of both internal and external risk factors; instead, diagnosis is based upon external observations. In using this approach for the assessment of the older patient, there is an increased risk of **iatrogenic** symptoms not being identified. For example, when a 42-year-old male begins complaining of chest pain, the symptom most likely is the result of a cardiac complaint; however, if an 82-year-old male complains of chest pain, the spectrum of likely possibilities increases, as this may be a sign of a cardiac event, respiratory event, or a combination of the two. For this reason, a holistic approach should be utilized to assess both internal and external influences currently experienced by the older patient.

To understand the multiple factors that affect the health of the older patient, it is important to consider what happens as a person ages and why this process makes a person susceptible to illness. As a person ages, a constellation of deteriorative changes produce a reduction in organ function, a decrease in the ability to maintain homeostasis, and an increase in disease susceptibility. Additionally, an older adult has longer exposure to elements that increase their susceptibility to illness and, therefore, their resilience to diseases may be weakened. For example, the 70-year-old individual whose chronic disease started at age 40 is likely to have more organ damage than that of the 70-year-old whose illness started at the age of 60 (**Figure 4-1**).

Assessment of the older patient follows the same approach used in younger adults: detect and treat immediate life threats and determine the patient's priority of care. However, there are a few unique considerations that should be taken into account:

1. An older patient is more likely to have more complex problems compared to a younger adult, whose problems tend to be less multi-dimensional.

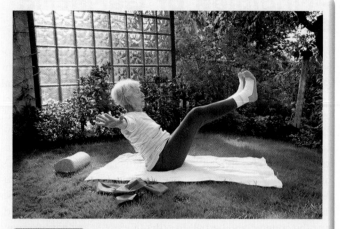

2. An older patient's evaluation of quality of life and functional status is an integral part of determining their independence.
3. A frailty level determines an older person's physiological ability to maintain homeostasis.[1]

The EMS provider's assessment approach should be built upon EMS training for emergent care. In addition to this foundation, assessment of the older patient must take into account a broader spectrum of symptoms, subtle detection of instability, and nonspecific generalized complaints. When the situation permits, utilizing a multitude of assessment tools may be useful. This chapter discusses the different techniques to use during assessment of the older patient, as well as the common complaints of the older population, including shortness of breath; chest pain; abdominal pain; fever; generalized pain; and nausea, vomiting, and diarrhea.

CASE STUDY 1

On a Sunday morning you are called to a local church for someone who has "passed out." On arrival, you find a short white-haired female sitting in a wheel chair in the church's gathering space. You are told the patient is 99 years old and very hard of hearing. She appears pale and does not respond to your initial questions; however, she is alert and looking around. Her skin is dry; her pulse is irregular at about 100; and her respirations are about 24. You see no obvious signs of trauma and no facial droop. The patient moves both hands equally to grasp at her friend's hand. Her friend tells you the patient has had several similar spells and that she recently saw her doctor for low blood pressure.

- How do you proceed?
- Does the patient need to be transported?

Principles of Geriatric Assessment

Before performing assessment of the older person, the EMS provider must remember that the clinical presentation of the patient may consist of a wide range of symptoms, such as altered mental status, behavioral changes, incontinence, gait disturbances, weight loss, and falls. The complexity of these symptoms may result from a multitude of factors. Assessment principles should include the patient's chief complaint, chronic conditions, polypharmacy categorization, and mental and physical status (including the patient's functional ability to perform activities of daily living [ADLs] or instrumental activities of daily living [IADLs]). Assessment should also include review of the patient's current medication list (prescribed, over the counter, and herbal) in order to identify any adverse reactions that may be contributing to the presenting symptoms.

The Five I's of Geriatrics (Intellectual impairment, Immobility, Instability, Incontinence, and Iatrogenic disorders) describes the specific challenges of assessing the older adult. These challenges can be addressed through a number of different assessment techniques:

1. Intellectual impairment: Based on the patient's first response, does he or she appear awake, alert, and attentive? Is dementia present?
   - The Mini-Cog tool can be used to detect cognitive impairment with initial triage and only takes a few minutes to administer. This tool, which can be administered in about 3 minutes, allows the EMS provider to quickly assess numerous cognitive domains, such as cognitive function, memory, language comprehension, visual-motor skills, and executive function.
   - No special equipment is required and the outcome of the test is relatively uninfluenced by the patient's level of education or language. To assess the patient, say three words (i.e. apple, fish, table) and ask him or her to repeat them back to you and remember them. Then ask the patient to draw a clock face with the hands of the clock indicating a certain time (i.e. 11:10). After the patient has drawn the clock face, ask him or her to repeat the three words that were given at the beginning of the assessment. The test is scored as follows:
     - Recall of 0 items indicates cognitive impairment.
     - Recall of 1–2 items with an abnormal clock face indicates cognitive impairment.
     - Recall of 1–2 items with a normal clock face indicates no cognitive impairment.
     - Recall of all 3 items indicates no cognitive impairment.
2. Immobility: How steady are the patient's gait and balance?
   - The Get Up and Go test can be used to assess the patient's mobility. This test begins with the older person sitting in a chair with his or her arms resting on the arm rests. The person is then asked to stand up and walk a distance of 10 ft (3 m), turn around, walk back to the chair, and sit down. Timing begins when the person starts to rise from the chair and ends when the person sits back down in the chair. The person should be given one practice trial and three actual timed trials. Score is given based on the average of the three timed trials. Predictive results are rated in seconds: <10: mobile; <20: independent most of the time; 20–29: variable mobility; >29: impaired mobility.
3. Instability: What does the older patient look like (frailty or failure to thrive [FIT])?
   - Is there evidence of muscle wasting or unplanned weight loss of 10%
   - Are there any signs of dry mucosa, dehydration, or poor dentition or denture fit?
4. Incontinence: As the body ages, the balance between urethral closure, **detrusor** instability, and sphincter weakness may interfere with urethral and bladder pressures, thus contributing to episodes of incontinence.
   - Resnick's DIAPPERS is a mnemonic for causes of urinary incontinence that are suddenly experienced by an older patient who does not have a history of incontinence: **D**elirium, **I**nfection, **A**trophic **urethritis**, **P**harmacy-induced, **P**sychological, **E**xcess urinary output, **R**estricted mobility, and **S**tool impaction.[2]
5. Iatrogenic disorder: Could the older patient be experiencing an adverse reaction from interactions among prescribed medications or over-the-counter medications, or from a previous medical procedure?

In all cases, the EMS provider must conduct a scene size-up and initial assessment of the patient. Findings in the initial assessment, as well as the patient's overall condition, will dictate how the assessment proceeds. Unresponsive medical patients and trauma patients with a significant mechanism of injury must receive a rapid assessment in order to further identify and manage immediate life threats. Conversely, patients with non-significant mechanisms of injury and those who are responsive should receive a focused history and physical exam based upon chief complaint. The decision to perform a detailed physical examination is also guided by the patient's condition. Generally speaking, if the patient is in need of a rapid assessment (medical or trauma) at the scene, a detailed physical examination will need to be performed while en route to the hospital.

 ## Scene Size-Up

Assessment begins with the scene size-up, during which access to the patient is gained and the general condition of the patient's surroundings, including factors related to the safety of the EMS provider and that of the patient, is assessed. Access to the older patient may be limited and assistance may be required. If the patient has fallen and is unable to come to the door, you may need to find other routes of access, which may require assistance from the fire or police department. Residential care or nursing homes may also pose access issues. For example, you may be delayed by front desk or admitting personnel or you may need to retrieve directions to the patient from the staff. You may also need to summon a nurse from another patient's room to provide a report or answer questions regarding the patient's status. Nursing home caregivers are a resource that should be routinely used, as they are often the best source of information on these patients.

In addition to normal scene size-up, you must assess the environment for hazards when responding to a call for an older patient. Is the environment well maintained? Is there concern over environmental hazards? For example, is the environment too cold or too warm? Is there exposure to carbon monoxide or other toxins (**Figure 4-2**)? This information, which may only be accessible to the EMS provider, is critical to the ongoing care of the patient.

Personal protection for the EMS provider is important. After you secure your own personal safety, do the same for your patient. Residents in long-term care facilities have an increased chance of being infected with resistant bacteria. Additionally, older persons have a weakened immune system, and a simple cold or flu could lead to a serious health problem such as pneumonia. If you are ill, wear a mask and gloves to keep from contaminating the frail older patient.

 # Initial Assessment

The first two goals of initial assessment are to detect and treat immediate threats to life and to determine the patient's priority of care based on the immediate

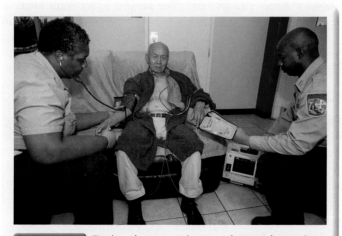

assessment of the patient's environment and chief complaint. Assessment of the scene should include the following considerations:

- Is the home or institution clean or dirty?
- Is there food in the house?
- What medications are in the house? (Bring the medication bottles to the emergency department.)
- Is the patient at risk of abuse or neglect?
- Is there evidence of drugs, alcohol, or an altered mental status?

As you assess the older patient, take note of his or her general appearance. If you notice a hospital bed in the living room or absorbent pads, suction equipment, or bandaging materials in the home, the patient likely has serious or chronic health issues. Home oxygen connected to the patient may also be a sign of chronic pulmonary problems. An ashtray next to the patient's chair is an equally important finding, as it is a sign that the patient still uses tobacco. Often, you are the only person with access to the patient's environment, so be sure to gather as much scene-specific information as possible.

 ## Mental Status Assessment

The history of a patient's current illness or injury may be hindered if cognitive impairment is not recognized during the initial interview. Establishing a patient's cognitive baseline is essential for ongoing assessment and should be accomplished for every confused older patient. Aging alone does not cause mental status changes, and confusion should NEVER be accepted as "normal." Many older patients have significant cognitive impairment that is undiagnosed. It would be a grave error to assume that an altered mental status presentation is normal for a patient without first investigating the potentially life-threatening medical or traumatic conditions that may exist.

The most common causes of cognitive impairment in older patients are dementia, depression, and delirium (the "3 D's"). With your initial patient interview, identification of any of the "3 D's" and an altered mental status establishes the need for assistance from the patient's caregiver. Always interview the patient first, but don't forget to listen to the patient's caregiver. A medical history of a patient's current illness may be hindered by not recognizing cognitive impairment at the initial interview. Caregivers may be instrumental in providing information crucial to establishing the onset of illness, medication nonadherence, or poor compliance with medical treatment.

During assessment, observe the older patient for head or face injury. If there is a possibility for head injury, a neurological assessment is required. Establish the patient's mental status baseline and level of cognitive function, and assess for origin of injury. Determine the patient's chief complaint and when the symptoms began. If the patient has two or more neurological complaints (such as back pain and a headache), consider neurological injuries. Associated complaints include the following:

- Dizziness or vertigo
- Weakness or incoordination
- Loss of consciousness
- Visual disturbances (such as blurred or double vision)

A functional assessment may also assist with determining the cognitive status of an older patient. The two key divisions of functional ability that should be assessed are ADLs and IADLs (**Table 4-1**).

Attitude Tip

Listen to the patient's caregiver, recognize and report concerns expressed about the patient, and note any signs of caregiver stress or frustration. Caregivers often need help as well.

When you approach the older patient, record what you observe. Is the patient alert, responsive, making eye contact, and speaking in a clear voice? What resting position has the patient chosen—is he or she sitting or lying down? Is the patient's response appropriate to the questions being asked? Is the patient in pain? Determining whether the patient's mental status impairment is chronic or acute may indicate the severity of the condition. For an acute situation, the AVPU (Alert, Verbal, Painful, Unresponsive) mnemonic may be utilized. A new change may be the sign of a stroke, meningitis, an iatrogenic disorder, or another serious life-threatening illness.

Determining the patient's orientation to person, place, time, and event also may be useful in determining cognitive impairment. Only the most severely altered patient will be unable to recall his or her own name. Ask if the patient knows where he or she is right now. "At home," "At work," "In the street," or "In an ambulance" would all be acceptable answers. To determine the patient's orientation to time, consider asking if he or she knows what day of the week it is. Many institutionalized patients will not know the answer to this question, however, so asking if they know the time of day (morning, noon, or night) may be more useful. Lastly, orientation to the event can be determined by asking the patient what happened to cause the call for EMS today. After the assessment, ask a family member or caregiver to confirm the patient's usual ability to recall the elements of person, place, time, and event in order to determine the reliability of the history gathered from the patient. (Use family members, caregivers, and the patient's chart to recover important facts about medical history if the patient is an unreliable historian.)

In early stages of dementia, older patients are aware of and often embarrassed by the loss of their cognitive abilities. They will often attempt to cover up or make light of their confusion. You may need to gently explore further if the older patient's response is vague. Do not accept answers like, "Of course I know what day it is. Don't bother me with stupid questions when I am in pain" (**Figure 4-3**). Obtain complete answers through firm, but kind, repeated questioning.

Attitude Tip

Patients in the early stages of dementia may be embarrassed by the loss of their cognitive abilities. If a patient resists your questioning, do not be rude in an effort to get a straight answer. Instead, continue to question the patient in a gentle manner, explaining that you are there to help.

Circulatory Assessment

Circulation is produced by cardiac output (cardiac output = stroke volume x heart rate). The normal aging adult heart is less responsive to stimulation from the nerves that adjust the

Table 4-1 Assessment of Functional Abilities

Activities of Daily Living (ADLs)	Instrumental Activities of Daily Living (IADLs)
Does the patient have the ability to participate in daily self-care activities, such as: - Eating - Dressing - Bathing - Using the toilet - Controlling bladder and bowel functions - Transferring between the bed and a chair	Can the patient live independently and perform functions at a higher cognitive level, including: - Doing housework - Preparing meals - Taking medications properly - Managing finances - Using a telephone

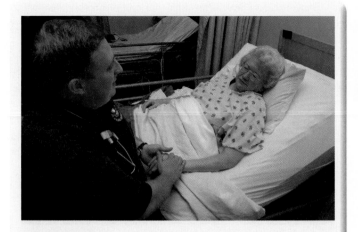

Figure 4-3 You may have to be patient and gentle to obtain the detailed information necessary to distinguish new mental status changes from usual functioning.
© Jones & Bartlett Learning. Courtesy of MIEMSS.

heart rate and strength of contraction, which can result in a lower heart rate and weaker pulse than expected. Always check pulses on both sides (bilaterally) to confirm that your findings are due to reduced heart function and not a blockage of flow to a specific extremity. An irregular pulse is also more common in the older patient. Knowing the patient has a history of **arrhythmias** or other problems is important when assessing circulatory status.

If you suspect hemodynamic compromise in an older patient, determine the patient's mean arterial pressure (MAP). A MAP of about 60 mm Hg is necessary to perfuse the coronary arteries, brain, and kidneys. The usual range of MAP is 70 mm Hg to 110 mm Hg; a patient whose MAP is less than 70 mm Hg should be further evaluated. Gently check the pulse of one of the carotid arteries and feel for a peripheral pulse. The pulse check may need to be adjusted for older patients, as peripheral pulses can be difficult to feel due to vascular changes and poor circulation. Also consider auscultating an apical pulse, using a stethoscope to listen to the heart in the left chest 5th intercostal space and counting the heart beat (S1/S2) for 60 seconds. This technique is useful for determining heart rate and rhythm or cardiac arrhythmias.

Heart rate, blood pressure, capillary refill (< 2 seconds), and mental status are all indicators of circulatory status. Heart rate may be affected by medications commonly taken by older people, especially **beta-blockers, calcium channel blockers**, or **antiarrhythmic medications**. You should be familiar with these medications and take extra care in the assessment of patients who are taking them. The heart rate of a patient who is volume depleted from blood loss or dehydration usually increases in order to compensate; however, patients who are taking cardiovascular medications such as beta-blockers are often unable to increase their heart rates due to the effects of the medication. In these cases, a normal heart rate can be misleading, causing signs of shock to be missed.

Low blood pressure is an indicator of hypoperfusion. When a symptomatic older patient develops hypotension (systolic pressure less than 90 mm Hg), the EMS provider should determine if there are contributing factors, such as inducement from prescription medications, hypovolemia post-gastrointestinal symptoms, vasovagal stimulation from vomiting, or **postprandial hypotension** following a meal. (Postprandial hypotension occurs in up to one third of older persons). A very high blood pressure, on the other hand, may signal an impending stroke. However, if an older patient normally has a very high baseline blood pressure, then a blood pressure that is considered normal in younger patients could indicate shock in the older patient. This is an example of why establishing a baseline is crucial: A change from baseline will be the best indicator of a problem.

Older patients may have chronic skin conditions that decrease the ability to assess capillary refill. Consider using alternate sites for evaluation of perfusion, including the lips and the conjunctiva (inner lining of the eyes). Again, establish the patient's baseline and determine if there has been a recent change. Poor perfusion is a serious problem. Patients who begin with circulation that is already compromised will deteriorate more quickly. Provide supplemental oxygen and consider administering IV fluids early if no contraindications exist.

Assessing volume status, or dehydration, is also different for the older patient. Look for signs of dehydration, such as dull eyes, poor urine output, low blood pressure, and dry mucous membranes. With these combined findings, formulate a treatment plan around aggressive fluid boluses and assess the lungs after each fluid bolus. Consider medication-induced iatrogenic complications leading to hypovolemia from blood loss. For example, an older patient taking amiodarone (an antiarrhythmic agent) in combination with warfarin may experience a prolonged **international normalized ratio (INR)**, thus increasing the risk of bleeding.

Airway Assessment

Airway management in the older adult can be compromised by several anatomic changes common with age. For example, dentures are commonly used by older patients and can help or hinder airway patency. If ventilation assistance with a bag-valve mask device is needed, attempt to leave the patient's dentures in place; dentures will help create a good seal by supporting the soft tissues of the patient's face so they do not collapse inward. However, if the patient needs to be intubated, removal of dentures is suggested in order to prevent damage to the patient's mouth, as well as to prevent the possibility of fracturing the dentures and risk aspiration or ingestion of the fragments.

An older patient's ability to protect his or her own airway may be compromised as the result of a prior disease. For example, stroke or severe dementia can lead to a loss of gag reflex and normal swallowing mechanisms. Patients who are on soft or liquid diets should alert you to the possibility of airway compromise and risk of **aspiration pneumonia**.

Be suspicious of a potential cervical spine injury when evaluating the older patient's airway. Bony changes, such as increased fragility and fracture susceptibility, occur in the jaw and cervical spine of older persons; because of this, the jaw-thrust maneuver, and especially the head tilt-chin lift maneuver, can be difficult to accomplish and should be performed gently to prevent damage. The jaw thrust results in the least amount of cervical spine motion, while the head tilt-chin lift results in a large amount of motion, which can further damage an injured spinal cord. In addition, spinal degenerative changes, such as kyphosis and scoliosis, may be present in the older patient. Due to these changes, the cervical, thoracic, or lumbar sections of the spine have a stiffness and exaggerated curvature, making positioning a challenge. The EMS provider must take the necessary precautions to prevent injury by appropriately padding to ensure airway patency and patient comfort, even when there is no concern of cervical trauma.

Breathing Assessment

In assessing the effectiveness of breathing in older patients, recall that the normal range for respiratory rate is the same as that of the young adult—12 to 20 breaths/min. Chest rise may be more difficult to assess due to increased chest wall stiffness; therefore, it is important to expose part of the chest to ensure adequate chest expansion. Additionally, a stethoscope may be needed to assess rate and depth of respiration (**Figure 4-4**). The astute EMS provider knows that a more involved exam is often necessary in the older patient. Be sure to take the time needed to perform it.

The patient's clinical presentation determines the severity of pulmonary compromise. The symptoms observed and voiced by the patient may assist the EMS provider in determining whether a respiratory condition is affecting the upper or lower airways. Listen for audible respiratory wheezes and, if heard, determine if they are present during inspiration or expiration. Additionally, note if the patient is speaking in one-word answers or conversing in breathy short sentences, and consider if a cough is present. The characteristics of a cough can assist you with determining which disease process is present:

- Does the patient cough only when lying down or upon waking, or is the cough harsh with chest discomfort?
- Is the cough productive? If so, what are the expectorate characteristics (consistency, color, and odor)?
- Does the patient have a temperature or low SpO2? Is he or she tachypneic?

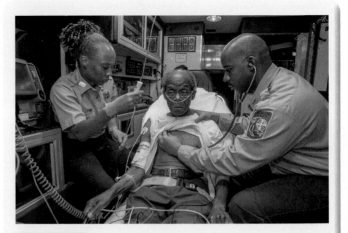

Figure 4-4   Assess the chest for adequate expansion. This may require exposing the chest or using a stethoscope.
© Jones & Bartlett Learning. Courtesy of MIEMSS.

- When did these symptoms begin? Has the patient been around anyone who has been ill or traveled out of the country?
- Does the patient smoke cigarettes? If so, how many per day, and for how many years?

Acute upper respiratory conditions are considered more severe when symptoms indicate croup, epiglottitis, or acute asthma exacerbation. Lower pulmonary symptoms may indicate conditions such as pneumonia, bronchitis, or chronic obstructive pulmonary disease (COPD).

Patient Medications

The World Health Organization identified that irrational use of medicines has become a worldwide risk, increasing the percentage of drug-related problems. The older population accounts for approximately 30% of all prescriptions written in the United States, with the typical older patient taking four or five prescription drugs and two over-the-counter medications.[3]

As the number of medications prescribed to an older patient increases, so does the risk of iatrogenic drug-related adverse reactions. As an EMS provider, understanding the principles of pharmacokinetics (absorption, distribution, metabolism, elimination) in the older patient will assist with identifying medication-induced conditions. (A complete discussion of the principles of pharmacokinetics in older people is presented in the *Pharmacology and Medication Toxicity* chapter.) Due to physiological changes that occur with aging, the kidneys decrease in renal mass, blood flow, glomerular filtration, and tubular secretion and absorption. Thus, the plasma concentration of medications is not eliminated as quickly and the risk of side effects (altered mental status, confusion, delirium, etc.) is increased.

A thorough medication history is essential. As you gather patient information regarding medication use, remember to also obtain information about the older person's use of over-the-counter medications and herbal remedies. It is especially important to determine if the patient is taking a new medication (prescription or nonprescription) or has had a recent change in medication dosage that may have contributed to the reason for the call. **Nonadherence** with medications can produce adverse effects, often causing the patient's condition to deteriorate. The same is true for nonadherence to other treatment plans, such as failing to comply with a diet for diabetes, which may cause hyperglycemia, or failing to restrict salt intake, which may worsen congestive heart failure (CHF).

Medication errors can occur from nonadherence, underdosing, and overdosing (accidental or purposeful). If medication is not taken appropriately, the patient can experience a variety of side effects from mild headaches and nausea to seizures and respiratory arrest. EMS providers can determine medication compliance by evaluating prescription bottles for the date, dose, and quantity prescribed. If there are too many or not enough of a specific medication, the provider should inquire further.

Medication Tip

As people age, they tend to use more over-the-counter medications and herbal remedies. Do not forget to ask patients about these.

Medication Tip

As an EMS provider, you have an opportunity that many other health care providers do not—observing the older patient first hand. If the patient is not transported to the emergency department, you may be the only person who interacts with him or her. You can affect how well older patients keep track of their medications by recommending the use of a weekly pill box reminder. This measure takes only a few minutes but may save a life.

Trauma Assessment

Mechanism of Injury

At the scene, you must determine whether the patient is injured, ill, or both. This requires determining the applicable mechanism of injury and/or nature of illness. Be cognizant of the fact that the patient's injury may be secondary to a medical problem.

Conversely, you should also be aware that medical conditions can be exacerbated by an injury.

In cases of trauma, it is important to keep in mind the differences between older and younger patients. Rapid initial evaluation of circulation, airway, and breathing must be accomplished, followed by a detailed history and physical exam as appropriate (**Figure 4-5**). The goal of assessment is to gather as much information about the patient as possible while minimizing the time necessary for transfer to definitive care. Because of the complexity of the older patient, taking a thorough history is crucial. Collect information from the patient and bystanders, if possible. Obtain as much information as you can, in the time you have, and be sure to consider environmental safety and elder abuse. (Elder abuse is discussed at length in the *Elder Abuse* chapter.)

When there is a question of injury, immediately inspect the older patient's physical appearance and assess for any abnormality. Start with the head and face; are there any obvious bleeding, wounds, or deformities? With a suspected head injury, cervical spinal precautions should be immediately instituted. As you assess the neck, inspect for bruising, tracheal deviation, or distended neck veins. Inspect the chest, abdomen, and pelvic area, observing for indications of guarding with limited movement, ecchymotic areas around chest or umbilicus, or muscle rigidity.

Determining the mechanism of injury for an older patient involves asking more questions than with patients in any other age group (**Figure 4-6**). For example, if an older patient falls, the EMS provider should consider the fall to be a symptom produced by a system failure within the body. Falls are NOT a simple trauma call for older patients. Falls caused by weakness, dizziness, or palpitations most likely have a very dangerous underlying cause. When a medical cause does exist, it can be more life

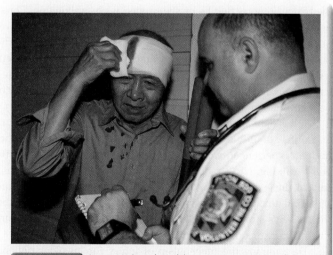

Figure 4-5 In assessing the older trauma patient, the goal is to gather the most information possible while minimizing the time required for transfer to definitive care.
© Jones & Bartlett Learning. Courtesy of MIEMSS.

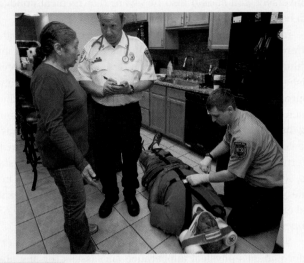

Figure 4-6 Determining the mechanism and cause of injury for an older patient involves asking more questions than with patients in any other age group.
© Jones & Bartlett Learning

threatening than the injury from the fall itself. Therefore, in every "trip and fall" call, the EMS provider must establish three things:

1. Did this older person really trip and fall?
2. Could this fall be the result of a medical condition or a reaction to a medication?
3. If the patient really did trip, was there an environmental hazard associated with the cause?

Some older patients will say they tripped, even if they did not, for fear of being labeled "frail." The expert EMS provider evaluates the patient's mental status and the surrounding environment to determine if the mechanism that was stated is plausible. For example, if the patient reports that he or she tripped while walking on a broken sidewalk, determine if the sidewalk is in fact broken. Are there other factors that could have contributed to the fall, such as a poorly lit hallway or a loose area rug? Identifying and reporting hidden hazards may save the patient from a future injury. If appropriate, a mobility assessment, such as the Get Up and Go test, should also be performed to assess the patient's gait and balance (**Figure 4-7**).

If it is determined that what was stated is not plausible, then questions should be targeted at determining whether or not the patient experienced weakness, dizziness, loss of balance, difficulty walking, chest pain, shortness of breath, or palpitations. Any of these symptoms can signal a serious medical condition requiring advanced life support (ALS) care. It is better to doubt the patient's story and discover a serious medical problem, than to be unaware and miss a potential life threat.

Determining the mechanism of injury for an older patient injured in an automobile collision is also extremely important, as research has shown that these patients have a higher fatality risk due to their frailty.[4] The mechanism of injury associated with a rapid forward deceleration can typically be attributed to the seat

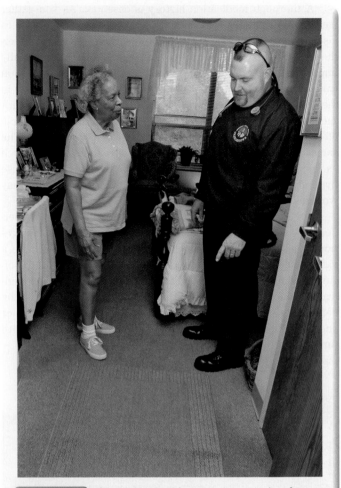

Figure 4-7 The EMS provider can impact the future health of an older patient by reporting fall risks noted at the scene and assessing the patient's mobility.
© Jones & Bartlett Learning. Courtesy of MIEMSS.

belt, even when correctly fastened. As you arrive on the scene, assess vehicle impact. Then, assess the body impact and organ impact of the patient. Note any obvious bruising, and consider compression injuries that may have been generated on impact. The older accident victim should be assessed for injuries involving soft tissue, as well as injuries to the neck, larynx, or trachea. If there is a question of steering wheel impact, assess for the following:

- Fractured sternum
- Pericardial tamponade
- Pneumothorax
- Flail chest
- Intra-abdominal injuries such as a ruptured spleen, liver, or bowel

Be especially suspicious of single-vehicle collisions. The older person experiences age-related physical changes that contribute to underlying limitations, which increase the risk for traffic accidents. For example, an older driver may experience a slower reaction time, lower visual acuity, decreased mobility, or suffer from a chronic condition that leads to driving impairment. However, there could also be a metabolic reason why the patient lost control of the car. For example, is there a chance the patient had a syncopal episode prior to the collision? When a person passes out, blood flow to the brain shuts off and the memory of passing out is not recorded. Therefore, even if the patient answers "no," he or she may have had syncope but just not remember clearly. The EMS provider must be a medical detective. Ask the patient, "What is the last thing you remember?" Was there a period of time when the patient experienced decreased mental alertness, making the patient unaware that time had passed? A major cause for syncope in the older patient has been attributed to polypharmacy interactions.[5] Do not miss a life-threatening problem because you are unaware of the common lack of recall that is associated with syncopal episodes.

In many EMS systems, age alone is a reason to bypass to a level-one trauma center. The older patient will likely require more interventions than the younger patient, including emergency department evaluation and treatment, surgical care, intensive care services, and rehabilitation. If you are concerned about the level of injury that has occurred to an older patient, err on the side of early triage to a level-one trauma center.

Immobilization Concerns

For older patients, the spine should be immobilized earlier and for lesser indications than younger patients. Older patients, especially those with arthritis, may sustain spinal injury with a lesser mechanism than younger, more flexible patients. Additionally, be sure to pad the area behind the patient's head and neck. If a patient's spine is **kyphotic**, modify your immobilization technique to prevent motion and maintain patient comfort. It is quite a challenge to immobilize older patients; because their risk of injury is greater, practice is important.

The older patient has thin skin that can quickly be damaged simply by the weight of the body on a hard surface (**Figure 4-8**). As a person ages, the characteristics of skin undergo intrinsic changes that cause the dermis layers to become thin with a loss of underlying fat cells, and wrinkled, transparent, and saggy due to bone loss. Due to these changes, pressure ulcers are more likely to occur when an area of the older person's skin is compressed between a bony prominence and an external surface, causing the flow of oxygen and nutrients to the skin's cells to decrease.

To prevent the formation of a pressure ulcer or worsening of one that already exists, place folded towels, wash cloths, or other soft padding material under areas where the skin comes in pressure contact with the backboard (**Figure 4-9**). Specifically, ensure the mid-back, shoulders, sacrum, heels, and occiput are cushioned; ask the patient about any additional areas where pressure is felt. Also, pay special attention to areas where arthritis or curvature of the spine creates a space between the patient's body and the backboard; fill in this space with towels or blankets so the patient is well supported and truly immobilized. As soon as the patient is cleared, take them off the backboard to avoid

skin breakdown. Commercial backboards with padding are also now available from various manufacturers. If you routinely transport many older patients, your service should consider investing in these boards.

Attitude Tip

Proper padding during immobilization is much more than a comfort issue for older patients. Lack of padding under "empty" spaces can lead to unnecessary spinal injuries, and inadequate skin protection at bony contact points can produce pressure sores that occasionally lead to life-threatening infections.

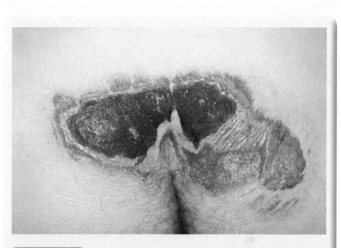

Figure 4-8 This photo shows a sacral pressure ulcer from a backboard. Be sure to pad older patients especially well at the mid-back, shoulders, sacrum, heels, and occiput.
© Mediscan/Alamy

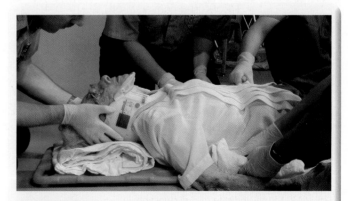

Figure 4-9 Provide padding at bony prominences to prevent damage caused by backboard pressure on fragile skin.
© Jones & Bartlett Learning. Courtesy of MIEMSS.

Physical Exam

If indicated, a rapid neurological examination of the patient should include the following:

- Glasgow Coma Scale (**Table 4-2**)
- Level of consciousness
- Pupil response
- Extremity movement
- Response to pain

Head/Neck

Caution must be used when assessing and palpating the neck of an older patient. Arthritic changes in the neck make cervical vertebrae more prone to fracture; manipulation of the older person's cervical spine should never be attempted in the field. Assess the neck for tracheal position, observe for flat or distended jugular veins, palpate the thyroid for size and symmetry, and assess the carotid impulse for strength and bruits.

Musculoskeletal

In order to address potential injuries to the older patient, the EMS provider must identify the normal and abnormal pathophysiological changes that occur with age. For example, bone deformities may occur with age or they may be induced by injuries. When the body ages, bones become less dense, more porous, and more fragile.

Muscle or ligament injuries will result in reduced movement due to swelling and tendon damage. To assess for joint mobility, tenderness, effusion, erythema, or deformity, evaluate the older patient's range of motion (ROM):

- Active ROM: Assess for pain or tenderness upon movement.
- Shoulder ROM: Assess flexion, extension, abduction, and adduction, observing for bilateral symmetry of shoulders or arms upon movement.
- Hand and forearm ROM: Assess hyperextension and extension of thumb/fingers, and forearm pronation with supination.

Document the joints assessed and any complaints of pain or signs of stiffness, spasm, and/or weakness. Generally, older patients with kyphosis and arthritis of the spine are in some sort of discomfort. Determine how the level of discomfort differs following the trauma. Remember that even a minor impact to the chest can fracture ribs in the older patient.

Lungs/Heart

Assess the chest for symmetry, rise, and expansion. Assess the lungs via auscultation. Watch for the use of accessory muscles, asymmetrical chest rise, or trachea shift for pneumothorax. Because the chest wall becomes stiffer with age, it may be difficult to identify a flail chest in the older patient by visualizing paradoxical chest movement. Patients may take shallow breaths due to the pain associated with deep breaths. Chest wall pain may be the only clues to significant chest trauma. The EMS provider should also be aware that loss of elasticity of the chest wall means that injury to the underlying lung requires less force in older people. These patients are more likely to develop pulmonary contusions with serious respiratory compromise and, therefore, also more likely to require level-one trauma center support when available.

Assess the heart, noting the apical impulse, rate, and rhythm, as well as any heart sounds, murmurs, rubs, or gallops. As you assess the chest, observe for bruising, tenderness, or radiating pain to the neck, shoulders, or back to rule out cardiac tamponade.

Abdomen

Assess the liver, spleen, and kidney area for ecchymosis, shape, and pain or tenderness when palpated. Aging blood vessels lose elasticity, so tears of the aorta are more common in older patients who sustain rapid deceleration. Due to the higher likelihood of the older patient needing computed tomography (CT) scans or angiograms for evaluation of a possible aortic injury, or thoracic surgery to repair one, a trauma center is the appropriate destination when available.

Table 4-2	Glasgow Coma Scale	
Test	**Response**	**Score**
Eye opening response	Spontaneous	4
	Voice	3
	Pain stimulation	2
	None	1
Verbal response	Oriented conversation	5
	Confused conversation	4
	Inappropriate words	3
	Incomprehensible sounds	2
	None	1
Motor response	Obeys commands	6
	Localizes pain	5
	Withdraws from pain	4
	Abnormal flexion (decorticate)	3
	Abnormal flexion (decerebrate)	2
	None	1

Score: 15 indicates no neurologic disabilities.
Score: 13–14 may indicate mild dysfunction.
Score: 9–12 may indicate moderate dysfunction.
Score: 8 or less is indicative of severe dysfunction.

Extremities

Deformity of the extremities may be the result of aging or disease, rather than injury. EMS providers should be familiar with the typical deformities that occur to fingers in the case of severe arthritis and not confuse these with fractures or dislocations (**Figure 4-10**). The **rule of symmetry** is an important consideration, especially for the older patient. A physical finding on one side of the body that is present on the other side of the body is more likely to be normal. Bruising found on one arm may be the result of trauma; however, if present on both arms, it may be due to age-related thinning of the skin and weakness in the capillary walls that supply the skin (**Figure 4-11**). Be sure to thoroughly question the patient in these cases.

Putting It All Together

The death of an older patient can occur in the first few minutes, hours, or days following trauma. The highest risk of death occurs within the Golden Hour, the 60 minutes immediately following the traumatic event. As the initial health care provider at the scene, the EMS provider's highest priority is to provide a rapid patient assessment while preparing to initiate resuscitation. For trauma patients, it is also vital to preserve body heat. This is especially important in older trauma patients who have decreased body fat.

Upon arriving at the scene, determine if the scene is safe. Once scene safety is established, begin to gather information regarding the incident. It is essential to gather as much information as possible about the patient's medical history from the patient and, when possible, those familiar with the patient. Based upon this initial assessment, further neurological and physical evaluations should be periodically performed throughout your assessment and compared to your original findings in order to assess for subtle changes.

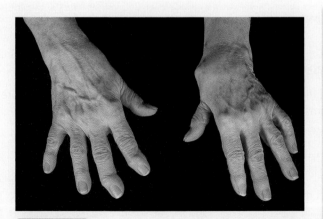

Figure 4-10 Do not confuse typical deformities of the fingers, caused by severe arthritis, with fractures or dislocations. Keep the rule of symmetry in mind.
© Joel Gordon Photography

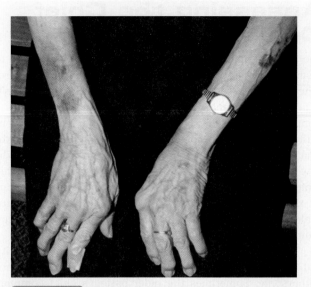

Figure 4-11 Check for symmetrical bruising on both sides of the body. Symmetrical bruising may be the result of age, not trauma.
Courtesy of Baltimore County Police Department, Baltimore, Maryland

Certain medical conditions and medications may influence treatment decisions, as well as decisions about whether or not to transfer the patient to a trauma center. Medical conditions such as heart disease and COPD can greatly reduce the body's ability to respond to trauma, and baseline hypertension can result in misleading findings regarding the patient's perfusion status. The use of an anticoagulant, such as Coumadin (warfarin), is of particular concern in the older trauma patient because it can cause prolonged bleeding from a relatively minor injury. Over-the-counter remedies such as aspirin, garlic, and ginkgo can also act as anticoagulants.

As with any trauma patient, the physical exam should be conducted in the most efficient manner to minimize on-scene time. Keep in mind that the physical exam should be performed systematically to ensure completeness, yet should be dynamic so that it may address the needs of individual patients. An important misconception is to assume that a decreased level of consciousness is the baseline mental status of an older patient. If people familiar with the patient are available, ask questions regarding the patient's cognitive baseline function. For example, "What was he like an hour ago? What was he like yesterday? Does he usually talk like this? Can he usually move his arms and legs?" This approach will provide a point of reference for the patient's cognitive evaluation. When in doubt, triage an older trauma patient to a trauma center.

Remember that hip fractures are serious injuries, and be sure to assess the hip or femur for an expanding hematoma. A patient may lose a liter of blood or more due to a hip or femur fracture. The hip can be supported by taping the patient's knees together, with a pillow or blanket between the thighs. Support the fractured leg in a position of comfort with additional pillows or blankets. Management of the older trauma patient is covered in more detail in the *Trauma* chapter.

Assessing the Chief Complaint

The chief complaint is the reason why the patient called for assistance and should be written in the patient's own words. Determining the chief complaint in the older patient may be difficult due to multiple disease processes and multiple or vague complaints. The signs or symptoms the patient presents with on-scene may be present every day, so consider asking what is different about what is bothering them today, what new problems they have today, or what is worse about their symptoms today. The history of the present complaint should be a chronological narrative that includes onset, location, quality, severity, and factors that both aggravate or relieve symptoms.[6]

When patients or caregivers list multiple complaints, it is helpful to ask them to identify the one thing that is the most bothersome. Sometimes the older patient's chief complaint may not be the most life-threatening issue. For instance, you may interview a patient whose complaint is inability to ambulate due to swelling in the feet but determine, based upon assessment, that the presenting problem is CHF, which is causing **pedal edema** and, thus, difficulty in getting around.

If the symptoms described by the older patient do not fit into a single category of complaint or presenting problem, ask targeted questions related to the most prominent or life-threatening complaint or finding; then, if time permits, move on to other assessment questions. For example, chest pain is usually a much more serious complaint than nausea. Therefore, if both are offered as complaints, begin by asking questions specific to chest pain assessment, and then move on as needed to the questions specific to nausea. In addition, do not focus only on the principal symptom; also note the absence of certain symptoms.

Attitude Tip

Attend to the emotional needs of the patient by asking directly if the patient is frightened, reassuring the patient, asking about previous history of emotional disturbances, and managing any emotional condition as professionally as possible.

Identifying Priority Patients

The EMS provider must understand how the assessment of the older patient differs from that of the younger adult and apply these principles during calls. The initial assessment should conclude with the identification of priority patients. These are patients who have conditions associated with higher risks of morbidity (illness) or mortality (**Table 4-3**). If your patient has one or more of these conditions, expedite transport and consider calling ALS if available.

Table 4-3 Identifying Priority Patients

Priority Patients	Considerations for Older Patients
Poor general impression	The patient has overall less reserves and, therefore, is more likely to deteriorate rapidly.
Unresponsive, no gag or cough	Gag response is less sensitive.
Responsive, not following commands	Determine if this is a change from the baseline mental status.
Difficulty breathing	The patient may fatigue earlier (run out of reserves).
Shock (hypoperfusion)	Early shock may be more difficult to identify because the heart rate and blood pressure compensatory mechanisms may be compromised by the patients prescribed medications.
Chest pain with blood pressure of <100 mm Hg systolic	Baseline systolic blood pressure may be higher; watch for a decrease from baseline blood pressure.
Uncontrolled bleeding	Gastrointestinal bleeding is more common.
Severe pain anywhere	The patient has less pain perception in general; therefore, moderate pain may be a priority.

Detailed Physical Exam

The decision to perform a detailed physical exam is based on the patient's condition. Similar to history, this part of the assessment may be a challenge with the older patient. Treating the older patient with respect and dignity is a high priority. Protect privacy by keeping undergarments intact if possible, and covering the patient with a sheet or blanket (**Figure 4-12**). Additionally, because thermoregulatory function is often impaired in older patients, they are frequently cold and prone to shivering. They may also have a diminished body temperature. The risk of heat loss is increased due to a decrease in body fat deposition and the ability to perspire. If possible, use blankets that have been warmed to cover the older patient. Make sure your ambulance compartment is warm, and take care to cover the patient's head when it is cold outside.

Table 4-4 lists some of the common physical findings of older patients that may be noted during the exam.

Attitude Tip

Covering the patient with a blanket to protect privacy and keep the patient warm shows the patient respect and will ultimately improve your exam.

Ongoing Assessment

As the body ages, there is a natural decline in organ function and physiologic reserve. As a result, a patient who is initially stable may become unstable in a short period of time. An older trauma patient with a systolic pressure of <90 mm Hg has an 82% mortality rate; in the presence of low cardiac output due to poor perfusion, the severity of a patient's injury escalates intervention priority.[7] If careful attention is not given to the appropriate areas of the ongoing assessment, the EMS provider could miss a patient's deterioration.

Ongoing assessment is made up of four steps: (1) repetition of the initial assessment, (2) repetition of the vital sign check, (3) repetition of the focused assessment (tailored to the patient's complaint or injuries), and (4) evaluation of the interventions that have been implemented.

Repetition of the initial assessment should take place at least every 15 minutes for a stable patient and at least every 5 minutes for an unstable patient. This step includes reevaluation of mental status, airway, breathing, circulation, and patient priority. Reassess and record the patient's vital signs, looking for trends toward improvement or deterioration. With frequent vital sign checks, remember to calculate MAP, which assesses the patient's coronary arteries, brain, and kidney function; if MAP is dropping below 70 mm Hg, intervention is needed.

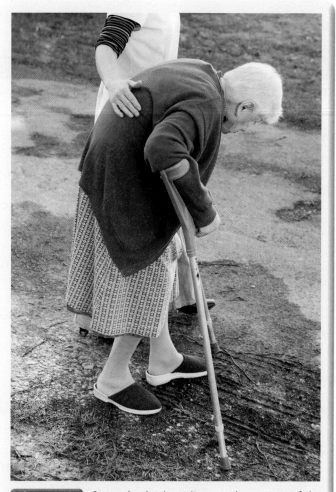

Figure 4-12 Severe kyphosis, or increased curvature of the spine, is not uncommon with older people.
© Phanie/Alamy

Repeat the focused assessment. In the medical patient, this means asking the patient how he or she feels now compared to before. In the trauma patient with a significant mechanism of injury, it will mean repeating the pertinent parts of the detailed physical exam. Check the interventions performed (**Figure 4-13**). Is the patient still receiving oxygen? If receiving ventilation, how well is the patient's chest rising? Has any bleeding resumed from a wound that was bandaged, or has bleeding started in a new area? How is the neurovascular function of the extremity that was splinted? Is spinal immobilization adequate?

Performing the ongoing assessment depends on the patient's condition. You may not have time to perform all of it or, sometimes, any of it. Occasionally you will not get past the initial assessment because the patient has life-threatening injuries that demand constant attention. Fortunately, these patients are uncommon; most EMS calls allow time to reevaluate the patient before arrival at the hospital.

Table 4-4 Physical Changes in Older Patients

Body Part	Finding
Head	■ Thinner scalp; less hair overall ■ Brown spots from sun exposure
Face	■ Skin wrinkles ■ Nose may enlarge due to cartilage changes ■ Brown spots from sun exposure
Ears	■ Hearing loss ■ Ears may develop small lumps or contain a hearing aid
Eyes	■ Decreased visual acuity ■ Smaller pupils ■ Opaque white ring of fatty deposits circling the cornea ■ Sunken appearance of the eyes due to loss of **periorbital** fat ■ Cataracts clouding the lens ■ Prior surgery may result in irregular pupils or a hole in the iris
Mouth	■ Dentures ■ Tooth loss, gum shrinkage ■ Less-white teeth ■ Varicose veins of the tongue
Neck	■ Decrease in range of motion; increased spinal curvature ■ Stiffness and chronic pain to touch and movement
Chest	■ Less chest expansion with breathing ■ Bilateral crackles on inspiration that clear with subsequent deep breaths
Abdomen	■ Decreased muscle tone ■ Loss of ability to become rigid with internal bleeding or infection
Pelvis	■ Decreased range of motion ■ Frail bones that fracture easily
Extremities	■ Decreased range of motion ■ Symmetrically decreased muscle strength ■ Varicose veins; symmetrical bruising; edema, especially in lower legs/feet ■ Decreased capillary refill, loss of muscle mass
Back	■ Increase in curvature of the spine ■ Frail bones that fracture easily ■ Chronic pain ■ Loss of flexibility (**Figure 4-14**)

Common Complaints of the Older Patient

Shortness of Breath

Shortness of breath is a common complaint in the older population. The sensation of being unable to breathe can be extremely frightening and potentially life threatening. With age, both lung performance and chest wall compliance decrease, and senile emphysema occurs with alveoli enlargement. As these natural physiological changes occur, functional residual capacity increases, thus increasing the older person's work of breathing and risk for respiratory failure following an injury or disease process (**Figure 4-15**).

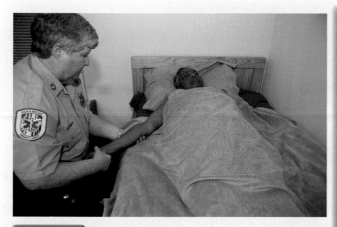

Figure 4-13 The older patient is often very modest and uncomfortable with being exposed. Protect privacy by keeping undergarments intact, if possible, and covering the patient with a blanket.
© Jones & Bartlett Learning. Courtesy of MIEMSS.

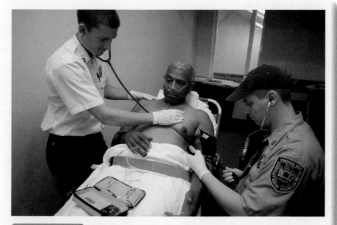

Figure 4-14 Ongoing assessment concludes with checking the interventions that have been performed. for example, is the patient still receiving oxygen? If so, is the oxygen having the intended effect?
© Jones & Bartlett Learning. Courtesy of MIEMSS.

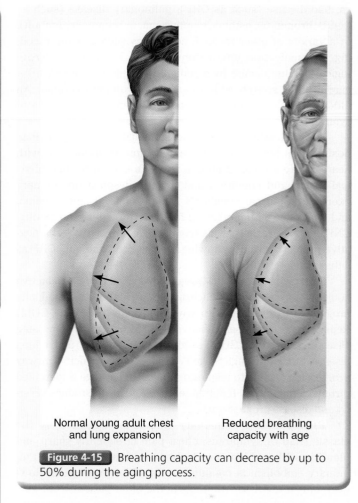

Normal young adult chest and lung expansion

Reduced breathing capacity with age

Figure 4-15 Breathing capacity can decrease by up to 50% during the aging process.

Potential Causes

In the older population, shortness of breath may be a symptom of anxiety associated with the older patient's disabilities, impairments, and/or inability to provide self-care. Situational anxiety disorder often goes undiagnosed and can lead to depression.[8] Shortness of breath may also be a symptom of

CASE STUDY 2

© 123dartist/Thinkstock

You are called to the local senior center for an older male complaining of weakness. Upon your arrival, you find the patient sitting in a chair in the senior center's dining area. You are told he walked to the dining room using his walker and are a full meal without any problem but when he went to stand, he suddenly felt weak and nauseated. The symptoms started about 10 minutes ago and have not improved. He appears pale and sweaty. He has not vomited but he complains of pain in his abdomen and between his shoulder blades. His breathing is slightly labored with a respiratory rate of 24 with oxygen saturation of 89%. You are able to palpate a radial pulse but it is slow (45 beats per minute) and weak.

- What additional information do you want to obtain about this patient?
- What should you do to manage this patient?

cardiac disease (such as CHF); pulmonary disease (such as COPD, bronchitis, asthma, emphysema, or pulmonary emboli); or a variety of other medical conditions such as pain, bleeding, or medication interactions. As the heart ages, physiological decline occurs by a reduction in ejection force, myocardial fiber stretch which can cause volume overload. An older patient's history is critical in determining the origin of symptoms.

RED FLAGS: There is no standard "red flag" in diagnosing CHF. Significant signs and symptoms associated with heart failure are based upon a patient's overall history, physical exam, and condition and include dyspnea on ordinary exertion, nocturnal cough, S3 gallop, bilateral ankle edema, and lung rales with increasing fatigue.[9] In the hospital setting, BNP and NT-proBNP levels have a high sensitivity and a negative predictive value, allowing their use to "rule out" CHF as a diagnosis.

RED FLAGS: COPD presents as a chronic productive cough and dyspnea with wheezing upon exertion that gradually progresses to dyspnea with wheezing upon rest.[10] The GOLD Report from the Global Initiative for Chronic Obstructive Lung Disease released the GOLD staging criteria for obstructive lung disease. Stage I through Stage IV produce an obstructive airway progression leading to respiratory failure. The stage is identified through a pulmonary function test (PFT) that determines severity and disease progression.

RED FLAGS: Pulmonary emboli is suggested by the classic triad of symptoms: chest pain (frequently sharp and pleuritic with sudden onset), dyspnea, and hemoptysis. Pulmonary embolism is common in the older population; however, one of the first symptoms in the older patient will likely be an altered mental status, and some older patients with pulmonary emboli will only present with syncope. In addition, massive pulmonary emboli could present with hypotension, tachycardia, syncope, or cardiac arrest. Important physical findings such as tachycardia, tachypnea, hypoxia, and fever are frequently misdiagnosed as pneumonia in the older patient. The EMS provider should assess for high-risk factors such as a sedentary lifestyle, blood clot in the legs, cancer, vascular injury, long-bone fractures, or a period of immobility.

RED FLAGS: When pulmonary edema is suspected, look for dyspnea, tachypnea, and respiratory distress. With this disease process, the patient's alveolar flood because the heart no longer pumps effectively. Cardiogenic origin is indicated by a history of paroxysmal nocturnal dyspnea or progressive orthopnea. Recent medical history for noncardiogenic pulmonary edema would be preceded by a specific predisposing clinical condition such as pneumonia or sepsis, or multiple blood transfusions. Noncardiogenic pulmonary edema is characterized by a productive cough of frothy pink sputum.

Table 4-5 shows a list of distinguishing features to aid in the differentiation of an older patient with COPD versus an older patient with CHF.

Medication Tip

The older patient is frequently prescribed many more medications than the younger patient, multiplying the risk of interactions and side effects, including breathing difficulty.

Assessment

Remember that the patient may have multiple disease processes or past medical problems. Determine if a chronic condition could be causing the breathing difficulty (**Figure 4-16**). If so, ask what made the patient call for help or what makes the breathing more difficult today. Attempt to learn which signs and symptoms are chronic and which are new or acute. Never withhold oxygen from a patient complaining of breathing difficulty, regardless of origin or onset.

Chest Pain

Chest pain is common in older patients, and can often be life threatening, with cardiovascular disease being a leading cause of death in the older population. Clinical presentation may be atypical due to altered sensitivity resulting from a comorbid illness such as diabetes or undiagnosed hypertension. A chief complaint of chest pain in the older patient should always be taken seriously and treated aggressively; identification of cardiovascular risk factors is significant, as a cardiac condition in the older patient may produce lethal afflictions if not treated immediately.

Potential Causes

Cardiac problems can present atypically in older patients—for example, with only a feeling of weakness or shortness of breath. Furthermore, pain may not occur in the chest at all, but instead may be felt in the shoulder, neck, arm, back, or jaw. This type of pain presentation may easily be mistaken for a toothache, a pulled muscle, or arthritis. History and the results of the physical exam will be helpful in ruling out or confirming a cardiac condition.

Chest pain is very commonly caused by **ischemia** (lack of blood supply to the heart muscle), which causes heart pain. When this is the case, the patient is usually aware of the diagnosis and may already take nitroglycerin. Often, the patient can tell you if the pain is different from the usual type of pain; that information can be a critical clue to the cause of the pain. The problem, however, is that chest pain is often attributed to **angina** when it is actually a heart attack in progress.

RED FLAGS: Assessment findings that should raise suspicion of a more serious etiology include abnormal vital signs and cardiac arrhythmias such as tachycardia or bradycardia.

Other significant signs include hypoperfusion that produces symptoms of confusion or skin changes such as ashen color or diaphoresis. Other indications for cardiac abnormalities include irregular heart sounds, such as new heart murmurs or S3 or S4 with a **pulsus paradoxus** >10 mm Hg, and/or MAP >70 mm Hg.

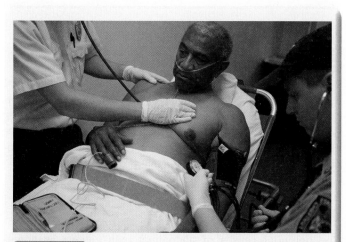

Figure 4-16 Determine if the patient's shortness of breath is caused by a chronic condition or if the problem is new.

© Jones & Bartlett Learning. Courtesy of MIEMSS.

Assessment

There are several questions that can help determine the cause of chest pain in the older patient. For example, ask where the pain is located. Substernal chest pain (located beneath the sternum) may be a sign of heart attack, while pinpoint chest pain may indicate a pulled muscle. **Epigastric pain** may be abdominal in nature. It is also important to ask what the pain feels like. Older patients may experience chest pain differently (or not at all) compared to younger patients. The older patient who had cardiac surgery in the past may not have the typical mid-sternal chest pain symptom. In addition, atypical chest pain may occur in postmenopausal women or older patients with comorbidity for peripheral vascular disease or diabetes neuropathy.

During cardiac assessment, it is very important to expose and examine the chest of a patient with chest pain. Inspection of the chest may reveal old scars from previous cardiac surgeries, indicating a patient history of cardiac problems. A pacemaker, defibrillator, or left ventricular assistive device (LVAD) may also be present under the skin on the upper chest (**Figure 4-17**). These devices are common in the older patient and provide clues about past arrhythmias. The upper torso may also reveal trans-dermal medication patches, such as a nitroglycerin patch. It is possible that the patient's complaint is caused by too much or too little of this medication. (If the patient is hypotensive and wearing a nitroglycerin patch, remove the patch and begin fluid

Table 4-5	Chronic Obstructive Pulmonary Disease (COPD) versus Congestive Heart Failure (CHF)	
	COPD	**CHF**
History	Long-time smoker Known emphysema or bronchitis On oxygen, inhalers, or steroids Made worse by upper respiratory infection Chronic hacking morning cough	Prior heart attacks/angina Prior coronary artery bypass graft, angioplasty On nitrates, cardiac medications, furosemide (Lasix) **Orthopnea**, nocturnal dyspnea New cough or frothy sputum
Physical	More trouble getting air out Pink Puffer* or Blue Bloater† Wide, round, barrel chest Swelling at the base of the nails (clubbing)	More trouble getting air in Jugular vein distention (JVD) and pedal/leg edema Generally normal chest Point of maximal impulse displaced to right
Treatment	Oxygen Inhaled beta agonists No morphine—bad for respiratory rate Intubation if severe	Oxygen No beta agonists—bad for heart Nitrates, aspirin (if chest pain) CPAP if severe

* *Pink Puffer:* Thin, frail, reddened complexion. Breathing fast, using accessory muscles. Has a prolonged expiratory phase with cheeks puffed out to force air out.

† *Blue Bloater:* Fat, bobust, cyanotic complexion. Breathing fast, using accessory muscles, but hard to see due to thick, short neck. Has a prolonged expiratory phase, leaning forward.

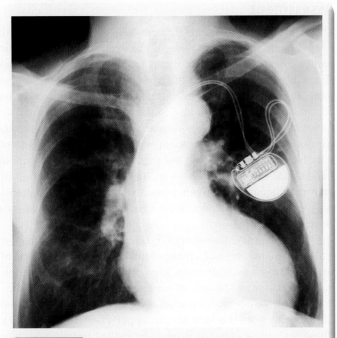

Figure 4-17 Presence of an implanted pacemaker or cardioverter-defibrillator (automated implantable cardio defibrillator [AICD], pictured) beneath the skin provides clues regarding past arrhythmias.

resuscitation!) At the very least, the patch will indicate a medical history of angina, heart attack, or arrhythmia.

Another extremely dangerous condition that is more common in older patients than in younger patients is an aortic **aneurysm**, or bulging of the blood vessel. An aortic aneurysm can lead to blood leakage or major bleeding if the vessel tears open. If undetected, a torn aorta can cause death in minutes. Classically, these patients will report a tearing chest pain that spreads to the back.

RED FLAGS: Physical findings (once dissection occurs) will include chest pain with neurological deficits, significant differentials in blood pressure and pulses in both arms (20% of the time), aortic regurgitation, and aortic murmur heard in the left upper sternal border (LUSB). Other signs and symptoms may include limb ischemia or back pain. Diagnostic tests include chest X-ray (60% show widened mediastinum), ECG with nonspecific ST and T wave changes, and computer-aided tomography (CAT) scan of the chest.

Medication Tip

If your patient is hypotensive and wearing a nitroglycerin patch, remove it. It is possible that the patient's complaint is caused by too much or too little of this medication.

Medication Tip

Numerous medications and other ingested substances can lower or raise the heart rate. Ask patients if they are taking beta-blockers or calcium channel blockers (lower), or if they are taking respiratory medications, caffeine, tobacco, or other stimulants (raise).

Abdominal Pain

The older patient who presents with abdominal pain is more likely to be hospitalized, have surgery, or die from the cause of pain compared to the younger patient. Early determination of the cause results in a higher chance of successful treatment. The care given by the EMS provider is often the first vital step in that process.

Potential Causes

The potential causes of abdominal pain change as a person ages. For example, appendicitis is common in younger patients, but uncommon in older patients. When it does occur in the older patient, the appendix is more often ruptured and the patient is sicker. Older patients also suffer from different disease processes than younger patients, including the following:

- Vascular problems
  - Abdominal aortic aneurysm (AAA)
  - Mesenteric ischemia/infarction
- Diverticulitis
- Gallstones
- Peptic ulcer disease
- Intestinal obstruction from hernia, tumor, or adhesion

Assessment

RED FLAGS: Take special note of abdominal pain of undetermined origin that includes the following symptoms:

- Acutely systemically unwell, abdominal distension, and dehydration
- Posttrauma guarding or rebound tenderness
- Abdominal distension with severe pain and/or signs of peritonitis
- Signs of shock (e.g., tachycardia, hypotension, diaphoresis, confusion)

While assessing the older patient with abdominal pain, remember: patient history is the key to successful care. The expected signs and symptoms associated with a particular abdominal problem may be altered or absent in the older patient. Having the patient show you the location of his or her abdominal pain may help in indicating the cause:

- Diffuse abdominal pain may indicate acute pancreatitis, mesenteric ischemia, peritonitis, gastroenteritis, or sickle cell crisis; abdominal distension with nausea and vomiting may be associated with alcohol abuse or a history of gallstones.
- Epigastric pain may indicate dyspepsia, peptic ulcer, or gastric ulcer. Nausea, vomiting, belching, bloating, and heartburn are more commonly associated with gastric ulcers in persons over 50 years old, whereas dyspepsia is more commonly associated with duodenal ulcers in persons 30 to 50 years old.
- Right upper quadrant pain may indicate cholecystitis, biliary colic, congestive hepatomegaly, or a perforated duodenal ulcer. The older patient may feel a sudden right upper quadrant pain that radiates to the right scapula and experience anorexia, nausea, and vomiting.
- Right lower quadrant pain may indicate appendicitis, cecal diverticulitis, or Meckel's diverticulitis. For the critically ill older patient showing signs of hemodynamic instability, observe for symptoms of vomiting, diarrhea, and shock associated with a ruptured appendicitis. Because of comorbidities and a decrease in sensory perception, the older patient with appendicitis experiences a 5% higher incidence of mortality.[11]
- Bilateral right and left lower quadrant pain may indicate abdominal abscess, abdominal hematoma, cystitis, endometriosis, incarcerated hernia, inflammatory bowel disease, pelvic inflammatory disease, renal stone, ruptured AAA, or torsion of ovarian cyst or testis.
- Left upper quadrant pain may indicate gastritis or splenic disorder or rupture and associated shock. For the critically ill older patient showing signs of hemodynamic instability, assess quickly!
- Left lower quadrant pain may indicate ischemic colitis or sigmoid diverticulitis. The older patient with acute diverticulitis may also experience symptoms of fever and constipation.

The approach of assessment is the same for the older patient as it is for the younger patient: observe, auscultate, and palpate. However, the abdominal organs of an older patient will not necessarily be in the same location as a younger patient; your knowledge of anatomy will help guide physical assessment (**Figure 4-18**).

When assessing abdominal pain in the older patient, use the acronym OLD CART (Onset, Location, Duration, Characteristics, Aggravating factors, Relieving factors, Treatment). Older

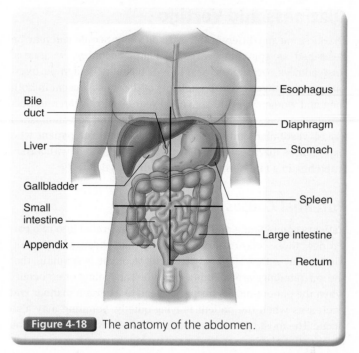

Figure 4-18 The anatomy of the abdomen.

patients have a blunted immune response, meaning they do not develop inflammation or an increase in sensory perception like a younger patient. Therefore, they often do not have the typical symptoms or physical findings associated with abdominal complaints.

A hard abdomen is a very serious sign in the older patient and signals the need for ALS care and rapid transport. A distended abdomen may indicate dilated loops of bowel due to an obstruction or blood due to a ruptured aneurysm. A whooshing sound (**bruit**) heard in the abdomen with each heartbeat may indicate an aneurysm. The absence of bowel sounds could suggest a serious abdominal problem; the patient with this condition should be frequently reassessed during transport, and findings should be reported to the emergency department.

Medication Tip

Medications, including over-the-counter medications, can alter a patient's response to the examination of an abdominal pain complaint. Keep medications in mind during examination.

Tachycardia or hypotension, even if transient, can indicate the presence of a life-threatening process such as gastrointestinal bleeding, an AAA, a perforated ulcer, spreading infection from diverticulitis, or a nonabdominal process such as heart attack. Recent mental status changes are often the earliest sign of a serious illness in the older patient.

Dizziness and Vertigo

Dizziness means different things to different people and may be described as spinning (**vertigo**), lightheadedness, weakness, unsteadiness, wooziness, or a loss of balance. Benign paroxysmal positional vertigo or complaints of dizziness present in both men and women over the age of 50 years, and is often multifactorial secondary to adverse effects of drugs and age-diminished visual, vestibular, and proprioceptive abilities. The patient who experiences dizziness and falls may wind up injured, with a fractured hip, in a long-term care facility, or even dead.

Potential Causes

Patients complaining of dizziness can be separated into two categories: those who experience vertigo and those who do not. The patient with vertigo may feel that he or she is spinning, that the surroundings are spinning, or both. The feeling often occurs when the patient moves his or her head in a certain manner and decreases when the patient is lying quietly. Vomiting may also occur. The most common causes of dizziness with vertigo in the older patient include conditions affecting the peripheral vestibular system (inner ear):

- Benign paroxysmal positional vertigo
- Meniere's disease
- Labyrinthitis

Brain injury patients may also develop vertigo. Make sure to assess for this condition, as it can be a very helpful indicator.

> **Communication Tip**
>
> Dizziness means different things to different people. You can separate these patients into two categories by asking whether the patient experiences vertigo.

Patients with dizziness but no vertigo can be further divided: those with dizziness when resting and those with dizziness when active. Possible causes of dizziness at rest include an irregular heart rate, severe hypotension, and hypoxia. Constant hypotension can be the result of shock or a heartbeat that is irregular, too fast, or too slow. The EMS provider should determine if the patient has a heart problem or pacemaker, and what medications he or she takes. Certain heart medications can make the heart beat too slowly, and some over-the-counter medications, such as certain cold compounds and herbal medications, can cause an increase in blood pressure, potentially causing dizziness.

Assess if the dizziness occurs with a simple activity such as sitting up from bed or getting out of a chair. If dizziness occurs, consider low blood pressure, dehydration, or anemia as a possible cause. Transient hypotension can be the result of mild dehydration, intermittent heart rhythm irregularities, or effects of medication. Determine if the patient has been eating and drinking fluids on a regular schedule, and ask if he or she took any medication before the onset of dizziness, as medicines that are used to treat high blood pressure (antihypertensives) can cause dizziness. Additionally, determine if the patient has diabetes and whether there are signs of low blood sugar, such as tremors or sweating.

Other possible causes for vertigo or dizziness include non-neurologic disorders that involve inadequate oxygen or glucose delivery as a result of hypoxemia or hypoglycemia; certain hormonal changes (e.g., thyroid disease); the effects of CNS-active drugs; and, occasionally, panic disorder, hyperventilation syndrome, anxiety, or depression.

> **Medication Tip**
>
> Certain heart medications can make the heart beat too slowly and some over-the-counter medications can cause the blood pressure to increase. Either of these effects can cause dizziness.

Assessment

Normal vital signs, oxygen saturation, and blood sugar should help rule out most potentially life-threatening causes of dizziness such as hypotension, heart rhythm problems, or hypoglycemia. Orthostatic (postural) vital signs may identify a low circulating volume that causes dizziness when the patient is standing. To obtain this measurement, take the patient's blood pressure and heart rate when he or she is lying quietly. Then, have the patient stand; observe for unsteadiness and ask if the patient feels unsteady. Recheck after approximately 1 minute of standing. If the systolic blood pressure decreases by 20 mm Hg or more or the diastolic blood pressure decreases 10 mm Hg or more, or if the pulse increases by 20 beats/min or more, the patient has orthostatic hypotension.

Is **nystagmus** present? These jerky eye movements can be seen with dizziness that is caused by problems in the balance mechanism of the inner ear or brain. Auscultate for bruits (whooshing) over the carotid arteries and gently palpate for a decrease in pulsatile force. These may be signs of decreased blood flow to the brain. Check for evidence of a previous stroke, such as facial droop, arm drift, or slurred speech. Check for scalp tenderness, bruising, or swelling from a recent trauma; note any difficulties with standing or walking.

Patients with dizziness due to hypotension, abnormal heart rhythm, evolving stroke, or a recent history of head injury are priority patients. Hypotension may be due to simple dehydration, but it may also indicate significant shock. Similarly, the abnormal heart rhythm can be the result of a simple decrease in heart rate or an unstable rhythm such as ventricular tachycardia. Patients with an evolving stroke are a priority because of the potential for treatment with clot-busting drugs. Changes in assessment after a head injury may indicate a worsening condition, and these patients also require priority transport and treatment. Nonpriority patients with dizziness are at risk for becoming priority patients from falls due to dizziness.

Fever

The approach to identifying the underlying cause of the febrile older patient should encompass both history taking and physical examination. Normal temperatures can range from 96°F to 100°F (35.6°C to 38.2°C). A fever can be defined as an oral temperature that is greater than 100°F or, in the older patient, a rise of 2°F from the person's baseline temperature. Because older individuals often have a lower baseline body temperature and are less able to develop a fever when infected, the presence of a fever in an older patient is a significant finding that requires immediate attention.

For an iatrogenic cause without the presence of a rash, consider pulse-temperature disassociation drug fever. Most commonly, this occurs when the older patient has been taking a new medication for about a week; however, this reaction does not pertain to patients with an underlying cardiac arrhythmia or those who are taking beta-blockers. If a patient has an elevated temperature, confirm that their apical pulse is tachycardic. In order to do this, subtract 1 from the last digit of the Fahrenheit reading, and then multiply by 10 and add to 100; so, for example, if the patient has a fever of 104° F, the formula would be the following: $(4 - 1) \times 10 + 100 = 130$ apical beats per minute. Medications that can cause an iatrogenic effect include barbiturates, penicillin, NSAIDS, salicylates, and atropine.[12]

Potential Causes

When fevers of an unknown origin are present in an older person, research has shown that several disease processes prevalent in the older population may exist; these include autoimmune rheumatologic disorders or malignancies (particularly, non-Hodgkin lymphoma). When an older patient presents with a fever and the secondary symptom of a severe headache, the EMS provider should consider meningitis. A stiffer-than-normal neck flexion is also a sign of meningitis. When shaking chills and dyspnea are secondary symptoms, pneumonia should be considered. The older patient has a higher risk of developing pneumonia; despite antibiotics, pneumonia is a common cause of death. Diminished breath sounds or crackles on one side that do not clear after several inspirations may indicate a pulmonary source for the fever. Infections of the urinary tract are also common. Other causes of fever include infection in the blood, gastroenteritis, and soft-tissue infections, especially those resulting from pressure ulcers. Although much less frequent, temperature elevation may also be caused by noninfectious problems such as heat stroke, **thyroid storm**, and aspirin overdose.

Assessment

The diagnostic approach to a febrile patient should be guided by the severity of the patient's symptoms. History must include origin, duration, residence, and past travel to determine exposure risks. Begin by asking about the patient's baseline temperature. The older patient may not have an elevated heart rate with temperature increase; instead, the patient may have an altered mental status change. If this is the case, suspect a serious infection. Even if the temperature is normal or only slightly elevated, recent mental status changes are suggestive of infection. Other commonly associated symptoms may be diminished or absent.

The older patient with pneumonia may not have a cough, and respiratory rate will normally stay in the higher range of normal. Low oxygen saturation may be the first indication of a pulmonary infection. Are there signs of increased work of breathing, or is the patient taking an over-the-counter medication? The patient may admit to using cough syrup, but forget to tell you about the cough. Ask about the patient's immunization status. Viral infections such as the common cold do occur in older people, and influenza can be devastating; thus, a yearly flu vaccination in the fall is very important. Pneumovax, the pneumonia vaccine, is generally only administered once and provides protection from the bacteria *Pneumococcus*, one of the most common causes of bacterial pneumonia.

Burning on urination may be absent in the older patient with a urinary tract infection. Instead, ask the patient or caregiver if daily activities have recently changed. The patient's eating habits may be altered, or the person may be less active or more fatigued. Additionally, ask if the patient is on medication that is known to alter the fever response (such as acetaminophen [Tylenol], aspirin, or NSAIDs) or alter the ability to fight infection (such as steroids like prednisone).

> ### Medication Tip
>
> If the patient with little or no fever is taking medications that are used to treat a possible infection (such as cough syrup), or used to alter fever response (such as acetaminophen [Tylenol], aspirin, or NSAIDs) or the ability to fight infection (such as steroids [prednisone]), it may be a sign of infection.

Determine the presence of any other diseases or conditions that may elevate the risk of infection, such as diabetes, kidney stones, or gallstones. Pneumonia and bronchitis are frequently seen in patients with COPD, and pressure ulcers often grow a variety of bacteria that can result in local or blood-borne (system-wide) infection.

The focuses of the physical exam for the febrile older patient are finding immediate life threats and helping determine the source of infection. Often, the older patient with a fever will lack the typical signs of infectious disease as seen in the younger adult. As previously noted, the patient's heart rate may not increase as expected with temperature increase, and the patient may be sicker than he or she appears on initial contact.

As you perform the head-to-toe exam, note any red, warm, tender, or swollen skin areas, which may indicate infection. Specifically, look for pressure ulcers that may have developed over high-pressure areas such as the heels, sacrum, or buttocks. Do these wounds look clean or dirty? Are they red, swollen, and/or draining? What is the color of the drainage? Is there an odor associated with the wound? Local or generalized abdominal tenderness upon palpation may also be the result of infection; tenderness upon percussion (tapping) of the back over the kidneys in the patient with a fever is consistent with a urinary tract infection involving the kidney.

Remember, fever in the older patient means serious infection until proven otherwise. Although the older febrile patient may not appear severely ill and may have fewer associated signs and symptoms of infection, older people die from infection more often than younger adults. In addition, the presence of chronic disease and use of routine medications may increase the potential for infection in the older patient, while simultaneously confusing the assessment process. Older patients with fever must be assessed for the existence of sepsis and septic shock; if found, make the patient a priority for ALS care and give fluids for hypotension. The course of infectious disease in the older patient is typically longer and more severe. Early detection in the field allows for early treatment and a better outcome.

Generalized Pain

Pain is whatever, wherever, and whenever the individual determines it to be. On any given day, older people experience pain about twice as often as younger adults. Surveys indicate that pain occurs in 25% to 50% of older people who live in the community and 45% to 85% of older people who live in nursing homes. Pain can be long-standing (chronic) or of recent onset (acute). The cause may be obvious (as in a deformed extremity after a fall) or a bit cloudy (as in, "I hurt all over"). In either event, intervention can help decrease the patient's pain or response to pain.

Potential Causes

The causes of acute pain in older people are the same as in younger people, and generally are the result of acute illness or injury. On the other hand, chronic pain in older people tends to result from the normal wear and tear of aging or the effects of chronic disease. Some of the more common causes are musculoskeletal and neurologic disorders, cancer, and depression. Examples of musculoskeletal disorders that may cause pain include arthritis, bone disorders (such as brittle bones [osteoporosis] or

soft bones), compression fractures, and narrowing of the spinal canal. Examples of neurologic disorders include shingles (herpes zoster infection) and nerve damage from diabetes (**diabetic neuropathy**). Cancers occur more frequently in older people and can result in pain due to the tumor or its spread, or the various cancer treatments. Psychiatric problems such as depression can cause pain or worsen a patient's existing pain. Conversely, pain can cause a patient to feel depressed, which may make the pain worse. It is important to remember that pain is an emotional experience.

Attitude Tip

Pain can cause a patient to feel depressed, which can make the pain worse. It is important to remember that pain is an emotional experience.

Assessment

With decreasing sensory perceptions, older persons often do not have the typical symptoms seen in younger patients, and history is key to pain evaluation. Use open-ended questions to hear about the pain in the patient's own words and follow up with appropriate direct questions, completing the familiar OPQRST (Onset, Provocation/Palliation, Quality, Radiation, Severity, and Time) mnemonic. The OLD CART mnemonic can also be used to assess the older patient's generalized pain.

An accurate history will reveal the most information concerning the patient's pain. If the patient cannot provide a history, it is important to enlist the assistance of family, friends, or caregivers. If minimal history is available, assume pain is present and manage accordingly. Older people often live with daily pain; however, their outward expression may be muted or they may hesitate to complain of the pain for several reasons. For example, they may believe that pain is a normal part of aging, they may fear they will not be believed, or they may fear the pain is caused by a serious illness such as cancer and worry about lengthy hospitalization. Cultural differences may also alter an older person's response to pain. It is important for the EMS provider to recognize these differences when providing services to a diverse population, and to believe the older patient's complaint of pain. Pain is a very personal experience. To be successful in the assessment of the older patient with pain, the EMS provider must demonstrate empathy and interest in the patient's problem.

The initial assessment should determine if the pain is the result of an immediate threat to life. The outward expressions of pain, such as grimacing or groaning, may be diminished or absent and vital signs may or may not be altered in the older patient, despite significant pain experience. Interpret altered vital signs as secondary to an illness or injury, and not pain, until proven otherwise. For example, the older person with gastric ulcer pain has tachycardia due to blood loss, not due to pain. If the patient is stable and the pain is acute and localized, a focused exam is indicated (**Figure 4-19**). For more generalized or chronic pain complaints, the head-to-toe or detailed physical exam is performed but may not provide an abundance of information.

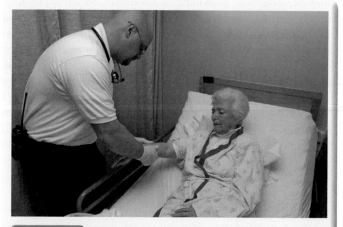

Figure 4-19 If the patient is stable and the pain is acute and localized, a focused exam is indicated.

© Jones & Bartlett Learning. Courtesy of MIEMSS.

> ### Attitude Tip
>
> To be successful in the assessment of the older pain patient, the EMS provider must demonstrate empathy and interest in the patient's problem.

Nausea, Vomiting, and Diarrhea

The EMS provider should automatically assess any older patient experiencing nausea, vomiting, and/or diarrhea for dehydration. Research has indicated that normal homeostasis declines with age: the ability to respond to thirst decreases and the kidney's ability to concentrate urine decreases. The result is a negative water balance in the body, which leads to dehydration and loss of **euvolemia**. Dehydration in the older patient can cause an altered mental status, rapid weak pulse with hypotension, systolic <90 mm Hg, and an increased risk for stroke or transient ischemic attack (TIA).

A detailed history of symptom onset will assist in determining the origin. For example, the older person with a sudden onset of loose watery diarrhea should be assessed for infectious disease. Foods contaminated with *Escherichia coli*, staphycoccal bacteria, or clostridial bacteria can cause toxin-induced diarrhea with vomiting within 6 hours of ingestion. *Campylobacter*, *Salmonella*, and *Shigella* are other frequent or well-publicized bacterial causes of food poisoning. Viral gastroenteritis accompanied by nausea, vomiting, and watery, nonbloody diarrhea occurs within several days following generalized body aches and low grade fever.

Because older people take more medication than younger people, medication-induced nausea, vomiting, and diarrhea can also be expected. Research has indicated that 20% to 40% of gastrointestinal symptoms are produced by iatrogenic drug-induced reactions.[13] Frequent offenders include antibiotics and cancer medications.

> ### Medication Tip
>
> Antibiotics and cancer medications are frequent offenders among the causes of nausea, vomiting, and diarrhea.

Everyone reacts to stress differently and, with many individuals, the gastrointestinal tract is sensitive to emotions. Thus, nausea, vomiting, and diarrhea may also be the result of the body's response to stress or extreme emotional experience. Additional causes of nausea and vomiting include an obstructed, distended, or twisted bowel; motion sickness;

CASE STUDY 3

© 123dartist/ThinkStock

You are called to the home of an 85-year-old female. When you arrive at the residence, you find the patient sitting in a recliner, alert but quite anxious. The patient is obese and complains of having shortness of breath for the last two days. She states it gets worse with exertion. Her skin is flushed and dry and her ankles appear swollen. Her vital signs are: BP: 168/90; HR: 100; and R: 24 with oxygen saturation of 97% on room air. Lung sounds are clear and equal.

- What additional information will be helpful in this case?
- What should you do?

inner ear infection; poisoning or overdose; diabetes; previous surgery; cardiac ischemia or brain irritation from increased intracranial pressure; and infection of the brain (encephalitis) or the brain coverings (meningitis). Additional causes of diarrhea include inflammatory bowel disease, traveler's diarrhea, and constipation. Constipation is a common problem in older people and can result in diarrhea when liquid stool moves past the fecal obstruction. Lactose intolerance is another cause with an increased incidence in older people. The decreased ability to digest milk sugar, or lactose, can produce diarrhea when milk products are ingested.

Assessment

Initially determine if the nausea, vomiting, or diarrhea is acute or chronic. Determine the onset, frequency, appearance, color, and odor of the vomit or stool. If acute, has there been any recent change in diet or medication? Has the patient traveled to a foreign country prior to the onset of symptoms? Ask if anyone in the home or long-term care facility has experienced an onset of the same complaints. If chronic, has there been any change in the usual pattern of symptoms? Are there any new symptoms such as bleeding, abdominal pain, dizziness, or chest pain?

Remember to prioritize patients with life-threat indicators such as a poor general impression, an altered mental status, or abnormal vital signs (low temperature, tachycardia, hypotension, etc.). Determine the presence of dehydration through vital signs and dry mucous membranes. Use the detailed physical exam to determine the need for further field treatment and to provide clues as to the cause of the problem. If the patient has been vomiting, listen closely to the breath sounds for evidence of aspiration, such as fine or coarse crackles. Note the characteristics of any observed vomitus or stool such as the consistency, color, odor, or presence of blood.

Recall that nausea, vomiting, and diarrhea can be the result of a problem inside or outside of the gastrointestinal system and can lead to significant fluid loss; alterations in the acid–base balance; or abnormal levels of body sodium, potassium, chloride, and bicarbonate (electrolytes). Determine whether the patient has signs or symptoms of gastrointestinal bleeding: bright red blood in the vomit (hematemesis) or stool (hematochezia) indicates active bleeding, while digested blood in the vomit (coffee-ground emesis) or dark, tar-like stools (melena) indicate previous bleeding in the stomach or small intestine. The importance of being familiar with nongastrointestinal causes for nausea, vomiting, and diarrhea is recognizing any serious underlying problem, such as cardiac ischemia, that would merit immediate EMS treatment.

Summary

The assessment of the older patient is more complicated and requires a greater level of knowledge from the EMS provider than does the assessment of the younger adult patient. A more comprehensive history and physical exam will lead to a better assessment and improved care to the older patient population.

References

1. Fried, Ferrucci, Darer, Williamson, & Anderson: Untangling the concepts of disability, frailty, and comorbidity: implications for improved targeting and care. *J Gerontol A Biol Sci Med Sci* 2004:59(3):255–63.

2. Resnick NM: Urinary incontinence in the elderly. *Medical Grand Rounds* 1984:3:281–290.

3. Galavis J & Wooten J: Polypharmacy: Keeping the elderly safe. *Modern Medicine*, 2009. Available at: http://www.modernmedicine .com/managed-healthcare-executive/news/polypharmacy-keeping -elderly-safe

4. Li G, Braver ER, Chen LH: *Exploring the high death rate per vehicle-mile of travel in older drivers: fragility versus excessive crash involvement.* Arlington, VA, Insurance Institute for Highway Safety, 2001.

5. Barker LR, Burton JR, Zieve PD (eds): *Principles of Ambulatory Medicine, ed 6.* Philadelphia, PA, Lippincott Williams & Wilkins, 2003.

6. Lynn S Bickley MD, Fiona R, Prabhu MD: *A Guide to Physical Examination and History Taking,* Philadelphia, PA, Wolters Health Kluwer 2005.

7. Jacobs D, Plaisier B, Barie PS, et al.: Practice Management Guidelines for Geriatric Trauma: The EAST Practice Management Guidelines Work Group, *J Trauma* 2003:54:391–416.

8. Hassan S. Anxiety Disorders in the Elderly. Nova Scotia, Dalhousie University.

9. Barker LR, Burton JR, Zieve PD (eds): *Principles of Ambulatory Medicine,* ed 7. Philadelphia, PA, Lippincott Williams & Wilkins, 2007.

10. Cash J, Glass C:. *Family Practice Guidelines, Second Edition.* New York, NY, Springer Pulishing Company, 2012.

11. Elangovan S. Clinical and laboratory findings in acute appendicitis in the elderly. *J Am Board Family Pract* 1996:9:75–78.

12. Barker, Burton, Zieve, 2007, p 460.

13. Ghahremani GG. Gastrointestinal complications of drug therapy. *Abdomen Imaging* 1999: 24:1.

CASE STUDY SUMMARIES

Case Study 1 Summary

You realize the patient is able to respond to your questions if she can see your lips moving. She tells you that she feels slightly weak and a little dizzy. She has no pain and had none prior to or during the episode. Additionally, she did not feel the episode coming on and there was no seizure activity. She has no lateralizing weakness or numbness. The patient's speech is clear, her grasp is equal, and she denies shortness of breath. She tells you she has an implanted pacemaker/defibrillator and that her blood pressure medication was recently changed. The patient's vital signs are: BP: 104/56; HR: 112 irregular (atrial fibrillation on the monitor); and R: 20 and clear with an oxygen saturation of 95%. The 12-lead ECG is non-diagnostic and finger stick glucose is "normal."
Additional questions to ask the patient include the following:

- What is her normal BP? Is a systolic BP of 104/56 actually hypotensive for her?
- What medications is she taking? Does she have a nitro patch affecting her pressure?
- Did she eat or drink prior to church?
- Has she had a recent volume loss via vomiting/diarrhea/bleeding?
- Is she orthostatic?

Syncopal Sunday episodes typically require an extensive work up and are often attributed to a variety of causes. Obtain IV access, monitor the patient, and transport her to a hospital. The patient's pacemaker/defibrillator will most likely be interrogated and the hospital may keep the patient overnight to run a variety of tests. Collecting scene and immediate post-event data about the patient and identifying any changes that occur en route to the hospital will assist in the overall management and treatment of the patient.

Case Study 2 Summary

There are a variety of possible causes for this patient's pain. You should obtain and monitor his blood pressure reading to determine if he is normotensive or hypotensive. Additional questions to consider include: What is the patient's normal heart rate and blood pressure? Is he on any other medications that affect heart rate or blood pressure? Has the dose been changed or have other medications been added to his regimen? Is he a dialysis patient that skipped dialysis and is now hyperkalemic and bradycardic as a result of a high potassium? Is the abdominal pain/nausea a symptom of an early bowel obstruction, ruptured diverticulum, or other abdominal issue? A low blood pressure reading could be the result of postprandial hypotension (the diversion of blood to the stomach to digest food). Patients with postprandial hypotension sometimes even develop chest pain. The pain also could be due to a myocardial infarction (MI) with atypical symptoms; a possible aortic aneurysm/dissection; an allergic or adverse reaction to a food he ate; or a reaction to a new medication, such as a calcium channel blocker or beta blocker that causes bradycardia and hypotension.

Placing the patient into a position of comfort will be important. Lying flat may not be the best position for this particular patient; instead, a semi-Fowler's position may make him feel better. The patient's heart rate may be caused by vagal stimulation related to the nausea or the nausea may be due to something else. Obtain a 12-lead ECG and look for a heart block of some sort. Consider if the patient actually needs to be treated for his heart rate, recognizing that he may only need monitoring if he remains alert and his symptoms diminish now that he is no longer sitting upright. Ask about the location, quality, and radiation of the patient's pain. Additionally, ask about the patient's last bowel movement and the color of the stool. Sometimes severe abdominal cramps occurring shortly after eating can be caused by the bowel attempting to move constipated stool. Palpate for rigidity and pain location.

The key to managing this patient is monitoring, IV access, and transport to the hospital. Further treatment will most likely depend on how the patient changes with repositioning. Does his oxygen saturation remain low? Was it low due to poor perfusion? Has it improved without supplemental oxygen? If not, does it improve with supplemental oxygen? In the hospital the patient's vital signs will continue to be monitored, lab tests will be run, and chest/abdominal x-rays or a CT scan will be taken. Abdominal pain in the older adult can be difficult to diagnose and typically requires hospital admission to determine final diagnosis.

Case Study 3 Summary

Ask the patient about any coughing, pain, fever, and/or chills. If she is coughing, is the cough productive? What color is the sputum? Is she infectious? Ask about medications and allergies, and assess the patient's work of breathing, looking for accessory muscle use or retractions. You note her nail beds and lips are pink. Her monitor shows a sinus tachycardia at 110. The 12-lead ECG has no ST elevation and there are no extra heart tones.

Other questions to consider include those related to her normal and recent activities. Is this patient possibly suffering from a pulmonary embolism? (Tachypnea and tachycardia with shortness of breath are common symptoms of this problem.) Is she anxious about something going on in her life? Does she have a history of lung problems (COPD, asthma, tuberculosis, CHF)? Clear and equal lung sounds seem to rule out asthma, COPD, CHF, and pneumonia, but may still be produced with a pneumothorax if the area collapsed is not large.

The patient's symptoms may only be a reaction to anxiety; however, she will need to go to the hospital for testing to make this determination. Start an IV and monitor cardiac rhythm, vital signs, oxygen levels, respiratory status, and mental status while en route to the hospital.

Psychosocial Aspects of Aging

LEARNING OBJECTIVES

1. Describe the epidemiology of depression, suicide, and substance abuse in older people, including incidence, morbidity/mortality, risk factors, and prevention strategies.

2. Identify the need for intervention and transport and develop a systematic treatment and management plan for the older patient experiencing a psychological emergency.

3. Discuss assessment findings and management considerations for older patients who have a history of substance abuse.

4. Describe the assessment and management of the older adult patient, when given a specific psychosocial scenario.

Introduction

For the majority of older adults, the later years are ones of fulfillment and satisfaction with a lifetime of accomplishments. Their children may be grown, they may be blessed with grandchildren, and it may even feel like life's work is mostly completed. For other older adults, however, later life may be characterized by physical pain, psychological distress, doubts about the significance of life's accomplishments, financial concerns, loss of loved ones, dissatisfaction with living conditions, and seemingly unbearable disability. When these factors lead to hopelessness about the possibility of positive change, depression, substance abuse, and even suicide are possible outcomes.

Substance abuse—particularly alcohol and drug abuse and misuse—is often underestimated, underdiagnosed, and undertreated among the older adult population. The EMS provider is often the first healthcare professional to have contact with an older adult suffering these afflictions. This chapter discusses the epidemiology, causes, recognition, and clinical management of depression, suicide, and alcohol or substance abuse to assist the EMS provider in recognizing the significance of identifying and caring for these specific psychiatric emergencies in the older adult.

Psychosocial Changes With Age

If an older person is viewed as more rigid and cautious than a younger person, is this an age-related change or a generational difference? Consider the older person who has lived through the Depression and is hesitant or resistant of a financial investment, even when the return is predictable and stable. This hesitation may be a cohort difference relating to an earlier time in life. The psychology of aging is complicated and influenced by many factors, including normal age-related psychological changes, disease processes (both physical and emotional), and society's views on the aging process.

One thing to keep in mind is that disease is not a normal part of aging. Do not assume that because someone is old that he or she cannot reason and discuss issues intelligently. Older people have a lifetime of experiences, and are often willing to share these experiences with younger people. Engaging an older person in conversation, even while providing prehospital care, can be rewarding (and therapeutic) for both patient and provider. The following sections briefly discuss cognition, memory, and personality, and how each is affected by the aging process.

Cognition

Disease processes and overall intellectual ability often have a bearing on cognition in later life. **Cognition** refers to the mental processes used for perceiving, remembering, and thinking. Cognitive abilities are the greatest when people are in their 30s and 40s. By the late 50s and early 60s, these abilities begin to decline, but only to a small degree. The effects of cognitive changes are not usually noticed until the 70s and beyond.

It should be noted, however, that these changes do not happen to everyone. Within each age group, there are wide variations in cognitive ability, and older people are the most heterogeneous of all cohorts.

Memory

Memory is a complex function that is divided into different types, and only some types are affected by age. Difficulties that occur with memory are usually minor and vary widely from person to person, making generalizations difficult. Further complicating the issue are the different methods by which researchers categorize memory.

One popular method for categorizing memory is dividing it into *implicit memory* and *explicit memory*. Implicit memory is the retention of skills and reflexes that have been acquired, such as the procedures for driving a car. This type of memory generally remains intact throughout life. Explicit memory is the conscious remembering of facts and events, and it is these memories that are more vulnerable to age-related decline. For example, older adults may have increasing difficulty with word retrieval—that is, recalling the name of a familiar person or object.

CASE STUDY 1

© 123dartist/Thinkstock

On a hot summer day you are dispatched to the parking lot of Bob's Big Burgers for a man slumped over in an automobile. The driver's side window of the vehicle is down and, as you approach the patient, you hear an occasional gasping breath. A law enforcement officer is standing beside the vehicle holding a pistol and an empty liquor bottle, which was found on the passenger seat. The officer advises you that the patient is a 68-year-old male and he has already spoken with the man's wife. She informed the officer of the recent loss of her husband's boss via suicide, which resulted in the loss of her husband's job. He has not been taking his medications as directed and keeps saying he is "worthless." As you initiate care, you note the patient is disheveled in appearance.

- What are your first priorities in caring for this patient?
- What additional concerns do you have?

It is widely believed that one type of memory—called working memory—is most affected by age. Working memory is the retention of information that must be manipulated or transformed in some way. Conscious mental processing goes on in working memory: Information must be taken from the environment and from the individual's memory stores in order to accomplish a mental task. For example, when a person is paying a restaurant check, the amount of the check is stored in working memory while the person figures out which bills should be used to pay the check, how much change is due, and how much tip to leave. Everyone has limits on how much information they can keep in working memory at one time. As a person gets older, complex mental tasks can become more difficult if they require too much information to be held in memory. Some researchers also postulate that reduced speed of information processing reduces the efficiency of working memory.

In general, memory tasks that are complex and require manipulating a lot of new information quickly become more difficult with age. However, knowledge that has been accumulated over a lifetime is generally retained, and well-practiced skills and abilities remain intact. In addition, vocabulary usually grows throughout life.

Personality

Personality, like intelligence, is complex, making it hard to measure. In general, personality is defined as the essence of a person—that is, the qualities that make an individual unique and recognizable. Longitudinal studies have found that personality traits remain relatively constant throughout one's adult life.

Depression

Depression is a common, often debilitating, psychiatric disorder, affecting an estimated 7 million adults aged 65 years or older in the United States.[1] Older adults with chronic illness and those residing in skilled nursing facilities are even more likely to be depressed, with as many as 25% to 50% suffering from some degree of clinical depression.[2] Depression is diagnosed three times more commonly in women than in men. In contrast to effectively coping with sadness, grief, loss, or temporary "bad moods," depression is persistent and can interfere significantly with an older adult's ability to function.

It is impossible to predict which older adults will develop depression, but studies indicate that substance abuse, isolation, prescription medication use, and chronic medical conditions all contribute to the onset of significant depression (**Figure 5-1**). The American Psychological Association lists nine symptoms of major depression[3]:

1. Depressed mood most of the day, nearly every day, as indicated by either the patient saying so (reports of feeling sad, empty, or hopeless) or observation made by others

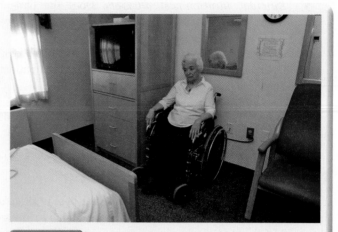

Figure 5-1 Isolation and chronic medical problems are among the factors that contribute to depression in older adults.
© Jones & Bartlett Learning. Courtesy of MIEMSS.

2. Markedly diminished interest or pleasure in all, or almost all, activities, most of the day, nearly every day
3. Significant unintended weight loss or gain (more than 5% change in body weight over 1 month)
4. Insomnia or hypersomnia nearly every day
5. Either physical agitation such as pacing, shaking, or rocking, or physical immobility nearly every day (observable by others, not merely subjective report of restlessness or lethargy)
6. Fatigue or loss of energy nearly every day
7. Feelings of worthlessness or excessive or inappropriate guilt nearly every day
8. Diminished ability to think or concentrate or indecisiveness nearly every day
9. Recurrent thoughts of death (not just fear of dying), recurrent suicidal ideation without a specific plan, or a suicide attempt or a specific plan for committing suicide

Symptoms of depression can also be remembered by modifying the popular mnemonic OPQRST (Onset, Provocation, Quality, Radiation, Severity, Time). This mnemonic is used during patient assessment to help providers remember key questions regarding the patient's chief complaint. When used for the assessment of depression symptoms, OPQRST stands for the following:

- *Orientation.* Is the patient oriented to time, person, place, and event?
- *Provokes/palliates.* What does the patient enjoy? Why were you called?
- *Quality of life.* Does the patient have a recent or pending loss?
- *Relationships/reassurance.* Does the patient have family, friends, or support groups?

- *Suicidal ideation/past attempts.* Does the patient make references to suicide? Does the patient have plans and the means to commit suicide?
- *Time/treatment history.* When did the symptoms begin, and how long have they lasted? Has the patient been treated?

Suspect depression when the patient has problems with four or more of these symptoms.

Red Flags: Possible Depression

Most of the signs of depression require a great deal of time, a quiet environment, and a well-established relationship to assess adequately. Other healthcare providers are rarely afforded the luxury of time or control over the older patient's environment, so it is vital that EMS providers are vigilant in making observations and aware of the "red flags" that indicate depression:

- *Frequent non-urgent EMS calls.* All EMS systems have clients who appear to overuse the system. These "frequent fliers" are a source of great frustration for many EMS providers and, more importantly, divert valuable resources away from more urgent patient needs. These habitual users also represent one of the most dangerous traps for EMS providers. A sense of complacency when caring for the same non-urgent patient multiple times is natural ("Oh, it's just Mr. Jones again; he's never really sick."), but very risky. For the older adult, frequent contact with caring, competent professionals may be an important part of the social support network. If an older adult begins to frequently call for EMS response, especially for non-urgent complaints, the healthcare team must assess for the presence of significant depression. Non-urgent complaints may be this person's desperate attempt to receive help, even if he or she is unaware of it.
- *Frequent visits to the emergency department or physician's office.* Many older adults are able to gain access to health care on their own. Any older adult who seeks contact with the healthcare system frequently, but has no chronic or complicated medical problem, must be evaluated for the possibility of depression.
- *Severity of complaint does not match physical findings.* Patient complaints of pain or discomfort that seem disproportionate to the amount of abnormality on physical examination can be troubling to EMS providers. In the older adult, these complaints may be a sign of depression. You must guard against discounting the patient's complaints of pain and remain cognizant of the personal, subjective aspects of pain perception.
- *Poor personal hygiene or neglect of home cleanliness and order.* Older adults suffering from depression often lose interest in keeping their environment clean and orderly. Personal hygiene is frequently neglected due to a lack of energy or a sense that "it doesn't matter."
- *Lack of social support network.* It is important for EMS providers to assess an older adult's support network. A patient who reports no contact with family, friends, or social or religious organizations is at a significantly higher risk of clinical depression than one who does have such contacts.
- *Anhedonia.* **Anhedonia**, or the sense that nothing is enjoyable anymore, is an important sign of significant depression that you can ask about. For a patient suffering from serious depression, a simple question like, "What do you do for fun?" may elicit an answer that alerts the provider to the condition.

Attitude Tip

Most EMS systems have "frequent fliers"—people who continually call upon EMS with seemingly non-urgent needs. It is natural to become frustrated when responding to these calls, but for the older adult, frequent contact with caring, competent professionals may be an important part of their social support network. If an older adult begins to call frequently for EMS response, especially for non-urgent complaints, the healthcare team must assess for the presence of significant depression. Do not become complacent in treating any patient.

Impact

Major depression, a significant predictor of suicide in older adults, is a widely underrecognized and undertreated medical illness. Emergency personnel who are astute and aware of the symptoms listed earlier can be instrumental in this identification, and can help prevent deterioration to suicidal intent. (Suicide in the older population is discussed in more depth later in this chapter.)

Suicide can be the ultimate, tragic outcome of untreated clinical depression, but the depressed older adult suffers from other problems as well. Several studies have found that a depressed older adult has a significantly higher mortality rate from *all* causes. Some of this increase in mortality may be due to the tendency of depressed older adults to be less adherent to health practices such as diet and medication regimens, but good evidence exists that physiologic changes associated with severe depression degrade both the immune system and the cardiovascular system. Studies of trauma victims also suggest that depressed older adults have a higher incidence of all forms of trauma, especially falls (**Figure 5-2**). Major depression will almost always lead to cognitive impairment, most markedly memory loss. Dementia, Alzheimer's disease, and "senility" have often been diagnosed in older adults when clinical depression was the real origin of their memory loss and inability to function independently.

Screening for Depression

The Geriatric Depression Scale can be used to assess an older adult's level of depression (**Table 5-1**). Although use of the full scale may not be practical in the prehospital environment, the concepts can still be valuable in spotting signs of depression during patient assessment.

Treatment

Treatment of severe depression in the older adult usually consists of psychological counseling and/or medication. For many older adults, simply reestablishing relationships with the community or with family is enough to lessen the severity of the illness. Senior citizen centers, community meeting places, social clubs, and other community outreach programs offer older adults a chance to build social networks that are extremely helpful in combating depression. Many older adults find participation in an organized religion to be especially helpful, and pet ownership is thought to significantly reduce the incidence of depression in older adults. It seems that any activity that increases

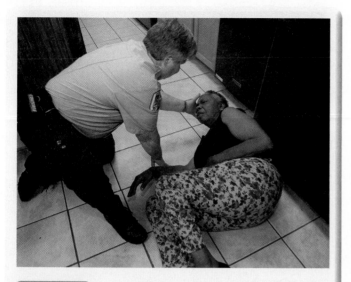

Figure 5-2 Depressed older adults have a higher incidence of trauma, especially falls.
© Jones & Bartlett Learning. Courtesy of MIEMSS.

Table 5-1 Geriatric Depression Scale	
1. Are you basically satisfied with your life?	Yes/**No**
2. Have you dropped many of your activities and interests?	**Yes**/No
3. Do you feel that your life is empty?	**Yes**/No
4. Do you often get bored?	**Yes**/No
5. Are you in good spirits most of the time?	Yes/**No**
6. Are you afraid that something bad is going to happen to you?	**Yes**/No
7. Do you feel happy most of the time?	Yes/**No**
8. Do you often feel helpless?	**Yes**/No
9. Do you prefer to stay home most of the time rather than go out and do new things?	**Yes**/No
10. Do you feel that you have more problems with memory than most?	**Yes**/No
11. Do you think that it is wonderful to be alive now?	Yes/**No**
12. Do you feel pretty worthless the way you are now?	**Yes**/No
13. Do you feel full of energy?	Yes/**No**
14. Do you feel your situation is hopeless?	**Yes**/No
15. Do you think that most people are better off than you are?	**Yes**/No

Scoring: Answers in **bold** indicate depression. Score 1 point for each bolded answer.
  A score >5 points is suggestive of depression.
  A score ≥10 points is almost always indicative of depression.
  A score ≥15 points should warrant a follow-up comprehensive assessment.

Source: Reproduced from Yesavage, J. (1986). Use of the self-rating depression scale in the elderly. http://www.stanford.edu/~yesavage/GDS.html.

social support and relieves isolation can be helpful in fighting depression. In addition, physical exercise may also combat depression.

Communication Tip

> Any activity that increases social support and relieves isolation can be helpful in fighting depression.

Antidepressant medications are widely used as effective treatments for depression (**Table 5-2**). Antidepressant drugs influence the function of certain chemicals (neurotransmitters)

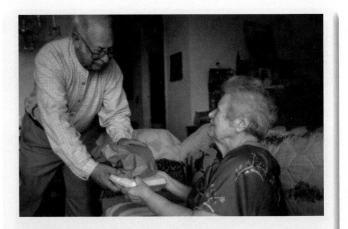

Figure 5-3 Social services with outreach programs provide contact that is valuable in preventing and treating depression.
© Joel Gordon Photography

Table 5-2 Medications (Antidepressants) Used to Treat Depression in Older Adults

Medication Type	Generic Name (Brand Name)
Monoamine oxidase (MAO) inhibitors	Isocarboxazid (Marplan) Phenelzine (Nardil) Selegiline (Emsam) Tranylcyopromine (Parnate)
Selective serotonin reuptake inhibitors (SSRIs)	Citalopram (Celexa) Escitalopram (Lexapro) Fluoxetine (Prozac) Fluvoxamine (Luvox) Paroxetine (Paxil) Paroxetine mesylate (Pexeva) Sertraline (Zoloft)
Serotonin and norepinephrine reuptake inhibitors (SNRIs)	Desvenlafaxine (Pristiq) Duloxetine (Cymbalta) Milnacipran (Savella) Venlafaxine (Effexor or Venlafaxine) Vilazodone (Vilibryd)
Tricyclic antidepressants	Amitriptyline (Amitriptyline) Amoxapine Clomipramine (Anafranil) Desipramine (Norpramin) DoxepinImipramine (Tofranil) Nortriptyline (Pamelor) Protriptyline (Vivactil) Trimipramine (Surmontil)
Other	Buproprion (Aplenzin, Wellbutrin, or Zyban) Maprotiline (Maprotiline) Mirtazapine (Remeron) Trazadone Nefazodone (Serzone)

in the brain. Tricyclic antidepressants and monoamine oxidase inhibitors are very effective drugs, but can have serious side effects. The newer antidepressants—selective serotonin reuptake inhibitors (SSRIs) and serotonin and norepinephrine reuptake inhibitors (SNRIs)—are also very effective in treating depression and are associated with much lower levels of side effects. The key to drug therapy is to encourage adherence, especially at the onset of therapy when effects are less noticeable.

EMS providers should become aware of the senior services available in their area of coverage. For example, most communities have outreach programs in place to keep older adults in contact with social systems (e.g., Meals On Wheels), which has been shown to be vital in both the treatment and prevention of clinical depression (**Figure 5-3**). Additionally, many resources are available for psychiatric counseling and treatment. In the event that the EMS provider finds the older patient in need of other services or resources, contact may be made to the local Area Agencies on Aging.

Suicide

The highest rates of suicide in the United States occur in the older population. In 2010, the reported rate of suicide for older people was 14.89 per 100,000.[4] For men, suicide rates rise with age, most significantly after age 65. The rate of suicide in men age 65 years and older is seven times that of females of the same age, with widowed white males being at particularly high risk. The suicide rates for women, on the other hand, peak first between the ages of 45 and 54 years, and again after age 75 years. It is estimated that as many as one-half of all suicides committed by older people go unreported and are mistakenly classified as death by accident, natural cause, or some other form of trauma.[5]

Table 5-3	Methods of Suicide in Older Adults in the United States
Method	**Percentage of Completed Suicides**
Firearms	71.6
Poisoning	11.9
Suffocation (hanging)	10.2
Falling	1.9
Drowning	1.0
Fire	0.3

Data from: Centers for Disease Control and Prevention, WISQARS. *Fatal Injury Reports, 2011*. 2013. Available from: webappa.cdc.gov/sasweb/ncipc/mortrate10_us.html

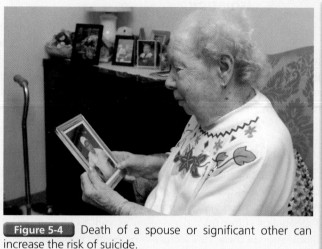

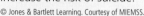 **Figure 5-4** Death of a spouse or significant other can increase the risk of suicide.
© Jones & Bartlett Learning. Courtesy of MIEMSS.

Older people who attempt suicide provide fewer warnings of intent and choose much more lethal means than younger victims (**Table 5-3**). For example, in 2011, more than 71% of completed suicides in older persons in the United States involved firearms, as compared to just over 50% in the general population.[6] Additionally, older people generally have diminished recuperative capacity to survive a suicide attempt. For the young, it is estimated that there are 100 to 200 attempts for every committed suicide; in the older population, that figure drops to four attempts to every completion.[7] Although women attempt suicide three times as often as men, males of all age groups are more than four times more likely to complete suicide than females. This discrepancy is due to the fact that the majority of males attempting suicide use firearms, whereas females often use other, less lethal means (such as an overdose).

Major depression is a significant predictor of suicide in older people, and is a widely underrecognized and undertreated medical disease. Compared to their younger counterparts, older people are more likely to suffer from a depressive diagnosis prior to their suicide. Several studies have found that many older people who commit suicide have visited a primary care physician very close to the time of the suicide: 20% on the same day, 40% within 1 week, and 70% within 1 month.[8]

Etiology of Suicide

Suicide can happen in any family, regardless of socioeconomic class, culture, race, or religious affiliation. Research suggests that some circumstances increase the risk of suicide in the older adult.

Death of a Loved One

As adults reach later years of life, loss of significant people in their lives, including family, friends, and spouses, becomes inevitable. Often the surviving person is left with feelings of abandonment, guilt, fear, and loneliness. Loss of a spouse or significant other who may have shared the person's life for decades can be especially devastating (**Figure 5-4**).

Physical Illness

Physical illnesses common in older adults can affect mood, self-esteem, independence, and sense of well-being. Along with the psychological pressures associated with physical illness often come economic insecurity and reliance on some form of public assistance (e.g., Medicare, Medicaid), which may deepen the feelings of diminished self-worth and dependency.

Depression and Hopelessness

As discussed earlier in this chapter, depression is a very common but serious problem for many older adults. Research shows that risk factors for suicide include depression and other mental disorders, or substance-abuse disorders (often in combination with other mental disorders). More than 90% of people who commit suicide have these risk factors.[9]

Although usually difficult to assess and even more difficult to quantify, hopelessness seems to be the biggest risk factor for suicide in all age groups. Multiple studies of suicide-attempt survivors have revealed almost universal feelings of hopelessness prior to the attempt. The older adult who truly feels that his or her life circumstances are hopeless is at an extremely high risk of imminent suicide.

Attitude Tip

The older adult who feels that his or her life circumstances are hopeless is at extremely high risk of suicide. Keep this in mind during your assessment.

Isolation

Many older adults have difficulty with mobility due to physical illness, which can lead to social isolation and feelings of diminished self-worth. Death of friends and relatives may further isolate older people. Loneliness resulting from social isolation has also been shown to contribute to suicidal thoughts.

Alcohol Abuse and Dependence

A direct relationship exists between alcoholism and suicide. Studies indicate that risk of suicide in alcoholics is 50% to 70% greater than in the general population. Between 40% and 60% of alcoholics suffer from depression as well as alcoholism; the combination of these risk factors is especially concerning.

Loss of Meaningful Life Roles

Significant changes in life roles often result in feelings of hopelessness and low self-esteem associated with suicide. Retirement, moving out of a long-time family home, the inability to continue to be involved in community projects, or the inability to work often contributes to a sense of isolation.

Suicide among Older People in Long-Term Care Facilities

Functional incapacity, loneliness, loss of control, lack of a strong family support network, limited visitation by friends and family, and social withdrawal are all factors that can lead to depression and suicide. Additional contributory factors for individuals in long-term care facilities include the following:[10]

1. *Loss.* Loss is a major contributing factor for suicide. Significant losses include loss of a spouse, friends, pets, money, control, independence, and physical mobility, as well as sensory/perceptual losses.
2. *Depression.* Environmental stress seems to be a primary factor in precipitating depressive symptoms. When older people are unable to control significant events in their environment, feelings of lowered self-concept and self-esteem result.
3. *Family dynamics.* Family rejection, abandonment, and lack of informal supports are important factors contributing to suicidal behavior among residents of long-term care facilities.
4. *Physical and functional loss.* Loss of physical function, especially sight, hearing, speech, mobility, and ability to perform activities of daily living, may contribute to a sense of helplessness and loss of control.
5. *Moves.* Frequent moves within and out of long-term care facilities serve to increase personal and psychological pain for vulnerable adults.

Screening for Suicide Potential

Frequently, the EMS provider is the first-line and, for some patients, only healthcare contact. Keep in mind that only a small percentage of older adults pursue medical treatment for psychological issues. Not only do many fail to seek care, they also frequently deny the problem when questioned. These conditions cross the entire socioeconomic spectrum. Afflicted older adults may be found in nursing homes, their own homes or apartments, prisons, homeless shelters, and on the street (**Figure 5-5**).

It is equally important to screen for suicide as it is to monitor for warning signs. The following sections discuss important warning signs every EMS provider should be aware of when interacting with the older patient. The easy-to-remember mnemonic, IS PATH WARM, may also be used (**Table 5-4**).

Talking About or Seeming Preoccupied with Death

It is common for older adults to contemplate the end of life and try to get their "affairs in order." However, when an older adult begins to talk excessively about death, especially at the expense of other topics that used to interest them, their risk of suicide must be assessed.

Giving Away Prized Possessions

The older adult contemplating suicide will often give away family heirlooms, photographs, and other keepsakes. EMS providers are seen as caring, concerned professionals who are always there to help, and therefore may also receive gifts. Gifts that are expensive or represent some significant personal event in the patient's life are the provider's clues to **suicidal ideation** (thoughts or plans). Distributing prized possessions to family members can also be a last attempt at maintaining some control over life circumstances and avoiding "causing trouble" for others with their suicide.

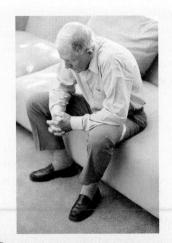

Figure 5-5 Substance abuse and depression cross the entire socioeconomic spectrum, affecting the older population in their own homes, in institutions, and among the homeless.
© Yuri Arcurs/ShutterStock, Inc.

Table 5-4		Mnemonic for Warning Signs of Suicide: IS PATH WARM
I	Ideation	Expressing or communicating suicidal ideation: ■ Threatening to hurt or kill him/herself; or talking of wanting to hurt or kill him/herself ■ Looking for ways to kill him/herself by seeking access to firearms, pills, or other means ■ Suddenly talking or writing about death, dying, or suicide
S	Substance abuse	Using substances (alcohol or drugs) more often
P	Purposefulness	Feeling no reason for living or no sense of purpose
A	Anxiety	Feeling anxiety or agitation, being unable to sleep or sleeping all the time
T	Trapped	Feeling like there is no way out
H	Hopelessness	Feeling hopeless
W	Withdrawal	Withdrawing from friends, family, and society
A	Anger	Feeling rage or uncontrolled anger, seeking revenge
R	Recklessness	Acting reckless or engaging in risky activities
M	Mood change	Having dramatic mood changes

Data from: American Association of Suicidology. *Know the Warning Signs.* Available from: web.archive.org/web/20111206024410/http://www.suicidology.org/web/guest/stats-and-tools/warning-signs

Taking Unnecessary Risks

Suicide carries a certain stigma among many people. One way to avoid an active role in one's own death is to put oneself at unnecessary risk through behavior. Walking alone in unsafe neighborhoods, driving with excessive speed without wearing a seat belt, and seeking confrontation with police or other imposing figures are all examples of behavior that may be an attempt to end life in a more "acceptable" way than suicide.

Increased Use of Alcohol or Other Drugs

In an attempt to lessen the feelings of hopelessness and depression associated with suicidal ideation, many older adults will turn to alcohol or other drugs as a means of escape. If you witness evidence of excessive alcohol or drug use at the scene of a response for an older adult, the patient must be assessed for suicide risk.

Nonadherence to Medical Regimens

Failure to take prescribed medications, follow special diets, or perform other basic healthcare needs may result in frequent EMS calls and generally poorer health. This is often also a sign that an older adult has "given up" and may be contemplating suicide (**Figure 5-6**).

Acquiring a Weapon

Most suicides committed by older adults involve firearms. If an older adult suddenly purchases a firearm but had no prior interest in guns, caregivers should be alerted to the potential for self-harm. Many who are not contemplating suicide acquire a weapon to protect their family and home, but any older adult who abruptly purchases a firearm should be questioned in regard to motivation.

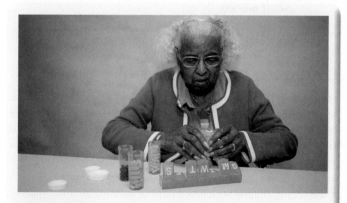

Figure 5-6 Failure to take medications or attend to other health needs can be a sign that an older adult has given up and may be contemplating suicide.
© Jones & Bartlett Learning. Courtesy of MIEMSS.

DOs and DON'Ts for Patients at Risk of Suicide

When managing a potentially suicidal older patient, EMS providers should be guided by the following list of DOs and DONT's:

1. DO transport any older adult whom you have concerns regarding suicide, regardless of your physical assessment findings.
2. DO voice your concerns to the emergency department staff, both verbally and in your documentation of the run.
3. DO take any verbal statements by the patient seriously and document them exactly as stated. Seemingly meaningless comments about suicide may be the only warning sign given before a serious attempt.

4. DO protect the patient from any further attempts. Secure potentially dangerous items in the home, the ambulance, and the emergency department.

5. DO ask the patient directly if he or she is thinking about suicide. Bringing up the topic of suicide will not "plant the seed" and cause a nonsuicidal person to consider it; on the contrary, a direct question and a professional response to any answer conveys trust and a genuine concern for the patient's welfare.

6. DO offer hope that alternatives are available.

7. DON'T be judgmental. Never debate whether suicide is right or wrong, or feelings are good or bad. Lectures on the value of life are not helpful to a suicidal patient.

8. DON'T let the mechanism of injury (suicide attempt) cloud your clinical judgment. Trust your training in the initial assessment and physical exam. Physical injury takes precedence over psychological intervention.

9. DON'T leave the actively suicidal patient unattended, even for a brief period.

10. DON'T be sworn to secrecy. Seek support from colleagues, emergency department staff, and outside agencies if needed.

Take Care of Yourself

Responding to a completed suicide is one of the most difficult tasks faced by an EMS provider. It is vital that some form of incident or stress debriefing be made available to allow the provider to deal with the normal feelings of frustration, anger, helplessness, and guilt associated with these cases. The professional stoicism often displayed by EMS providers serves them well while at the scene, dealing with loved ones or calming an upset patient, but the emotional stress resulting from responding to a suicide must be acknowledged and coped with. Staff in most hospitals that treat critically ill and injured patients have a mechanism in place to care for one another after stressful incidents. EMS providers at times need to avail themselves of these resources and constructively deal with the feelings normally generated by responding to disturbing calls.

Chemical Dependency and Substance Abuse

Chemical dependency and **substance abuse** are problems among the older population. As the number of people older than 65 years in our country increases, these problems are likely to grow. Chemical dependency can include addiction to alcohol, prescription or over-the-counter (OTC) medications, or unlawful street drugs. An **addiction** occurs when an older adult has an overwhelming desire or need to continue using a substance at whatever cost, with a tendency to increase the amount or dose.[11]

Epidemiology

Research estimates that approximately 10% of the older population, or up to 3 million people over the age of 60 years, suffer from chemical dependency—alcohol-related problems in particular—at a cost to hospitals of $60 billion annually.[12] One study noted the rate of alcohol-related admissions for older adults is comparable to that of cardiac events (heart attack).[13] Unfortunately, alcohol and drug abuse by older patients is often not identified, and thus underreported. Several factors contribute to this phenomenon. Symptoms of alcoholism or medication misuse or abuse may be mistaken by the EMS provider, physician, or family member as signs of dementia or depression. Surprisingly, some family members believe their older relative's drinking is the only "cure-all" to combat loneliness or depression. Family members may also be ashamed or embarrassed about their older relative's addiction and, as a result, fail to help the patient seek medical care.

Compared to younger adults, older alcoholics are less likely to have criminal records or difficulties with the police. They are seldom menacing or disorderly. They have lower rates of divorce, financial problems or bankruptcy, violence, and involvement in motor vehicle collisions while driving under the influence of alcohol. Many live alone, are isolated, and lack the assistance of a support system. As a result, the older person is less likely to be identified and referred for treatment.

Men are five times more likely than women to drink, become heavy drinkers, and become alcoholics.[14] Additionally, men are more apt to become heavy drinkers early in life, whereas women who drink are more likely to start later in life

CASE STUDY 2

© 123dartist/Thinkstock

You are at the residence of a 75-year-old male who has had a syncopal episode. On your arrival, he responds purposefully to painful stimuli and appears pale and diaphoretic. His wife states, "He has been doing this a lot lately. He really hurt his hip bad the one time. The pain seems to go away with a few shots of whiskey and several tablets of ibuprofen and Advil." During your examination, you note what appears to be blood on the front of the patient's shirt and the back of his pants. When asked, the patient's wife says, "He has had a lot of blood coming from both ends."

- What are your first priorities in caring for this patient?
- What do you feel may be the cause of this patient's condition?

Table 5-5	Characteristics of Early and Late Onset Drinkers	
	Early Onset	**Late Onset**
Age (in years)	<25, 40–45	>55
Gender	Males more than females	Females more than males
Response to stressors	Frequent	Frequent
Socioeconomic status	Tends to be lower	Tends to be higher
Age-associated medical problems aggravated by alcohol (e.g., diabetes, hypertension)	Frequent	Frequent

(**Table 5-5**). Substance abuse has the potential of affecting the older person's ability to care for chronic medical conditions, as the afflicted older patient may have difficulty keeping routine doctor appointments, complying with medication directions, or seeking medical help when it is needed. Most disturbing is the fact that alcohol abuse and depression correlate closely with suicide in the older adult.

Medication Misuse and Abuse

Medication or substance misuse and abuse may be considered by some to be interchangeable terms; however, they have very different meanings. **Medication misuse** is an unintentional or willful use of a medication in a way that differs from its prescribed dose or intent. Prescription and OTC medication misuse is the most common form of substance abuse by the older adult. Examples of misuse include the following:

- An individual with a sore throat taking several old or unused antibiotic pills from last year's prescription for strep pharyngitis, with the thought that the sore throat is also strep pharyngitis
- An individual ingesting double or triple the dose of over-the-counter Tylenol for a headache, thinking a higher dose of the medication will improve symptoms more quickly
- An individual failing to take an entire course of antibiotics

Medication or substance abuse is a deliberate use of a drug for nonmedicinal reasons. Most often, it occurs because the individual is trying to produce the desired effect of the drug. This is common with the use of alcohol and illicit drugs.

To understand the potential for medication problems, consider the variety of medications prescribed to treat chronic medical problems in older adults. Cardiovascular medications, tranquilizers, diuretics, sedatives, antidepressants, and anti-inflammatories are all frequently prescribed to manage conditions including hypertension, depression, elevated cholesterol levels, heart disease, arthritis, and diabetes. Five out of six patients older than 65 years take at least one prescription medication; almost one-half of all older persons take at least three.[15]

Medication Tip

Thirty percent of patients older than 65 years take eight or more prescription medications daily, a reminder of the potential for misuse and abuse.

Medication Tip

Cardiovascular medications, tranquilizers, diuretics, sedatives, antidepressants, and anti-inflammatories are frequently prescribed to treat chronic medical problems in older adults.

Risk Factors for Substance Abuse
Alcohol

Several factors make the older person vulnerable to alcohol and medication misuse or abuse. Depression, caused by physical ailments, limited financial resources, loss of a job, or loneliness, can place the older adult at risk. Shifting from a busy, productive career to a time of unwanted or unplanned retirement can produce boredom and stress. Alcohol and medications may be used to suppress the anxiety caused by inactivity. Older women who are alcoholics often have or had alcoholic spouses or suffered the loss of a spouse, triggering problem drinking.

Medications

Many factors place the older patient at significant risk for medication misuse or abuse. A significant number of older persons take medications on a continual basis for conditions such as sleeping problems, chronic pain, and mood disorders, including depression or anxiety. This chronic use opens the door for drug tolerance and potential abuse. For example, many older adults require two or more medications that strengthen or counteract one another. Often, these adults "doctor shop," acquiring the same medication from different physicians who may not know the medicine has already been prescribed to the patient. Other patients are unaware of the hazards of mixing alcohol with mood-altering, pain-relieving, or muscle-relaxing medications. This is especially dangerous and potentially fatal if alcohol is mixed with sedative-hypnotic drugs, including benzodiazepines and barbiturates.

Some older adults with visual impairment may not be able to read prescription directions properly. These patients may fear loss of independence or may simply be embarrassed, and, therefore, may be reluctant to ask family, friends, and their medical provider for help in clarifying medication directions, thus further increasing risk of abuse or misuse. Other patients may suffer short-term memory loss, having difficulty recalling if and when they took their last dose. Given that most medications are prescribed to older adults, it is not surprising that more than 50% of medication overdoses and adverse reactions requiring hospitalization occur in older persons (**Figure 5-7**).[16]

Alarmingly, one must consider that some older adults know exactly what they are doing when abusing their medications. Medication abuse with true intent to do self-harm may be a cry for help or an actual suicide attempt. A list of medications and their potential side effects (signs and symptoms) secondary to overdose appears in **Table 5-6**.

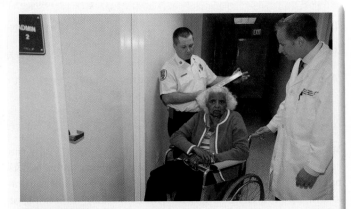

Figure 5-7 More than one-half of medication overdoses and adverse reactions that require hospitalization occur in older patients.
© Jones & Bartlett Learning. Courtesy of MIEMSS.

Table 5-6 Toxidromes: Typical Signs and Symptoms of Specific Drug Overdose

Drug Class	Examples of Drug	Signs and Symptoms of Overdose
Opioid	■ Butorphanol (Stadol) ■ Codeine ■ Fentanyl derivatives ("China White") ■ Heroin ■ Hydrocodone (Hycodan) ■ Hydromorphone (Dilaudid) ■ Meperidine (Demerol) ■ Methadone (Dolophine) ■ Morphine ■ Oxycodone (Percodan) ■ Pentazocine (Talwin) ■ Propoxyphene (Darvon)	■ Hypoventilation or respiratory arrest ■ Pinpoint pupils (miosis) ■ Sedation or coma ■ Hypotension
Sympathomimetics	■ Albuterol ■ Amphetamines ■ Benzadrine ■ Cocaine ■ Crack Cocaine ■ Ecstasy ■ Epinephrine ■ Methamphetamine ("ice") ■ Phenteramine (Adipex-P, Fastin, Ionamin)	■ Hypertension ■ Tachycardia ■ Dilated pupils (mydriasis) ■ Agitation or seizures ■ Hyperthermia
Sedative-hypnotics	■ Diazepam (Valium) ■ Secobarbital (Seconal) ■ Flunitrazepam (Rohypnol)	■ Slurred speech ■ Sedation or coma ■ Hypoventilation ■ Hypotension

Anticholinergics	<ul><li>Atropine</li><li>Diphenhydramine (Benadryl)</li><li>Jimson weed</li><li>Some tricyclic antidepressants (Amitriptyline [Elavil], Imipramine [Tofranil])</li></ul>	<ul><li>Tachycardia</li><li>Hypertension</li><li>Hyperthermia</li><li>Dilated pupils (mydriasis)</li><li>Dry skin and mucous membranes</li><li>Sedation, agitation, seizures, coma, delirium</li><li>Decreased bowel sounds</li></ul>
Cholinergics	<ul><li>Pilocarpine</li><li>Bethanechol (Duvoid, Myotonachol, Urecholine)</li><li>Neostigmine bromide (Prostigmin)</li></ul>	<ul><li>Excess defecation</li><li>Muscle fasciculations</li><li>Pinpoint pupils (miosis)</li><li>Excess lacrimation or salivation</li><li>Airway compromise</li><li>Nausea or vomiting</li></ul>
Selective serotonin reuptake inhibitors (SSRIs)	<ul><li>Citalopram (Celexa)</li><li>Escitalopram (Lexapro)</li><li>Fluoxetine (Prozac)</li><li>Fluvoxamine (Luvox)</li><li>Paroxetine (Paxil)</li><li>Sertraline (Zoloft)</li></ul>	<ul><li>Confusion, agitation, or restlessness</li><li>Dilated pupils</li><li>Headache</li><li>Changes in blood pressure or temperature</li><li>Nausea or vomiting</li><li>Diarrhea</li><li>Rapid heart rate</li><li>Loss of muscle coordination or twitching muscles</li><li>Shivering or goose bumps</li><li>Perfuse sweating</li><li>Severe symptoms such as high fever, seizures, irregular heartbeat, and unconsciousness</li></ul>
Calcium channel blockers	<ul><li>Amlodipine (Norvasc)</li><li>Diltiazem (Cardizem, Tiazac)</li><li>Felodipine</li><li>Isradipine</li><li>Nicardipine (Cardene SR)</li><li>Nifedipine (Procardia)</li><li>Nisoldipine (Sular)</li><li>Verapamil (Calan, Verelan, Covera-HS)</li></ul>	<ul><li>Syncope</li><li>Lightheadedness</li><li>Chest pain</li><li>Palpitations</li><li>Diaphoresis</li><li>Flushing</li><li>Weakness</li><li>Peripheral edema</li><li>Dyspnea</li><li>Confusion</li><li>Seizure</li><li>Dizziness</li><li>Headache</li><li>Nausea</li><li>Vomiting</li><li>Slowed heart rate</li><li>Hypotension</li><li>Decreased level of consciousness</li><li>ECG showing:<ul><li>Bradycardia</li><li>First-, second-, or third-degree atrioventricular (AV) block</li><li>Any type of bundle-branch block</li><li>Nonspecific ST–T wave changes</li></ul></li></ul>

(continues)

Table 5-6	Toxidromes: Typical Signs and Symptoms of Specific Drug Overdose (*continued*)	
Drug Class	**Examples of Drug**	**Signs and Symptoms of Overdose**
Beta blockers	▪ Acebutolol (Sectral) ▪ Atenolol (Tenormin) ▪ Bisoprolol (Zebeta) ▪ Metoprolol (Lopressor, Toprol-XL) ▪ Nadolol (Corgard) ▪ Propranolol (Inderal LA, InnoPran XL)	▪ Hypotension ▪ Hypothermia ▪ Hypoglycemia ▪ ECG changes: 　▪ Progressively worsening sinus bradycardia 　▪ Increased PR intervals 　▪ Loss of atrial activity 　▪ Atrioventricular junctional rhythm 　▪ Widening of the QRS complex 　▪ Atrioventricular block 　▪ Idioventricular rhythm 　▪ Asystole

Adapted from American Academy of Orthopedic Surgeons, *Emergency Care and Transportation of the Sick and Injured*, 10th ed. Sudbury, MA: Jones and Bartlett: 2011: 670

Pathophysiology of Substance Abuse in Older Adults

As the body ages, several physiological changes occur throughout the body's organ systems, which make the older adult much more vulnerable to the harmful effects of drugs and alcohol. It is important to remember that alcohol is a powerful CNS depressant. It is both a **sedative**, a substance that decreases activity and excitement, and a **hypnotic**, a substance that induces sleep. Alcohol and several prescription medications dull the sense of awareness, slow reflexes, and reduce reaction time.[17] Abuse of alcohol or other substances can impact most of the major organ systems (**Figure 5-8**).

Cardiovascular System

Not only does alcohol depress an older person's reactions, it also reduces cardiac muscle and decreases cardiac output (the amount of blood pumped out of the heart in 1 minute). It elevates the level of fatty acids in the bloodstream, and worsens high blood pressure, or **hypertension**. Most importantly for the EMS provider, alcohol has the potential to mask more serious medical problems, including **angina pectoris** (chest pain caused by **ischemia**). Older persons unable to interpret the warning sign that heart muscle needs additional oxygen are at greater risk for **myocardial infarction** (heart attack).

Respiratory System

The natural drive to breathe is slowed by alcohol. Inadequate oxygenation of the brain may result in marked mental confusion, especially in patients already afflicted with respiratory disorders such as chronic obstructive pulmonary disease (COPD) or psychological conditions such as anxiety and depression.

Hepatic System

The function of the liver is greatly impaired by chronic alcohol use. Because the damaged liver will not metabolize alcohol and drugs, these substances may circulate through the body for an extended period of time, prolonging their effects. Heavy drinking also increases the risk of bruising and significant bleeding, as the liver controls essential blood clotting factors.

Cirrhosis, a chronic disease of the liver resulting in degenerative changes and death of functioning liver cells, causes an increased resistance to the flow of blood through the liver, resulting in a dangerous condition known as **portal hypertension**. As the blood continues to back up in the portal venous system, fluid is displaced into the abdomen, the liver enlarges, and **esophageal varices** (enlarged venous channels in the esophagus) may develop. Esophageal varices put a patient at increased risk of esophageal cancer and internal hemorrhage.

Medication Tip

Alcohol and medications unable to be metabolized by the liver or excreted in the kidneys can build to toxic levels and may even be life threatening in the older adult.

Gastrointestinal System

Long-term alcohol use results in inflammation or erosion of cells lining the esophagus and stomach. Abdominal pain and diarrhea from gastritis, **peptic ulcer disease**, or **pancreatitis** may be common complaints verbalized by the older patient. Bright red blood in feces, or dark tarry stools known as **melena**, indicates bleeding somewhere in the gastrointestinal tract. Continued alcohol abuse may result in cancers of the upper digestive tract.

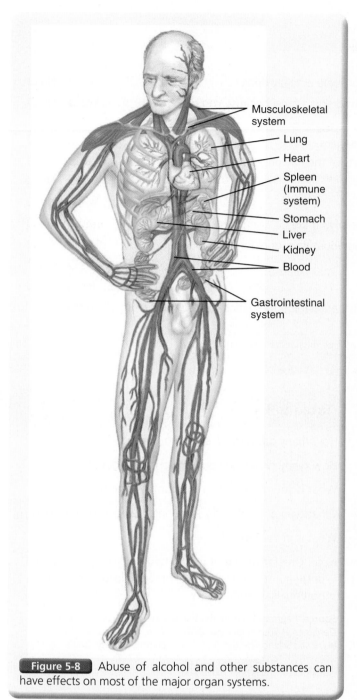

Musculoskeletal system
Lung
Heart
Spleen (Immune system)
Stomach
Liver
Kidney
Blood
Gastrointestinal system

Figure 5-8 Abuse of alcohol and other substances can have effects on most of the major organ systems.

Esophageal varices created by persistent portal hypertension have the potential to erupt, causing uncontrolled, life-threatening bleeding and possibly compromising the airway.

Musculoskeletal System

Bone density decreases with age. Muscle tissue, which is composed mostly of water, wastes away over time. The result of this decrease in body mass is that drugs and alcohol remain in the bloodstream for a longer period of time. The prolonged effects of drugs and alcohol magnify the risk of weakness, falls, and fractures.

Immune System and Blood Components

Long-term alcohol abuse impairs the immune response, making the body much more susceptible to infection and cancer. Severe alcohol ingestion may also cause low blood sugar, or **hypoglycemia**. Vitamin stores, including vitamin B_{12}, folate, and iron, are significantly depleted. Without these substances, essential nutrients are not absorbed, contributing to overall malnutrition. In addition, alcohol suppresses the functioning of the bone marrow, where most blood cells are made. These elements are essential in creating blood cells vital to oxygen transport. A lowered ability to transport oxygen can lead to confusion, falls, memory loss, or fatigue.

Screening for Substance Abuse or Misuse

Screening for substance abuse or misuse is a critical element of your encounter with the patient. The tools in the following tables may be useful to identify older patients at risk. The Michigan Alcoholism Screening Test helps to identify older patients at risk for alcoholism (**Table 5-7**). Two questions answered with a "yes" should prompt you to consider that the patient is abusing alcohol, and make appropriate referrals. If substance abuse or even possible overdose is suspected, the questions suggested in **Table 5-8** and **Table 5-9** can be used to guide your focused history and detect harmful drinking.

Approaching the Older Patient

A few key strategies can make the evaluation of the older adult easier. First, gain the patient's and family's trust by identifying yourself in a calm and reassuring manner. Be honest and direct with the patient, describing every intervention you want to perform. Communicate clearly and slowly—some older adults may have hearing impairments. Remain totally nonjudgmental and refrain from imposing your values or ideas on the patient or family. Remember, it may take additional time to thoroughly listen to and answer any questions posed by the older adult. Be ready to commit additional time on scene.

Assessment Goals

Using the GEMS diamond, you have the tools to properly assess environmental, medical, and social aspects that affect the health of older adults. Your objective is twofold: (1) recognize any major life-threatening condition, and (2) reduce any factors that may be contributing to unnecessary stress for both the patient and family.

Table 5-7   Michigan Alcoholism Screening Test—Geriatric Version

In the past year:

When talking with friends, do you ever underestimate how much you actually drink?	Yes ❑ No ❑
After a few drinks, have you sometimes not eaten or been able to skip a meal because you didn't feel hungry?	Yes ❑ No ❑
Does having a few drinks help decrease your shakiness or tremors?	Yes ❑ No ❑
Does alcohol sometimes make it hard for you to remember parts of the day or night?	Yes ❑ No ❑
Do you usually take a drink to relax or calm your nerves?	Yes ❑ No ❑
Do you drink to take your mind off your problems?	Yes ❑ No ❑
Have you ever increased your drinking after experiencing a loss in your life?	Yes ❑ No ❑
Has a doctor or nurse ever said they were worried or concerned about your drinking?	Yes ❑ No ❑
Have you ever made rules to manage your drinking?	Yes ❑ No ❑
When you feel lonely, does having a drink help?	Yes ❑ No ❑

Scoring: If the person answered "yes" to two or more questions, encourage the patient to seek counseling. You may have to help, or even make, the first contact for help.

Source: © The Regents of the University of Michigan, 1991. Reproduced with permission from Frederic C. Blow.

Table 5-8   Focused History Questions Pertaining to Substance Abuse or Possible Overdose

How much did you ingest?

What substance did you take?

What actions have you taken?

When did you take the substance?

If any injury resulted, when did it occur?

Source: American Academy of Orthopaedic Surgeons. Emergency Care and Transportation of the Sick and Injured. 8th ed. Sudbury, MA: Jones and Bartlett; 2002: 434.

Table 5-9   Detecting Harmful Drinking

How many days per week do you drink?

How many drinks do you have on those days?

What is your maximum intake on any one day?

What type of alcohol do you drink (i.e., beer, wine, liquor)?

What is in "a drink"?

Note: Greater than or equal to two drinks/day for women, or greater than or equal to three drinks/day for men, is potentially harmful.

Source: Reproduced from Reuben DB, Herr K, Pacala JT, et. al. *Geriatrics at Your Fingertips: 2002 Edition,* p. 14 Malden, MA: Blackwell Science for the American Geriatrics Society; 2002.

History

It is imperative to gather an accurate history. Avoid asking any questions in an accusatory or threatening manner; the interview is less likely to produce helpful information if you lose the patient's trust. Gather data from family members, friends, or caretakers, including questions about signs of substance abuse. Use the questions suggested in Table 5-8 to guide your focused history when substance abuse is a possibility.

Environmental Observations

Perform a scene size-up and ensure that the environment is safe for yourself and the patient. Carefully assess the older adult's surroundings (**Figure 5-9**).

Remember that many older adults at risk of substance abuse live alone, with limited financial resources. Look for unsanitary or dangerous home conditions that may place the patient at risk. This may include the presence of a gun or other weapon. Carefully document any findings that may support substance abuse.

Particular attention should be paid to the presence of alcoholic beverages, whether they are empty or full, and the presence of prescription or OTC medication bottles. Note the date of the initial prescription and the number of pills remaining in any of the bottles. This may be useful in determining if an overdose has occurred.

Observations you make of the older patient's home environment, along with your assessment of psychosocial status, may provide valuable clues to a history of depression, alcoholism, or other substance abuse. When such observations are reported to the staff of the emergency department (or other receiving facility), the patient's long-term outcome will most likely be improved and any associated risk of serious decline when the patient returns home will be reduced.

Older adults commonly self-medicate with similar classes of OTC drugs. Failing to understand that the drugs are the same type of medication increases the potential for overdose or adverse effects.

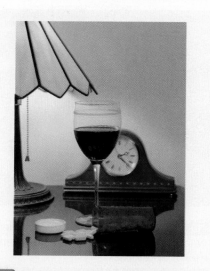

Figure 5-9 Carefully observe the patient's surroundings for dangerous conditions or signs of substance abuse.
© mg7/iStock/Thinkstock

Medical Examination and Care

If the scene is safe, perform an initial assessment of the older adult, as outlined in the *Assessment of the Older Patient* chapter, and give appropriate medical care where indicated. Clear, maintain, and protect the airway if the level of consciousness is altered from either drug or alcohol ingestion. Be prepared to provide additional oxygenation and possibly ventilatory support in anyone who shows signs of **cyanosis** (bluish skin color) or **dyspnea** (shortness of breath). Consider the need to mechanically clear or suction the airway if the patient vomits.

Evaluation of pupillary size may assist the emergency department professional in identifying potential drug overdose. For example, opiate narcotics (e.g., codeine, dilaudid, demerol, fentanyl, morphine, oxycontin, vicodin) cause pinpoint pupils. Several other drug types can produce pupillary dilation, such as amphetamines, antihistamines, atropine, cocaine, decongestants, eye drops, LSD, and marijuana.

Assess for any signs of physical trauma, such as altered mental status, fractures, or bruising; many older patients are at risk for falls, especially when compromised by alcohol or medication abuse. Older patients are also at higher-than-normal risk of **subdural hematoma** (intracranial bleeding between the dural layer and the brain). This risk generally rises with age, and increases in heavy alcohol users.

Be sure to assess hydration status. Alcohol and certain medications, including diuretics, remove fluids, thus dehydrating the patient. Evidence of self-neglect, a decline in personal hygiene, disheveled clothing, poor grooming, and weight loss are red flags indicating possible alcohol or medication abuse or misuse. In addition, findings of fatigue, difficulty concentrating, unexplainable confusion, incontinence, or insomnia may also be physical clues suggesting substance abuse.

Consider that the older adult who is withdrawing from chronic alcohol abuse may be suffering from a condition known as **delirium tremens** (DTs). DTs may occur 24 hours to 1 week following the cessation of alcohol ingestion, or when alcohol consumption stops abruptly. Objective findings on examination include fine tremors, sweating, agitation, hallucinations, and confusion. DTs is a life-threatening condition and is much more severe in the older adult than in younger patients. These patients require prompt evaluation and medical transport. In addition, an older adult experiencing DTs has the potential to experience seizure activity. Every attempt should be made to protect the airway and prevent accidental injury. Administer oxygen immediately following the episode, as the patient was likely deprived during the seizure. At no point should any type of physical restraint be used in an attempt to prevent physical harm.

Short-acting benzodiazepines such as lorazepam (Ativan) and oxazepam (Serax) can safely be used to treat DTs. These medications are not oxidized in the liver, which may be damaged due to long-term alcohol abuse.

Look for emotional factors that may point to substance abuse. During assessment, older adults may ask for a tranquilizer or an antianxiety medication. In addition, the patient may be withdrawn; exhibit feelings of hopelessness, worthlessness, or guilt; or demonstrate paranoid tendencies or thoughts of suicide.

Social Setting

Continuously observe interactions between the patient and family. You may notice **enabling behavior** demonstrated by family members that can indicate substance abuse. Enabling behavior is defined as actions

promoting continued self-destructive behavior of another individual. For example, a spouse who continues to make excuses for continued alcohol ingestion (e.g., "My husband needs his daily beer to keep him happy") is demonstrating enabling behavior. It is also important that the EMS provider observe for behavioral signs of neglect or abuse. A complete discussion of neglect can be found in the *Elder Abuse* chapter.

Management Considerations

The episodic, short-term nature of most EMS responses makes it difficult for providers to significantly affect the psychological well-being of older patients. As an EMS provider and patient advocate, you can intervene in a variety of ways to help the older adult afflicted with a psychosocial issue. Continuously treat the older patient with respect, compassion, and dignity. Remember, many have lost the independence or autonomy they have enjoyed for years and have become dependent on others for care.

The following are tips to help guide you:

1. Review all medication regimens with both the patient and family; clarify the drug, dose, and time of day the medication is to be taken. This practice may reveal multiple dosing or missed doses. It may also help identify expired drugs or medications that have been discontinued by the doctor but remain in the patient's medicine cabinet.
2. Ensure that your ambulance carries a current list of phone numbers and email addresses of helpful community contacts, including social service agencies, companion groups, drug and alcohol rehabilitation programs, and crisis intervention hot lines that can be provided on request to the patient or family.

3. For individuals whom you suspect want help, but are reluctant to seek it, consider initiating the first telephone contact for the patient while on scene (**Figure 5-10**). Your empathetic support and assistance through the interaction may be what the patient emotionally needs to seek treatment. The key to success in medically treating an older adult afflicted with substance abuse is their (and your) recognition that a problem does in fact exist. Studies have shown remarkable treatment success in older adults who began to abuse alcohol late in life.
4. The attention of a caring and competent professional can be enough reassurance to get a depressed or suicidal person through an acute crisis, while other agencies are marshaled for more aggressive intervention. It is of paramount importance that EMS providers report—verbally and in writing—their impressions or perceptions of potentially suicidal older adults. One explanation for the high suicide completion-to-attempt ratio is the fact that many

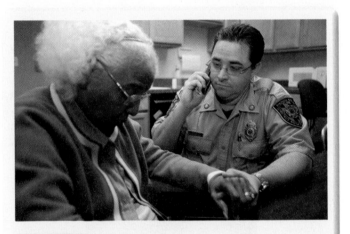

Figure 5-10 Offer to make the first telephone contact for a patient who you think wants help but is reluctant to seek it.
© Jones & Bartlett Learning. Courtesy of MIEMSS.

CASE STUDY 3

Mr. Pratt is an 83-year-old retired school teacher who, with his wife, lives independently in a continuing care retirement community. He is in excellent health, does not usually take any prescription or nonprescription drugs or herbal supplements, and still drives and enjoys golfing. Two weeks ago, however, he developed an itchy rash on his arm after retrieving his golf ball from the brush. Over the course of two days, Mr. Pratt self-medicated by taking a total of six doses of Benadryl (diphenhydramine), 25 mg. Additionally, he took a nonprescription sleep-aid pill containing diphenhydramine, 25 mg, at bedtime for those two days because he was having trouble sleeping due to the itching.

On day three, Mr. Pratt woke up with severe pain in his lower abdomen and the urge to urinate, but he was unable to empty his bladder. In addition, his vision was blurry. When he complained to Mrs. Pratt about these symptoms, she noticed that he sounded very confused. Fearing that Mr. Pratt was having a stroke, Mrs. Pratt called 911.

■ What are your concerns about this patient?
■ What are your assessment considerations?

suicidal older adults never ask for help. The EMS provider who is astute enough to recognize the warning signs for suicide is in a position to initiate referrals and assure that emergency department personnel are aware of the potential for self-harm.

5. Objective data gathered on the scene indicating substance abuse or medication problems should be conveyed to the patient's family physician or the emergency department. Substance abuse and medication problems are often unrecognized among this population group. The data from your "eyes and ears" assessment give other healthcare providers an accurate picture of what is occurring in the patient's environment.

6. Patients experiencing altered levels of consciousness secondary to drug or alcohol abuse, lack of oxygen (hypoxia), or even depression may be mentally incapacitated. These patients—although they require medical attention—may refuse your assistance, and may become violent. They should never be left unattended. Doing so endangers the patient and may constitute abandonment, placing the EMS provider in legal jeopardy.

Some psychosocial issues (such as suicidal acts [or threats], overdoses, depression, self-neglecting behavior, and even a lack of social support) that EMS providers encounter with older patients are, or can potentially become, life-threatening emergencies. The most important thing that prehospital providers can do is recognize the warning signs and circumstances that can result in a serious decline in an individual's physical and emotional states.

Summary

Fortunately, EMS providers infrequently interact with older adults suffering from substance abuse or serious suicidal intentions. When these patients are encountered, it is vital that all members of the healthcare team be aware of the issues and take appropriate steps to ensure patient safety and initiate effective treatment. On the other hand, older adults suffering from depression are frequent clients for almost all EMS providers. The challenge facing any professional concerned with care of the older adult is to recognize the signs of depression and aggressively intervene to prevent the ultimate failure of care—suicide.

References

1. Aldrich N, Benson WF. CDC Promotes Public Health Approach To Address Depression among Older Adults. Available from: http://www.cdc.gov/aging/pdf/CIB_mental_health.pdf

2. Geriatric Mental Health Foundation. *Late Life Depression: A Fact Sheet.* Available from: http://www.gmhfonline.org/gmhf/consumer/factsheets/depression_factsheet.html

3. American Psychiatric Association. *Diagnostic and Statistical Manual of Mental Disorders (DSM-IV-TR).* Washington, DC, Author, 2000

4. National Center for Health Statistics. (2009). As summarized by the American Foundation for Suicide Prevention. *Facts and Figures.* Available from: http://www.afsp.org/understanding-suicide/facts-and-figures

5. American Association of Suiciology. *Elderly Suicide Fact Sheet.* 2012. Available from: http://www.suicidology.org/c/document_library/get_file?folderId=262&name=DLFE-624.pdf

6. Centers for Disease Control and Prevention, WISQARS. *Fatal Injury Reports, 2011.* 2013. Available from: webappa.cdc.gov/sasweb/ncipc/mortrate10_us.html

7. Centers for Disease Control and Prevention. (2012). *Suicide: Facts at a glance.*

8. Conwell, Y. Suicide in elderly patients, in Schneider LS, Reynolds, CF III, Lebowitz BD, Friedhoff AJ (eds): *Diagnosis and Treatment of Depression in Late Life.* Washington, DC, American Psychiatric Press, 1994, pp. 397–418.

9. National Institute of Mental Health. *The Numbers Count: Mental Disorders in America.* Available from: http://www.nimh.nih.gov/health/publications/the-numbers-count-mental-disorders-in-america/index.shtml

10. Osgood NJ, Brant BA, Lipman A. *Suicide among the Elderly in Long-Term Care Facilities.* New York, NY, Greenwood Press, 1991, pp. 95–98.

11. American Academy of Orthopaedic Surgeons. *Emergency Care and Transportation of the Sick and Injured,* ed 10. Sudbury, MA, Jones and Bartlett, 2011, p. 679.

12. Adams WL, Cox NS. Epidemiology of problem drinking among elderly people. *Int J Addict* 1995:30(13–14):1693–1716.

13. Adams WL, Yuan Z, Barboriak JJ, Rim AA. Alcohol-related hospitalizations of elderly people: Prevalence and geographic variation in the United States. *JAMA* 1993:270(10):1222–1225.

14. Barry PP, Ackerman K. Chemical Dependency in the Elderly, in Hazzard WR, Blass JP, Ettinger WH, Halter JB, Ouslander JG

(eds): *Principles of Geriatric Medicine and Gerontology*, ed 4. New York, NY, McGraw-Hill, 1999, p. 1358.

15. U.S. Food and Drug Administration. Saving Money on Prescription Drugs. Available from: http://www.fda.gov/Drugs/EmergencyPreparedness/BioterrorismandDrugPreparedness/ucm134215.htm.

16. National Clearinghouse for Alcohol and Drug Information. Use and Abuse of Psychoactive Prescription and Over the Counter Medications. Available from: http://www.health.org/govpubsBK-D250/26t.htm.

17. American Academy of Orthopaedic Surgeons. *Emergency Care and Transportation of the Sick and Injured*, ed 10. Sudbury, MA, Jones and Bartlett, 2011, p. 680.

CASE STUDY SUMMARIES

Case Study 1 Summary

Scene safety (which was completed) and airway management are the initial priorities in managing this 68-year-old patient. During the assessment, you noted several suicide risk factors, including the following: loss of interest in self-esteem (disheveled appearance and stating he is "worthless"), increased alcohol use (the empty liquor bottle), acquired weapon (the pistol in his presence), the recent loss of his close friend and job (suicide by his boss), and not following his medication regimen. Completion of care would include further assessment and monitoring of the patient's vital signs, intravenous access, and rapid transport to the emergency department.

Case Study 2 Summary

Airway protection in the altered mental status patient is essential. Breathing and circulation are also vital once an open airway is maintained. Your initial findings on exam allude to a potentially poor hemodynamic status. Intravenous crystalloids should be initiated to maintain a systolic blood pressure of around 100 mm Hg. EMS should realize after the various statements from his wife that this patient's pain management regimen is probably the cause. A mixture of various nonsteroidal anti-inflammatory drugs (NSAIDs) with alcohol may cause gastric and esophageal irritation and erosion with subsequent bleeding. Misinformation has caused misuse of medication. Hemodynamic instability in this patient (as in all older patients) must be a treatment priority. The information that was learned from the patient's wife must be relayed to the hospital staff, as further education on NSAID usage and improved pain management can be discussed at the hospital once the patient is stabilized.

Case Study 3 Summary

Mr. Pratt is an otherwise healthy 83-year-old individual who usually does not take any prescription or nonprescription drugs or herbal supplements. As you gather information from Mrs. Pratt, you discover that Mr. Pratt self-medicated for two days with six doses of Benadryl (diphenhydramine), 25 mg, as well as a nonprescription sleep-aid pill containing diphenhydramine, 25 mg, at bedtime.

The symptoms Mr. Pratt is experiencing are a result of diphenhydramine use. Diphenhydramine can have serious, life-threatening effects in older people. Even with the recommended dosing, diphenhydramine can worsen or cause constipation, drowsiness, urinary retention, mental confusion or delirium, blurred vision, and dry mouth. In general, the signs and symptoms of diphenhydramine overdose include dry mouth, stomach pain, nausea, unsteadiness or difficulty in making normal body movements, rapid heartbeat, skin flushing, and extreme drowsiness. Neurological effects of diphenhydramine overdose include agitation or confusion. Hallucinations can also be present. Overdose can also result in seizures, which may get worse if the patient consumes Benadryl with drugs that enhance its effects (such as alcohol, antihistamines, and monoamine oxidase inhibitors). Cardiac symptoms include hypotension, sinus tachycardia, cardiogenic shock, decrease in myocardial contractility, ventricular tachycardia, and heart block due to slowing of sodium conduction.

The patient should be transported to the emergency department for evaluation. Prehospital treatment should include low-flow oxygen by nasal cannula, initiation of an intravenous line, ECG monitoring, and symptom-based care.

CHAPTER 6

End-of-Life Care Issues

LEARNING OBJECTIVES

1. Define death.

2. Define palliative and hospice care.

3. Discuss do not resuscitate (DNR) orders and other legal considerations as they relate to the care of the older person.

4. Understand the principles of effective communication with families and companions of deceased patients.

5. Discuss grief and loss.

Introduction

EMS providers will face many challenges when encountering a patient who is dying or has died. Death may occur as a sudden, unexpected event or as the inevitable result of continued clinical deterioration. When death is impending or occurs, EMS providers must balance a vast array of medical, legal, emotional, and operational concerns. After the patient has died and no longer requires EMS assistance, continued support of the patient's family and companions is often necessary.

Definition of Death

Death is the complete cessation of certain essential biological functions. Humans require respiration, circulation, and the ability to interact with the environment in order to be considered alive. Death is demonstrated in humans by the permanent cessation of both cardiac and respiratory function, or the complete loss of brain function. Patients who are unresponsive, with no spontaneous ventilation and no mechanical activity of the heart, are considered clinically dead. Clinical death becomes permanent if no resuscitation efforts are attempted, or if resuscitation efforts are determined to be ineffective and are discontinued.

Three separate events must occur once a patient is believed to have died: (1) determination of death, (2) pronouncement of death, and (3) certification of death. Individual state laws and regulations grant different types or levels of health care providers the authority to perform each event.

Determination of Death

EMS providers often make the initial determination that a patient has died. This is the least formal of the three events and is based upon patient physical examination. Patients must be completely unresponsive and without any cardiac or respiratory activity. The lack of cardiac activity is inferred in the prehospital setting by an absence of central pulses and heart tones. The presence or absence of organized electrical activity in the heart can be evaluated through the use of an electrocardiogram (ECG) by an advanced life support (ALS) provider.

Still, many factors make the determination of death difficult for prehospital providers. Adverse scene conditions such as noise, weather, bystander chaos, and movement can interfere with the physical examination and obscure subtle clinical findings. Loud noises and vibration make auscultation unreliable. Vehicle or stretcher movement may mimic or disguise the patient's respiratory effort. Movement and vibration can also cause artifact on the cardiac monitor, interfering with cardiac rhythm evaluation.

Clinical peculiarities blur the line between life and death. Gasping or **agonal** respirations may persist for several minutes after a patient has experienced a cardiac arrest. These unusual respiratory patterns often cause harmful delays in recognition of cardiac arrest and initiation of resuscitation efforts. Patients may also demonstrate electrical "escape" activity on the cardiac monitor for a significant period of time after other signs of life have ceased. Advances in medical technology, such as cardiac pacemakers or long-term mechanical ventilators, can also make determination of death challenging at times. These devices can continue to function independent of the underlying patient condition. EMS providers must carefully follow protocols when considering whether to disable life-sustaining equipment in a patient who appears to have died.

EMS providers are granted the authority to withhold resuscitation on certain patients who are found to be apneic and pulseless. This authority may be tied to certain obvious findings such as incineration, decapitation, **rigor mortis** (muscle stiffness following death), or **dependent lividity** (settling of blood in a deceased body; also known as **livor mortis**); this typically extends to situations in which a patient becomes apneic and pulseless, and resuscitative efforts are not permitted or indicated, such as when advanced health care directives or surrogate decision makers are present. By deciding to withhold resuscitative measures on these patients, EMS providers make the determination that death has occurred.

Signs of life may be subtle or unexpected, and are often difficult to adequately assess in a chaotic or uncontrolled scene. There have been events in the past in which EMS providers mistakenly determined that a patient had died. In these instances, funeral homes, medical investigators, and others discovered living patients who missed the opportunity for timely emergency medical treatment. Although these events are relatively rare, they will undoubtedly create embarrassment, liability, and jeopardy of professional licensure for the individual providers involved.

Conversely, patients may be declared legally dead, despite the presence of spontaneous circulation, if essential brain function is

CASE STUDY 1

© 123dartist/Thinkstock

You are called to a nursing home for a patient having an obvious stroke. You are told by nursing staff that the patient is typically the "life of the party," but that symptoms started about 15 minutes ago. The patient is still conscious, but has difficulty speaking, right-sided weakness, and facial droop. Her vital signs are within normal parameters, as is her blood sugar.

As you are about to take the patient out the front door and put her in the ambulance, several family members arrive and confront you. They tell you that the patient has a DNR and ask why you are taking her to the hospital.

- What should be your next steps in caring for this patient?
- What should be your response to the family members?

permanently lost. Physicians in a hospital setting may evaluate a patient for the determination of **brain death** if the patient remains in a persistent coma, without an identified reversible cause. Brain death is declared in comatose patients when underlying apnea is present accompanied by the loss of brainstem reflexes.

Pronouncement of Death

A pronouncement of death must be made following the determination of death. The pronouncement of death is a formal clinical conclusion, assigned a precise day and time, which allows movement of the body and other essential postmortem (after-death) activities to proceed. States grant this authority to physicians and other licensed independent providers, such as nurse practitioners or physician's assistants; in some states this authority extends to EMS providers, registered nurses, or medical investigators. Additionally, physicians in certain regions may provide the pronouncement of death through EMS providers utilizing online medical control.

Certification of Death

The final significant event following the death of an individual is the certification of death. The death certificate is an important document that has far-reaching legal implications. Physicians and licensed independent providers sign the death certificate, which is then used by government, business, and financial entities for a wide variety of actions pertaining to the deceased individual.

Epidemiology

Two important statistics indicate that the overall health in the United States continues to improve. In 2014, the average life expectancy in the United States was 79.56 years, up from 76.8 years in 2000.[1] Life expectancy increases are related to reductions in death rates from many common conditions such as cardiovascular disease, cancer, and respiratory conditions. Additionally, the infant mortality rate in the United States is at a record-low of 6.17 deaths per 1,000 live births.[2] Despite these notable statistical improvements, the overall death rate in the United States remains constant at 100%.[3]

The most common causes of death change as individuals grow older. In general, younger individuals more often die from external causes such as accidents, homicides, and suicides. Older individuals, on the other hand, die more often from health-related conditions such as heart disease, stroke, and cancer. Approximately one-quarter to one-third of deaths occur in hospitals, depending on the source. The remaining deaths usually occur either at home or at a long-term care facility. Deaths occurring outside the hospital setting have the potential to involve EMS.

Palliative Care and Hospice

EMS providers may be called upon to assist patients receiving either **palliative care** or **hospice** care. These treatment approaches focus on improving overall patient comfort, rather than aggressively treating the underlying disease process or processes. Palliative care is a medical specialty that utilizes various health professionals to assist with the physical, emotional, and spiritual needs facing patients who suffer from a serious or life-threatening disease (**Figure 6-1**). In many of these instances, the side effects of the medications and treatments worsen the impact of the disease process itself. Palliative care specialists focus on improving the patient's quality of life, while other specialists may simultaneously work to treat the underlying medical condition. In addition to symptom relief and social/emotional support, these patients often require assistance managing financial affairs, navigating the health care system, and implementing advanced health care directives. The palliative care team provides resources to help fulfill these patient needs.

Palliative care may evolve into hospice care when the underlying disease(s) can no longer be effectively treated and death is expected. Hospice care utilizes the same palliative care approach for individuals with a terminal illness. Depending on the circumstances, hospice may begin when the patient's death is expected within the next 6 to 12 months. The focus of both hospice treatment and palliative care are largely the same. Hospice programs utilize a variety of specialists to maximize the patient's physical, emotional, and spiritual comfort as death approaches. Hospice staff forego providing aggressive medical treatment and, instead, concentrate on interventions such as pharmacologic and nonpharmacologic methods of pain control, nutritional support, individual and group emotional support, and a vast array of related services. Depending on the patient's wishes and the individual situation, patients in hospice care may or may not receive interventions such as antibiotics, oxygen, or hydration.

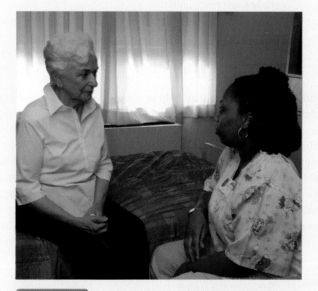

Figure 6-1 A patient in hospice care receives visits from physicians, nurses, home health aides, social workers, clergy, and therapists.
© Jones & Bartlett Learning. Courtesy of MIEMSS.

EMS providers may interact with hospice patients during interfacility transfers, hospital discharge transports, and when summoned through the 911 system. Distraught family members may request EMS assistance for hospice patients as the patient's death nears and emotions become overwhelming. EMS providers face a difficult dilemma when conflict exists between patient desires for end-of-life treatment and family members (surrogate decision makers) who insist on aggressive resuscitation measures.

Good Death

The concept of a "good death" is heavily analyzed in medical and social science literature, and frequently discussed after a person has died. In the report, *The Future of Health Care of Older People*, 12 "principles of a good death" have been identified:

- To know when death is coming, and to understand what can be expected
- To be able to retain control of what happens
- To be afforded dignity and privacy
- To have control over pain relief and other symptom control
- To have choice and control over where death occurs (at home or elsewhere)
- To have access to information and expertise of whatever kind is necessary
- To have access to any spiritual or emotional support required
- To have access to hospice care in any location, not only in hospital
- To have control over who is present and who shares the end
- To be able to issue advance directives which ensure wishes are respected
- To have time to say goodbye, and control over other aspects of timing
- To be able to leave when it is time to go, and not to have life prolonged pointlessly[4]

While these principles may help provide closure to a dying individual or comfort to grieving companions, they are far from universal. Many cultures, religions, and individuals hold different notions of what is considered to be a "good death." Some seek a quick, peaceful death. Others may find comfort when an individual has died during a treasured activity or in a special location. The possible variation among individuals and cultural groups is endless. When EMS providers provide care to a patient who is close to death, the simple principles of minimizing discomfort, demonstrating compassion, and allowing for patient and companion closure should be paramount.

Controversy

The meaning of a "good death" can vary from person to person.

Impending Death

Patients demonstrate certain physical changes that indicate death is rapidly approaching. Signs of impending death may appear unexpectedly in a matter of minutes or hours, or they may slowly evolve over many weeks or months as the health of an individual steadily declines. Regardless, EMS providers should recognize the patterns of change in patients nearing the end of life. These patients will demonstrate a decline in respiration, circulation, and perfusion, resulting in cool, often mottled, skin. Pulses may feel noticeably weak; capillary refill is often delayed; and breathing may become shallow, deep, irregular, or include long pauses.

Mental status often progressively deteriorates as death nears. Patients may sleep longer and more often; it may be more difficult to arouse these patients or obtain meaningful responses to questions. Patients can become disorientated or agitated. Moaning, groaning, or grimacing may be present, resulting from discomfort or part of the dying process. Normally interactive individuals may become withdrawn and less social. It is also common for these patients to stop eating or drinking. They may lose the ability to swallow, or lack the appetite for food or drink. Patients frequently become incontinent of bowel or bladder function, increasing discomfort and requiring greater assistance from others.

Death occurs as a medical condition or disease process ultimately overcomes the individual's ability to continue functioning. There may be an abrupt cessation of breathing and perfusion, such as after a sudden cardiac event. Patients may linger for what feels like an eternity with a slowly diminishing heartbeat, agonal breathing, and minimal signs of life. This slow transition can often be very disturbing for EMS providers and companions at the patient's bedside. During this tense period, prior decisions to withhold aggressive resuscitation are often questioned.

Ethical and Legal Considerations

Care of a dying patient presents many legal and ethical challenges for EMS providers. In a controlled hospital or long-term care setting, patients, their companions, physicians, and other involved individuals often have the opportunity for a meaningful evaluation and discussion of the patient's medical condition, treatment options, and desires for end-of-life care. In the prehospital setting, EMS providers rarely have this same luxury, often encountering patients for the first time as a critical event is rapidly evolving. In only a few moments, EMS providers must often decide whether to initiate or withhold aggressive resuscitation measures. This decision is often made with inadequate or conflicting information and documentation, at odd hours or in odd settings, and with any possible combination of companions or individuals on scene.

EMS systems are structured in a manner that encourages certainty over debate. This approach supports quick decision making in emergency situations, but often complicates delicate end-of-life matters if the proper preparation and documentation has not already occurred. EMS systems can mitigate this problem by obtaining support through online medical control or by implementing policies that recognize the role of surrogate decision makers and other manifestations of patient wishes regarding resuscitation. EMS providers must balance ethical responsibility, organizational policies, operational needs, state EMS regulations, personal beliefs, and the persistent threat of professional malpractice liability, all while making split-second decisions regarding whether to initiate resuscitation on a dying patient.

Autonomy and Consent

Autonomy is the ethical principle that states a patient should be able to make his or her own decisions regarding medical treatment. It is part of a larger group of ethical principles that provide the philosophical basis for many health care laws, regulations, practices, and the professional responsibilities of health care providers. The principle of autonomy is used as the basis for the **doctrine of informed consent** or implied consent, which must be present before EMS providers can provide medical care. State laws and EMS regulations allow patients to refuse medical treatment for themselves, even if the proposed treatment would ultimately be beneficial. In the context of this text, autonomy is the ethical principle that provides the basis for patients to refuse aggressive resuscitation measures when a critical illness or cardiac arrest occurs.

EMS providers must have some form of consent to provide any medical treatment to a patient. Without consent, EMS providers do not have any legal right to touch, move, transport, or perform any medical procedure. Actual consent may be given by a patient, if the patient: (1) has the ability to understand his or her situation (decision-making capacity), (2) has received enough information regarding proposed treatment options, and (3) is capable of communicating the decision to EMS or other health care providers. Without all three of these factors present, EMS providers must utilize an alternate form of consent.

Advanced Health Care Directives

Patients have the ability to demonstrate actual consent or refusal of medical treatment through the usage of an **advanced health care directive (AHCD)**. This document is completed by the patient while the patient has decision-making capacity, and provides instruction for health care providers in the event that the patient cannot make medical decisions or communicate for himself or herself. The patient may specify whether to permit or withhold a variety of medical treatment options or resuscitation measures, including artificial hydration or nutrition, diagnostic tests, surgical procedures, ventilator support, organ donation, etc.

A variety of different AHCD forms and formats are available. Depending on the particular state, the ACHD may require a physician's signature, one or more witnesses, or a notarized patient signature. The instructions specified in an AHCD may be utilized as the basis for a **do not resuscitate (DNR) order** or a **do not attempt resuscitation (DNAR) order** to be followed in health care facilities or during EMS transport between health care facilities. EMS providers face potential uncertainty when instructions contained in an AHCD do not meet the requirements of EMS statutes or regulations pertaining to DNR or DNAR documentation. Online medical control can often be utilized to resolve any conflict, ambiguity, or inconsistency between the AHCD and the local EMS statutes, regulations, or protocols.

The patient may also utilize an AHCD to designate a **power of attorney (POA)** to make health care decisions on behalf of the patient either before or after the patient loses decision-making capacity. (The appointment of another individual to make health-care decisions is often termed "durable," meaning it remains valid despite prolonged passage of time or subsequent incapacity of the patient.) A patient may designate a single individual or contingent (alternate) individuals to be the POA. POAs may be empowered either to make certain specified decisions or to make all health care decisions on behalf of the patient.

Surrogate Decision Maker

A surrogate (alternate) decision maker is often necessary when a patient is not capable of providing consent for medical treatment and an AHCD has not been completed. State laws typically specify the hierarchy of who may make decisions for an incapacitated individual when an AHCD or POA is not present; however, a court-appointed guardian (or custodian for minor children) would trump all other surrogate decision makers.

Unless a court has intervened, biological or adoptive parents would be the initial surrogate decision makers for minor children. These parents may also designate a POA to make decisions for their minor children, such as in situations of prolonged incarceration or when a relative-caregiver is present. As minor children approach the age of majority (typically 18), certain states give "mature minors" increased autonomy to consent or refuse certain medical or mental health treatments. For a married individual, the spouse is usually the primary surrogate decision maker if the individual becomes incapacitated, although this role may defer to an alternate if there is a pending divorce or legal separation. If no spouse is present, states may or may not recognize the role of a domestic partner. The remaining hierarchy typically involves adult children of the patient, parents of an adult patient, siblings, more distant relatives, and, in certain instances, a non-relative who is familiar with the patient's values and beliefs.

The identified surrogate decision maker is empowered to make any health care-related decisions on behalf of the patient, including the decision to permit or withhold resuscitation efforts. The individual may exercise either substituted judgment or a best interests approach when making health care decisions. In substituted judgment, the surrogate makes the decision based upon what he or she believes the patient would choose if that patient were capable of making or expressing a decision. In the best interest approach, the decision is more objective and based upon what the surrogate believes would ultimately provide the greatest benefit for the patient. Sometimes the conclusions of either approach are identical; other times the outcomes are vastly different, depending on the known values or beliefs of a particular patient.

Implied Consent

Implied consent can provide a valid basis for EMS providers to treat a severely ill or injured patient when no other methods of consent or refusal are present. The doctrine of implied consent is the assumption that individuals generally want to receive medical treatment in an emergency. Health care providers utilize this assumption to provide emergency care to a person who appears ill or injured and cannot provide actual informed consent. Implied consent is used in situations in which an individual is unconscious, severely intoxicated, in cardiac arrest, or has a severe neurological or psychiatric impairment that prevents the person from understanding or communicating information. In order for implied consent to be utilized, the following factors must be present:

1. There must be a true emergency situation.
2. EMS providers must have no indication that a patient would likely refuse a proposed treatment.
3. A surrogate decision maker must not be available.

These factors are the theoretical basis for implied consent. EMS providers must be careful to follow state EMS regulations and department policies when using implied consent to perform medical care.

Medical Orders for Life Sustaining Treatment (MOLST) or Physician Orders for Life Sustaining Treatment (POLST)

EMS providers may encounter an emerging practice known as **Medical Orders for Life Sustaining Treatment (MOLST)** or **Physician Orders for Life Sustaining Treatment (POLST)**. Physicians, nurse practitioners, and physician's assistants collaborate with patients to determine the patient's wishes, typically pertaining to resuscitation or life-sustaining treatments. The provider then completes the POLST or MOLST paper or electronic form on behalf of the patient (**Figure 6-2**). This document functions as a physician's order and is designed to remain valid and in effect as the patient travels through the health care system. The orders provide direction for health care providers in prehospital settings or various acute and long-term care facilities, allowing for greater continuity of care and theoretically greater implementation of the patient's health care decisions. In EMS systems that recognize POLST/MOLST order sets, the document can function as a valid DNR/DNAR form or as an authorization for a particular treatment, such as pain control, hydration, or initiation of resuscitation, which might otherwise require online medical control or an established protocol.

Do Not Resuscitate (DNR) and Do Not Attempt Resuscitation (DNAR) Orders

Many patients, particularly older patients, in the prehospital, hospital, and long-term care settings have DNR or DNAR orders in place. These orders are essentially identical. DNR orders evolved into DNAR orders in certain settings to underscore the reality that the majority of cardiac arrest resuscitation attempts are unsuccessful.

DNR and DNAR orders are written by a patient's physician, nurse practitioner, or physician's assistant to instruct other health care providers not to initiate cardiac arrest resuscitation (CPR) or certain other advanced treatments in the event of cardiac or respiratory arrest. Individual states may enact laws and regulations pertaining to DNR/DNAR use by EMS. Such laws and regulations often include exclusion criteria (such as suspected homicide or suicide), requirements for a periodic renewal, or allowance for symbolic indications of DNR/DNAR status such as bracelets or pendants. EMS providers should consult state or regional protocols for specific rules in a particular jurisdiction.

> **Attitude Tip**
>
> Remember that "DNR" *does not* mean "do not treat."

> **Controversy**
>
> There may be situations when the family disagrees with a DNR and the patient is unable to speak for himself or herself. The patient's wishes should be respected regarding resuscitation. If the family wants CPR started, but there is a DNR order stating otherwise, attempt to convince the family to honor the patient's wishes. If the disagreement continues, begin resuscitation while contacting medical control for direction.
>
> In some states, the DNR order can be revoked. A patient may revoke the order verbally or by physically destroying the directive. The legal spokesperson for the patient, known as the surrogate decision maker, may revoke the order by stating that they are expressing the patient's wishes. You will need to learn your local or state protocol.

Communication With Families and Companions of Deceased Patients

Effective communication becomes vitally important when EMS providers are with a patient who is dying or who has died. In many instances, EMS providers are the only medical personnel present to inform family members and other companions that the patient has died. Certain practices greatly impact how this crucial information is received and interpreted by those connected to the patient.

EMS providers rarely have the luxury of choosing or controlling the environment. Whenever possible, communication with family members should occur face-to-face in a location away from bystanders or nonessential personnel. The area should be away from the general public, but not so isolated that it places the EMS providers at increased risk if the individual(s) being notified have a violent outburst or engage in some other form of dangerous behavior. Consider a posture that can convey

MM 3 2013

Maryland Medical Orders for Life-Sustaining Treatment (MOLST)

Patient's Last Name, First, Middle Initial	Date of Birth	
		☐ Male ☐ Female

This form includes medical orders for Emergency Medical Services (EMS) and other medical personnel regarding cardiopulmonary resuscitation and other life-sustaining treatment options for a specific patient. It is valid in all health care facilities and programs throughout Maryland. This order form shall be kept with other active medical orders in the patient's medical record. The physician, nurse practitioner (NP), or physician assistant (PA) must accurately and legibly complete the form and then sign and date it. The physician, NP, or PA shall select only 1 choice in Section 1 and only 1 choice in any of the other Sections that apply to this patient. If any of Sections 2-9 do not apply, leave them blank. A copy or the original of every completed MOLST form must be given to the patient or authorized decision maker within 48 hours of completion of the form or sooner if the patient is discharged or transferred.

CERTIFICATION FOR THE BASIS OF THESE ORDERS: Mark any and all that apply.

I hereby certify that these orders are entered as a result of a discussion with and the informed consent of:

_____ the patient; or

_____ the patient's health care agent as named in the patient's advance directive; or

_____ the patient's guardian of the person as per the authority granted by a court order; or

_____ the patient's surrogate as per the authority granted by the Heath Care Decisions Act; or

_____ if the patient is a minor, the patient's legal guardian or another legally authorized adult.

Or, I hereby certify that these orders are based on:

_____ instructions in the patient's advance directive; or

_____ other legal authority in accordance with all provisions of the Health Care Decisions Act. All supporting documentation must be contained in the patient's medical records.

_____ Mark this line if the patient or authorized decision maker declines to discuss or is unable to make a decision about these treatments. **The patient's or authorized decision maker's participation in the preparation of the MOLST form is always voluntary.** If the patient or authorized decision maker has not limited care, except as otherwise provided by law, CPR will be attempted and other treatments will be given.

1

CPR (RESUSCITATION) STATUS: EMS providers must follow the *Maryland Medical Protocols for EMS Providers.*

_____ **Attempt CPR:** If cardiac and/or pulmonary arrest occurs, attempt cardiopulmonary resuscitation (CPR). This will include any and all medical efforts that are indicated during arrest, including artificial ventilation and efforts to restore and/or stabilize cardiopulmonary function.

[If the patient or authorized decision maker does not or cannot make any selection regarding CPR status, mark this option. Exceptions: If a valid advance directive declines CPR, CPR is medically ineffective, or there is some other legal basis for not attempting CPR, mark one of the "No CPR" options below.]

No CPR, Option A, Comprehensive Efforts to Prevent Arrest: Prior to arrest, administer all medications needed to stabilize the patient. If cardiac and/or pulmonary arrest occurs, do not attempt resuscitation (No CPR). Allow death to occur naturally.

_____ **Option A-1, Intubate:** Comprehensive efforts may include intubation and artificial ventilation.

_____ **Option A-2, Do Not Intubate (DNI):** Comprehensive efforts may include limited ventilatory support by CPAP or BiPAP, but do not intubate.

_____ **No CPR, Option B, Palliative and Supportive Care:** Prior to arrest, provide passive oxygen for comfort and control any external bleeding. Prior to arrest, provide medications for pain relief as needed, but no other medications. Do not intubate or use CPAP or BiPAP. If cardiac and/or pulmonary arrest occurs, do not attempt resuscitation (No CPR). Allow death to occur naturally.

SIGNATURE OF PHYSICIAN, NURSE PRACTITIONER, OR PHYSICIAN ASSISTANT (Signature and date are required to validate order)

Practitioner's Signature	Print Practitioner's Name	
Maryland License #	Phone Number	Date

Figure 6-2 A MOLST form identifies decisions a person has made regarding treatment preferences.

Courtesy of Maryland Department of Health and Mental Hygiene

empathy without jeopardizing safety; if the risk of danger is low, consider sitting next to the individual, rather than standing.

Communicating that a person has died is very challenging. It is often helpful to determine how much information the individual already understands regarding the situation. The patient's death may be expected, in which case the family and companions may have been given considerable opportunity to prepare. These individuals may have even recognized the patient's deterioration or otherwise become aware that the patient has died. If the patient's family or companions are not aware that the patient died, EMS providers should attempt to demonstrate compassion and empathy when informing these individuals. A careful combination of verbal and nonverbal communication is essential when conveying this information. Good eye contact creates a sense of trust and connection. Tone and posture dramatically impact how spoken information is received. It is tempting to use euphemisms such as "passed away" or "not with us anymore," as they may feel easier to say; however, these euphemisms frequently create confusion or uncertainty and ultimately complicate the conversation.

Once news of the death has been conveyed, family members or companions may have a wide range of questions regarding the manner of death, such as whether there is something else that can be done, or practical questions such as "What happens to the body?" EMS providers should be as prepared as possible for receiving these questions. An experienced colleague can be a great resource throughout this entire process. One thing to keep in mind when delivering death notification is that it matters less *who* delivers the information, but rather *how* the information is delivered. **Table 6-1** summarizes important points when delivering death notification. Be prepared to assist grieving family and companions to identify and connect with other sources of support such as other family members, neighbors, and clergy. Many obvious tasks or calls may be overlooked in this time of grief.

Communication Tip

When initiating communication with friends and family of a patient who has died, listen to their concerns and expect any reaction. The death of a loved one can be one of the most stressful experiences of a person's life.

Bereavement and Grief

It is possible for family members and companions of a deceased patient to have many different kinds of reactions to the person's death. The state of having had a loss is known as **bereavement**. The emotional process following the loss of something important is known as **grief** or the grieving process. Individuals who have felt an emotional loss with the death of the patient will present in different ways at different times. EMS providers should be prepared to encounter anything from ambivalence or relief to violent outbursts or uncontrolled behavior from those on scene. Personal and scene safety should always remain the top priority.

Death may occur as the final event in a long, painful clinical struggle. Depending upon the circumstances, death may represent the end of a person's suffering, rather than a horrible, tragic event. A patient's family and companions may have already started the grieving process months or years prior to the actual death of the patient, depending on the course of the condition or illness. Feelings of ambivalence or relief may alternate with sadness, loss, or many other possible emotions.

Grieving following a sudden, unexpected loss can be divided into different phases or stages. In 1969, these distinct stages were articulated by Elizabeth Kubler-Ross; they continue to be cited, with or without modification, in many professional resources pertaining to coping with death and dying. The initial reaction of the grieving person includes shock, disbelief, denial, or isolation. As the reality of the loss emerges, individuals then progress into some combination of the next three stages: anger, bargaining (an emotional attempt to rationalize the loss or situation), and depression. These powerful emotions are frequently accompanied by physical manifestations such as weakness, weight loss/anorexia, loss of sleep, hallucinations, etc. As these emotional conflicts slowly resolve, individuals transition towards a state of acceptance. Acceptance is the final stage, during which an individual adjusts to day-to-day existence without the deceased. Reaching some level of acceptance may take months or years, or may never fully be attained. Similarly, individuals may progress through the different phases from one to the next, or they may experience the phases to varying degrees at different times throughout the grieving process. It is not unusual for people to revisit the same stage multiple times as the grieving process continues.

Older adults express their grief in the same ways as younger and middle-aged adults. However, due to their age and life circumstances, older adults are more likely to experience several losses within a short period of time. This may result in the older person grieving the losses at the same time or grieving over a longer period of time. It may also cause them to feel overwhelmed, numb, or have more difficulty expressing their grief. They may feel sad and experience other signs of grieving without even realizing that they are grieving.

Older people also experience losses related to the natural aging process itself. They may need to give up roles within their family. They may lose physical strength, stamina, and societal standards of beauty. They may lose independence in areas that they previously mastered, such as the ability to drive a car, which is an especially difficult loss. Additionally, the older person may be unwilling to tell other people that they are grieving. They may also be unwilling to tell other people how sad they feel when they see or care for older loved ones who are ill or aging.

Older people may lack the support system they once had. An older adult who depended on his or her spouse or other family members for social contact may lack a support system after the spouse dies or other family members move away or die. Losing a spouse may cause the older adult to suffer many losses, including the loss of his or her best friend, financial security, and social contacts. The older adult may also feel anticipation that he or she is going to lose someone or something special due to aging or chronic

Table 6-1 Delivering Death Notification

Prepare yourself.

- Take off your gloves, tuck in your shirt, and wipe the sweat off your face.
- Switch from resuscitator to death notifier (from clinical to empathic).
- Direct yourself to the spouse, parent, family member, or friend.
- Put yourself on the same height level (sitting or standing).
- Make eye contact but do not stare.

Deliver death notification.

- Deliver the death notification by using the 'D' word: dead, died, death (this helps to avoid denial).
- Deliver the notification quickly; do not drag out the process.
- If applicable, reassure the survivor(s) that resuscitation efforts were performed: "We did every medical procedure possible, but were unable to revive him/her."
- Allow a pause for survivor response.

Support survivors.

- Attempt to touch the key survivor's hand, shoulder, or arm as a sign of closeness, and take the individual's lead from there.
- Describe what you did and why.
- Listen to how the survivor feels and what they need.
- Answer with honesty (not brutal) and in a nonjudgmental way. Omit clichés.
- Do not reinforce the survivor's denial of death.
- Restrain violent survivors only enough to protect them and you, and then involve the police.
- Offer to make tea or coffee, or to get drinks for the survivors.
- Offer to call relatives if needed.
- Do not feel you have to keep talking—just being there is usually sufficient enough.
- Offer the family the chance to say goodbye; this may include touching the deceased individual (consult with police).
- If allowed by the police and/or coroner, place the body in an appropriate location, such as on a bed.
- Have your partner clean up and prepare for the next call.
- Explain the local policy for certification of death and removal of body.
- Explain the role of the police, family physician, and coroner.
- Offer to call or, if necessary, call local victim/crisis services staff to respond to the scene and provide grief counseling.
- If you transport the deceased, do not leave the survivor behind without a ride to the hospital.

Use helpful phrases.

- "I can't imagine how difficult this is for you."
- "I know this is very painful for you."
- "I'm so sorry for your loss."
- "It must be hard to accept."
- "It's harder than most people think."
- "You must have been very close to him/her."
- "How can I help?"
- "Most people who go through this react just as you are."

Avoid hurtful phrases.

- "It was actually a blessing because…"
- "You shouldn't feel/act that way."
- "Aren't you lucky that at least…"
- "You must get a hold of yourself."
- "You must focus on your precious moments."
- "You don't need to know that."
- "I can't tell you that."
- "His/her death was for the best."
- "I know how you feel. My _____ died last year."
- "We all have to deal with loss."
- "At least he/she died in their sleep."
- "He/she had a very full life."
- "Everything is going to be OK."

Data from: Ontario Base Hospital Group. *Death Notification for Paramedics.*

illness. These adults may feel lonely and think that they have no one to confide in. Older adults are also more likely to become physically ill after experiencing a major loss. They may already have long-term physical illnesses or other conditions that interfere with the ability to grieve or become worse when they are grieving.

Because of these special grieving challenges, older adults are more at risk to develop unresolved grief or complications associated with grieving. As such, adjusting to change may be more difficult and contribute to emotional stress, which may lead to an overreaction to a minor loss that brings about memories and feelings from a previous, greater loss.[5] Older adults may need more time than younger adults to adjust to change.

Role of EMS on Scene

In the case of a dead or dying patient, the EMS provider will perform many critical roles on scene. In the 911 context, the EMS response typically originates as some request for medical assistance. Providers must ascertain whether the identified patient desires or requires medical treatment or transportation. If it appears that respiratory or cardiac arrest is imminent, EMS personnel must quickly decide what, if any, resuscitation measures are indicated. This decision may involve a focused conversation with the patient and/or his or her family members, health care providers, or other on-scene companions. It may be necessary to determine the validity of any DNR/DNAR, POLST/MOLST, or advanced health care directive documentation present with the patient. If information is conflicting or inadequate, EMS personnel must decide whether to initiate resuscitation measures or seek additional guidance through some manner of online medical control.

Additional responsibilities emerge if a patient dies or has died on scene or in an EMS vehicle. Once death is determined, a variety of laws, regulations, and department policies impact whether EMS personnel must remain on scene until custody of the body can be transferred to law enforcement or another entity. If death occurs during patient transport, similar laws, regulations, and policies will dictate where the pronouncement of death must occur or whether the transport of the body is allowed to continue. EMS providers must also remain alert for signs of abuse, neglect, or other criminal activity related to the patient's death. If any of these events are suspected, law enforcement involvement is essential.

Family and companions present with the patient will have a vast array of emotional and supportive needs. EMS providers should remain prepared for any responses or behaviors that jeopardize responder safety. EMS system characteristics will determine how long EMS providers can remain on scene or what assistance can be offered to the patient's family and companions.

Documentation is essential in the previously discussed scenarios. These literal life-and-death decisions have serious implications for the EMS provider and agency, and are based upon patient refusal, interpretation of critical documents, direction from a surrogate decision maker, or situations where death has occurred. Unfortunately, the split-second determinations that are made will be subject to intense scrutiny at a later time.

Critical Incident Stress Management

A massive emotional burden is placed on EMS providers responding to death. This burden may gradually accumulate after many repeated difficult EMS activities, or may emerge suddenly after even a single emotionally traumatic event. Critical Incident Stress Management (CISM) is a systematic approach to providing emotional support to EMS personnel and other emergency responders. CISM utilizes a variety of methods including educational programs, resources for families and responders, crisis intervention, and other services. A major component of a CISM program is educating individuals, coworkers, and family members to recognize dysfunctional reactions to emotionally stressful events. Stressful events during EMS calls can interfere with a responder's ability to function "normally" in everyday life and can lead to harmful physical, cognitive, emotional, and behavioral changes that adversely impact the EMS provider's life.

EMS agencies may utilize a Critical Incident Stress Debriefing (CISD) after a particularly gruesome or emotionally traumatic event. This debriefing facilitates "psychological first-aid" for responders who are experiencing powerful responses to an emotionally traumatic event, such as a pediatric death or mass-casualty event. Other calls that may cause massive emotional turmoil for responders include responding to the death of a colleague or family member or being unable to rescue an entrapped patient. CISD is a structured program, led by trained facilitators and designed to guide responders towards the start of the healing process. These programs typically highlight warning signs of further emotional deterioration and identify resources for peer and professional emotional support.

CASE STUDY 2

© 123dartist/Thinkstock

You are called to the home of a hospice patient. When you arrive, you are greeted by a family member that tells you he became scared when "grandma started to breathe funny." The patient is mottled, cold, and does not appear to be breathing when you arrive at the bedside. There are valid/signed DNR papers on the bedside table. The family member is distraught. You are checking for a pulse and breathing when several other family members enter the room. There is no palpable pulse or breathing.

- What should you do?
- What do you need to know?

Summary

Care of patients who have died or are on the verge of dying creates a significant ethical, legal, emotional, and operational challenge for EMS providers, beyond simply providing medical treatment. These complex concerns frequently overlap or conflict, forcing EMS providers to make difficult, split-second, life-and-death decisions that have an enormous impact on the patient, or the families and companions left behind.

References

1. Central Intelligence Agency. *The World Factbook.* Available from https://www.cia.gov/library/publications/the-world-factbook/geos/us.html
2. Ibid.
3. Ibid.
4. Smith, R. A good death. *BMJ* 2000:320:129–130.
5. National Center for Gerontological Social Work Education. *Grief, loss, and bereavement in older adults: Reactions to death, chronic illness, and disability.*

CASE STUDY SUMMARIES

Case Study 1 Summary

DNR does not mean "do not treat," and since neither the patient's heart nor breathing has stopped, the DNR does not apply. This patient is still well within the treatment window for stroke. She needs to be taken to a stroke center to determine if she meets criteria for thrombolytic therapy. Still, it should be determined if the patient actually has a formal set of advance directives in place, or if the family members have medical power of attorney, that states that she should not be assessed and treated for stroke.

Keeping in mind that "time equals brain," you should rapidly discuss options with the family members, explaining to them that patients can be successfully treated for stroke symptoms if treatment is started within 3.5 hours. Explain that the patient will most likely not require CPR for this problem. Stroke victims often can understand, even if they have trouble speaking; therefore, if you are able to communicate with the patient, explain the situation to her and obtain her consent to take her to the appropriate stroke hospital. Should the patient deteriorate en route, you will need to re-consider options, as some hemorrhagic stroke patients will stop breathing due to increased intracranial pressures.

Case Study 2 Summary

You need to tell the family their loved one has died. It can become challenging when family members suddenly change their mind or disagree with the DNR order, and the patient is unable to confirm his or her wish. Should someone insist that chest compressions, ventilations, or medications be given, or that the patient be transported to the hospital, you should try to convince the family to honor the patient's wishes. If that does not work, it would be better to start resuscitation and contact medical control.

If the family seems accepting of what is happening, it is a good idea to move them to a quiet place to convey the news to them. Take your gloves off, sit at eye level, and make good eye contact. Use a sympathetic tone and posture; and be empathetic and compassionate when telling them that the patient has died. Do not use phrases such as "passed" or "not with us anymore," as these may lead to confusion.

The family may ask about the death or if something else could have been done. If you provided care for the patient, let the family know that you did all you could, explaining what you did and that you could not revive the patient. Listen to what the family says and address their concerns. This is a tough part of the job and how the family responds to the news will depend on how prepared the family was for the death. They may be accepting, angry, quiet, loud, or violent. Make sure you are safe. Also, remember this death may affect you, your partner, or the other responders; it is okay to debrief and seek assistance from counselors.

CHAPTER 7

Trauma

LEARNING OBJECTIVES

1. Discuss the epidemiology of trauma in the older population, including the risk factors for falls, motor vehicle crashes, pedestrian accidents, and burns.

2. Describe the incidence, morbidity/mortality, risk factors, and preventive strategies for osteoporosis, osteoarthritis, and rheumatoid arthritis.

3. Discuss the assessment findings common in older patients with traumatic injuries, including orthopedic injuries.

4. Discuss assessment considerations of the older patient with traumatic injuries or complaints related to the musculoskeletal system.

5. Discuss the relationship between medical conditions and trauma in the older patient.

6. Discuss medical risk factors, medications as risk factors, and environmental risk factors that make older people particularly susceptible to falls.

7. Discuss intervention, management, and transport considerations of the older patient with traumatic injuries or complaints related to the musculoskeletal system.

8. Review immobilization, packaging, and splinting considerations in treating older patients, including those with physical deformities.

9. Discuss strategies for prevention of falls in older people.

Introduction

In general, older individuals tend to be less active than younger people and suffer from injuries less frequently. However, when an older person is injured, the injury tends to be more serious and involve more complications. Treatment of the older person should reflect the fact that the patient's body does not respond to injury in the same manner as that of a younger individual. The purpose of this chapter is to identify the changes associated with aging and to review how these changes should affect the decisions made by EMS providers who treat older trauma patients.

Although morbidity and mortality caused by major trauma is high in the older population, the vast majority of older patients survive through hospital discharge, and a significant percentage return to their previous levels of function. By identifying occult instability, resuscitating and stabilizing the patient, identifying important injuries and relevant comorbidities, and making an appropriate hospital disposition, prehospital care providers can positively impact the morbidity and mortality of older trauma patients.

Attitude Tip

Remember that older trauma patients *do* benefit from aggressive prehospital and in-hospital care! In related studies of patients older than 70 years of age with multiple injuries, it was found that after the trauma, 89% returned home rather than to long-term care facilities.

Epidemiology of Trauma in the Older Population

Trauma is the fifth-leading cause of death in patients older than 65 years, with this population sustaining a disproportionate share of fractures and serious injury. In addition, the older population accounts for approximately 34% of deaths caused by trauma, despite the fact that they only account for 14% of the overall trauma population.[1, 2]

There are many contributing factors associated with injuries in older people (**Table 7-1**). The most common cause of trauma in older people is ground-level falls (falls from a standing height). Complications resulting from falls are the leading cause of death from injury in men and women older than age 65 years in the United States, followed by motor vehicle collisions and suicide.[3]

Falls

Falls are a common reason for calls to 9-1-1, but the actual number of falls that occur far exceeds the number of times a patient is examined by a medical provider. It is estimated that about 30% of people older than age 65 years and living independently fall each year, and about one half of these patients have multiple falls. The rate of falls increases with age; however, because many older patients are reluctant to report falls and often do not recall having fallen, the true prevalence of falls in the community (as opposed to institutions) is difficult to accurately determine. It does appear that the prevalence of falls is even higher in institutionalized patients, with about 50% of ambulatory nursing home residents falling per year; however, it is also not clear whether nursing home residents truly fall more frequently, or falls are simply documented more often in a supervised setting.

Attitude Tip

A fractured hip can lead to a rapid decline in the patient's quality of life and/or death within the coming year or less. Do not treat these patients as "just another fractured hip."

People age 75 years and older who fall are four to five times more likely than those age 65 to 74 years to be admitted to a long-term care facility for a year or longer. Men are more likely than women to die from a fall. After taking age into account, the fall death rate in 2009 was 34% higher for men than for women; however, older women are more than twice as likely as older men to endure fall-related fractures. Falls are also the most common cause of traumatic brain injury (TBI), accounting for approximately 46% of fatal falls among older adults. Head injury

CASE STUDY 1

At 10:00 a.m., you are dispatched to a bicycle crash for a 75 year-old man named Mr. Parks. When you arrive, you find Mr. Parks lying on the roadway next to his bicycle. The weather is overcast, and it rained earlier in the morning. Your scene observations reveal no other vehicle involvement. Your initial assessment of Mr. Parks reveals that he appears to be confused and unaware of what happened. He has left-sided facial droop and also what appears to be swelling of the left humeral area.

- What was the likely reason for the crash?
- How should this patient be treated?

Table 7-1   Contributing Factors to Injuries in Older Patients

Chronic Medical Conditions	Acute Medical Conditions	Environmental Factors	Other
Osteoarthritis	Syncope	Rugs	Older age
Osteoporosis	Dysrhythmias	Lighting	Female gender
CVA	CVA/TIA	Stairs	Alcohol and drug abuse
Ischemic heart disease	Seizure	Bathtubs/showers	Elder abuse
Anemia	Acute renal failure	Footwear	
HTN	Infection	Uneven ground	
Gait and balance disturbances	Hypoglycemia	Weather	
Visual impairment	AAA	Walking aids	
Depression	New medication		
Polypharmacy	Dehydration		
Parkinson's disease	Acute fractures		
Dementia	Self-inflicted injury		

Abbreviations: AAA, abdominal aortic aneurysm; CVA, cerebral vascular accident; DM, diabetes mellitus; HTN, hypertension; MI, myocardial infarct; TIA, transient ischemic attack.

Reprinted from Emergency Medicine Clinics of North America, 24(2), Aschkenasy, Miriam T., Rothenhaus, Todd C., "Trauma and Falls in the Elderly", Page Nos. 413-432, Copyright 2006, with permission from Elsevier.

should be expected in any older patient with a history of blunt trauma (including ground-level falls) and any loss of consciousness, mental status change, history of direct impact to the head or neck, or signs of external injury to the head or neck. Those older patients who are anticoagulated are at even higher risk of intracranial hemorrhage.

Though most people consider the physical injuries associated with falls, it is also important to keep in mind that falls profoundly affect many other aspects of an older patient's quality of life. For instance, not only are falls a leading cause of death in the older age group, but about 50% of falls result in less severe injuries (such as soft-tissue trauma and lacerations) that still require treatment. Fortunately, only 1% of falls results in hip fractures; however, 5% of falls result in other types of fractures. Head trauma (including concussion and subdural hematoma) is also an uncommon but serious consequence of falls.

Perhaps most devastating of all are the psychological and social impacts of falls. About one half of fall victims report they were unable to get up after falling (**Figure 7-1**). Ten percent remain on the ground for over 24 hours, with resultant risk of pressure ulcers, deep vein thrombosis, **rhabdomyolysis** (disintegration of muscle fibers), compartment syndrome, and fluid and electrolyte abnormalities. The possibility of not being found certainly contributes to the fear of falling. In fact, 40% to 73%

of older people who have fallen report that they restrict their daily activities because of this fear, and a striking 20% to 40% of people *who have never fallen* report the same. In addition, older patients who fall tend to use healthcare resources more often. Falling is a very common reason that older individuals must give up their homes and move into a more supervised setting.

Motor Vehicle Collisions

There were 35 million licensed older drivers in 2011. That same year, 5401 people 65 years and older were killed and 185,000 were injured in traffic crashes. These older individuals made up 17% of all traffic fatalities, 16.3% of all vehicle occupant fatalities, and 19% of all pedestrian fatalities, with the majority of these fatalities occurring during the daytime, on weekdays, and involving other vehicles.

Of all adult drivers involved in fatal crashes in 2011, older drivers made up the lowest proportion of total drivers with a blood alcohol concentration (BAC) of 0.08 grams per deciliter (g/dL) or higher. In addition, over 75% of all older occupants of passenger vehicles involved in fatal crashes were using restraints at the time of the crash, compared to 63% of adults aged 18 to 64 years. In fatal two-vehicle crashes involving an older driver and a younger driver, the vehicle driven by the older person was nearly twice as likely to

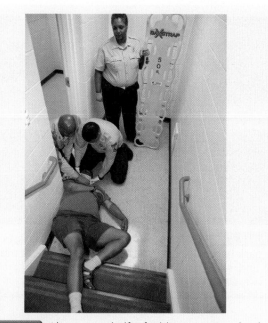

Figure 7-1 About one half of older persons who have fallen report not being able to get up afterward. Some of these patients may have been "down" longer than 24 hours.
© Jones & Bartlett Learning. Courtesy of MIEMSS.

be the one that was struck. Among all fatally injured adult pedestrians, older adults also made up the lowest proportion of pedestrians with a BAC of .08 g/dL or higher. In 2011, 69% of older pedestrian fatalities occurred at nonintersection locations, compared to 83% of fatalities in other pedestrians.

Older patients have an increased severity of injuries from motor vehicle collisions when compared with younger patients. However, the pattern of injury appears quite similar, with the exception being an increased incidence of sternal fractures from seatbelts in patients older than 65 years of age. Older pedestrians injured by automobiles are also at a high risk for very serious injury. Slow ambulation; impaired reflexes; misjudgment; and visual, auditory, and gait impairment may increase the risk of being struck while crossing the street. One study found a significantly increased mortality rate (greater than 25%) for older pedestrians struck by a motor vehicle compared to younger patients.[4] Fatal injuries tended to include severe head injury or major vascular damage, with the majority of deaths occurring at the scene of the accident or in the emergency department. Older patients struck by cars also sustained twice as many lower extremity injuries as their younger counterparts. Age plays a tremendous role in severity of injury to multiple body systems, as well as a dramatic increase in skeletal injuries and injuries to the brain, spine, and thorax.

Burns

The older population accounts for approximately 13% of all patients admitted to burn units. Total body surface area burned, mortality rate, and length of hospital stay are all higher in the older population. Factors that increase the morbidity

and mortality from burns in this population include physiologic changes associated with aging, acute and chronic medical conditions, and social isolation. As with other forms of trauma, burn treatment in the older patient is complicated by coexisting disease and impaired functional reserve; however, there is no available data to suggest that changes are warranted in initial burn treatment protocols, other than taking into consideration underlying medical conditions that may require additional care. Liberal transfer to a burn unit is recommended, particularly for patients with significant coexisting medical conditions.[5]

Physiological Changes Associated with Aging That Impact Trauma

Nearly every part of the body undergoes some type of change during the aging process. (These changes are reviewed in detail in the *Changes with Age* chapter.) Specifically, changes in the pulmonary, cardiovascular, neurologic, and musculoskeletal systems all significantly affect an older person's susceptibility to injury and response to trauma.

Changes in the pulmonary system, such as decreased pulmonary function due to the loss of lung and chest wall elasticity, commonly contribute to the cause of death in older trauma victims. These changes contribute to more broken ribs and a higher risk of **atelectasis** (partial lung collapse) and pneumonia, and must be considered in the management of ventilation.

Changes in the heart and blood vessels predispose older trauma victims to a reduced ability to maintain adequate circulation. These patients are less able to increase cardiac output, heart rate, and blood pressure in response to blood loss or increased peripheral oxygen demand and, similarly, do not adapt as well to increases in volume in the circulatory system. Because of this, cardiovascular collapse is often the cause of death in acutely injured older patients. This is particularly important to consider in an older patient with burns, because burns can be associated with marked fluid shifts. As a result of the normal and pathological changes associated with aging, the usual indicators of volume status, such as heart rate and blood pressure, may be unreliable in this population. An older trauma patient with a history of hypertension who presents with a normal blood pressure should be considered unstable until proven otherwise. The risk of a concomitant cardiac event must be considered, and a 12-lead electrocardiogram (ECG) is mandatory in these patients.

Changes in the brain and surrounding structures contribute to head injury being second only to profound shock as the leading cause of traumatic death in older patients. As a person ages, the brain shrinks, resulting in a higher risk of developing a subdural hematoma (venous bleeding between the dura matter and the brain). Older patients often do not show immediate signs or symptoms of a head injury because there is more space for blood to collect. Thus, examination of the neurologic system in an older trauma patient must be repeated frequently.

Numerous age-related changes that affect trauma and injury occur in the musculoskeletal system. Most notable are the loss of bone and muscle mass, though other common changes include:

- **Kyphosis**, a condition in which the back becomes hunched over (**Figure 7-2**)
- Arthritis, which reduces the flexibility of joints, decreases range of motion, causes pain, and may alter limb mechanics in a way that increases fracture risk
- Diminished strength, which results from changes in the composition of muscle fibers

All of these changes contribute to an increased propensity toward trauma and injury. Older people tend to become progressively less active for a number of reasons, including prior injury, medications, illnesses, and a decreased level of energy. In response to being less active, conditions such as arthritis and muscle weakness can be aggravated, leading to further reduction in activity.

With aging, the size, number, and function of muscle cells in the body decreases, resulting in a progressive loss of strength at a rate of approximately 10% per decade after the age of 40. The greatest loss of muscle mass occurs in the fatigue-resistant fast-twitch muscle fibers, such as those found in the calf, that are used for postural stability. Additionally, muscle fibers contract less forcefully in older patients. The result of these changes is that older people have a loss of strength and power. Exercise and strength training are necessary to restore and maintain strength in the older patient (**Figure 7-3**).

Musculoskeletal Disorders

Osteoporosis

Clinically, **osteoporosis** is a condition that affects both men and women, and is characterized by a decrease in bone mass, leading to a reduction in bone strength and a greater susceptibility to fracture. It is estimated that 52 million people in the United States are afflicted with osteoporosis. It is a major public health issue, leading to 2 million fractures annually and generating nearly 19 billion dollars per year in healthcare expenses.

Human bone is living tissue that is constantly being remodeled. Cells known as **osteoclasts** absorb bone, while **osteoblasts** deposit newly formed bone in areas where it is needed. The greatest bone mass is reached at approximately 35 years, after which an imbalance develops between the activity of these two types of cells, leading to a loss of bone mass. The extent of bone loss that an individual experiences is influenced by numerous factors, including genetics, smoking, level of activity, diet, alcohol consumption, hormonal factors, and body weight. The most rapid loss of bone occurs in women during the years following menopause because of decreased hormone production. Fair-skinned, thin women have the highest risk of developing osteoporosis.

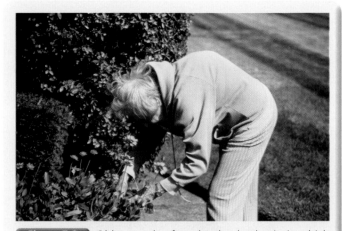

Figure 7-2 Older people often develop kyphosis, in which the back becomes hunched. This condition can contribute to falls and make spinal immobilization difficult.
© Larry Mulvehill/Science Source

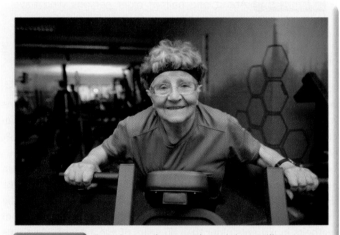

Figure 7-3 Exercise and strength training will restore a significant amount of an older person's strength.
© gilotyna/iStock/Thinkstock

Smoking is believed to cause a reduction in bone mass because it may affect the levels of hormones responsible for maintaining bone mass. A diet poor in calcium and vitamin D, or gastrointestinal problems leading to poor nutrient absorption, are additional contributing factors to osteoporosis. Finally, many medications can contribute to osteoporosis. People with a higher body weight and those who are physically active are likely to have less bone loss because mechanical stimulus helps the body to deposit new bone.

The most common fractures associated with osteoporosis are those of the spine, hip, and wrist. Fractures of the spine occur more frequently in women than in men, and are typically compression (or collapse) fractures. Nearly 50% of these fractures are asymptomatic; the others result in significant pain, disability, and physical deformities that affect breathing, digestion, and body image. Hip fractures are often markedly debilitating injuries that result in permanent decrease in function, potential loss of independence and, for 20% to 30% of individuals, mortality within the first year after the fracture. Wrist fractures, which frequently occur as the result of attempting to brace from a fall, generally only lead to short-term disability, but serve as an opportunity to identify and treat osteoporosis before more serious fractures occur.

Numerous measures may be undertaken to reduce the risk of developing osteoporosis or slow its progression. For example, many postmenopausal women use hormone replacement therapy as a means to reduce the loss of bone. Calcium and vitamin D supplementation is another common treatment for the condition, because it may retard the loss of bone in both men and women. Many other medications are now available to improve bone strength. Older people should also remain physically active by walking and performing low-impact exercises to maintain bone and muscle strength (**Figure 7-4**).

Osteoarthritis

Osteoarthritis is a progressive disease process of the joints that results in the destruction of cartilage, the formation of bone spurs in joints, and joint stiffness (**Figure 7-5**). This type of arthritis is thought to result from "wear and tear" and, in some instances, repetitive trauma to the joints, but there are also hereditary factors that influence the development of this condition. The disease affects approximately 35% to 45% of the population older than 65 years, and its prevalence is equal between men and women.

Typically, osteoarthritis affects several joints of the body, most commonly those in the hands, knees, hips, and spine.

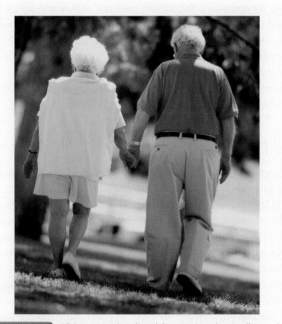

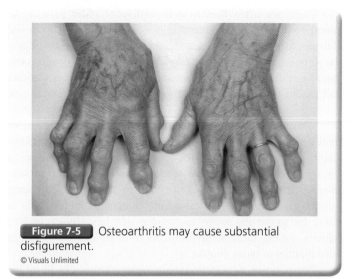

Figure 7-5 Osteoarthritis may cause substantial disfigurement.

Patients will complain of pain and stiffness that gets worse with exertion and tends to be worse at the end of the day. Ultimately, substantial disuse and disfigurement can occur. Most commonly, patients are treated with anti-inflammatory medications and physical therapy to improve range of motion.

Rheumatoid Arthritis

Unlike osteoarthritis, **rheumatoid arthritis** is a systemic inflammatory disease that affects the body's joints. Approximately 1% of the population is affected by this condition, and women are 3 times more likely to be affected. To date, no specific cause has been determined for rheumatoid arthritis; however, some consider it to be an autoimmune disease.

Patients affected by rheumatoid arthritis have a variety of symptoms, most commonly inflammation in and around the joints in the hands, wrists, ankles, and feet, and less often in the knees and spine. As a result of the inflammation, joints become stiffer. In addition, the tissues supporting the inflamed joint may become unstable, leading to dislocation or subluxation (sinking of the bone out of position). For this reason, one should always pay particular attention to the spine in an older trauma victim with rheumatoid arthritis.

Specific Injuries in the Older Patient

Cervical and Spinal Injuries

Most people think that injuries to the spinal column and spinal cord occur in isolation and to adolescents or younger adults. However, epidemiological studies of patients with spinal cord injury demonstrate a bimodal distribution, with the first peak occurring in adolescents and young adults and the second in those older than 65 years of age.[6] Falls are the leading cause of spinal column and spinal cord injury in older people, followed by motor vehicle crashes. The mechanism of injury often involves a much lower velocity than in younger patients.

There are many factors that predispose older patients to spinal column and spinal cord injuries, including osteoporosis; changes in bone density; **osteopenia**; the development of spinal stenosis, resulting in less room for the spinal cord within the spinal canal; and the propensity to fall due to sensory deficits and medications. Many medications taken by older people can cause postural hypotension and impair coordination and sensation. Chronic conditions in older people—such as diabetes with peripheral neuropathy, osteoarthritis, and Parkinson's disease—also contribute to risk factors. Older patients sustaining injury to the spinal column and spinal cord tend to present with incomplete neurologic injuries (as opposed to complete neurologic injuries that are more common in younger patients). This is likely due to the less severe mechanism of injury. Upper cervical injuries are the most common location for fractures and spinal cord injuries in older people.

Three types of injury occur more commonly in older patients: central cord syndrome, cervical extension/distraction injuries, and odontoid fractures.[7] Central cord syndrome is frequently associated with a cervical hyperextension injury. Older people are more prone to this type of injury because of **cervical spondylosis**, a degenerative condition resulting in narrowing of the cervical spinal canal. With hyperextension, the cord is pinched, resulting in injury involving more of the central portions of the cord rather than the peripheral areas. Patients with central cord syndrome tend to have a disproportionate weakness in their upper extremities as compared to their lower extremities. Many of these patients do not have any associated fractures of their cervical vertebrae.

Cervical extension/distraction injury is another injury type that occurs more commonly in older patients, as these patients tend to have stiffness in their spinal column from degenerative changes. In addition, many older patients have **osteophyte** formations that bridge the disc spaces, severely limiting motion in the cervical spinal column. With hyperextension of the neck, the osteophytes can actually fracture, resulting in instability at the involved disc space. If an older patient presents with abrasions to the forehead or face and describes a hyperextension mechanism, the EMS provider should be highly suspicious of an unstable cervical spinal injury. These fractures are also referred to as "open book" fractures because they are associated with an opening or lengthening of the anterior column of the spine.

Odontoid fractures are the third type of spinal fracture frequently encountered in older patients. An odontoid fracture is a fracture of the C-2 vertebral body, specifically the odontoid process, which usually occurs from falls. Although this type of fracture can cause neurologic deficit, the majority of patients present normal neurologically. Normal presentation is likely due to the generous width of the spinal column at this level, which allows for fracture displacement to occur without resulting spinal cord impingement. The goal in treating this injury is to protect the spinal cord while aligning the spinal column to promote stability and to decrease pain. In these patients, the first and most important concern is early establishment and maintenance of an adequate airway, oxygenation, and ventilation. Patients with spinal cord injury can be at risk for airway compromise.[8]

Torso Trauma

Torso trauma represents the second-leading cause of mortality in older people after brain injury. Older persons are at risk for the same thoracic injuries as are younger people. Treatment of some injuries, including pneumothorax and hemothorax, do not require specific age-associated considerations; however, others, including rib fractures, flail chest, and blunt thoracic injuries, do.

Rib fractures are the most common injury encountered in older patients with blunt trauma. The two predominant mechanisms of injury for rib fractures in older patients are motor vehicle crashes and falls. Rib fractures are a significant cause of morbidity and mortality in older patients. They have also been associated with intra-abdominal injury. Because many older people are prescribed medications that control heart rate (beta-blockers), tachycardia may not be present as a sign of ongoing hemorrhage.

Flail chest in older patients is a serious, life-threatening injury almost always associated with significant underlying pulmonary injury. Older people are vulnerable to flail chest following trauma due to their decreased muscle mass, bone density, and chest wall compliance. Advanced age is known to be associated with higher mortality rates for all blunt thoracic traumas, but particularly for flail chest injuries and pulmonary contusions. Traumatic aortic injury also occurs with relative frequency in older patients and is associated with high mortality. Factors contributing to the increased frequency of these injuries include the lack of physiologic reserve to compensate for severe multiple injuries, as well as age-related aortic wall changes. Aortic dilation, increased aortic stiffness, and elevated blood pressure contribute to the increased aortic fragility and susceptibility to injury in older people. Diagnosis of aortic rupture is challenging and requires a high index of suspicion. As many as 50% of older patients with aortic injury have a normal physical exam. Signs and symptoms are often nonspecific and unreliable: Some patients state that lying down causes severe back pain, while others present pale and clammy. Additionally, some patients may sound throaty or exhibit a difference in blood pressure between the right and left arm. Suspect traumatic aortic injury in patients who sustain a rapid deceleration injury.[9]

Hip Fractures

Hip fractures are the second-leading cause of hospitalization for older persons, with approximately 350,000 hip fractures occurring in the United States each year. These injuries occur predominately in older women with osteopenia or osteoporosis, and often result from minor trauma or a fall. Older literature suggested that the hip actually fractured as a result of the underlying osteoporosis prior to the patient falling; however, newer evidence suggests that mechanical falls are responsible for the overwhelming majority of injuries and that efforts to carefully monitor the environment for trip hazards are effective in preventing hip fractures.[10]

By definition, a hip fracture is a fracture of the head, neck, or proximal portion of the femur. This includes intertrochanteric and subtrochanteric femoral fractures. Even after successful treatment, patients often have decreased mobility and can require prolonged rehabilitation. An estimated 18% to 33% of older patients die within the first year following a hip fracture (13.5% die in the first 6 months).[11] Hip fractures can be physically and emotionally challenging for both the patient and his or her family.

Lower Extremity Injuries

Distal femur fractures are more common in older patients due to knee joint arthritis with associated stiffness, whereas increased mobility in younger patients may result in stresses being concentrated further up the shaft of the femur. Because of osteoporosis, however, low-energy twisting motions (such as from a low-energy fall due to missing a step) can also result in femoral shaft fractures in older patients. Proximal fractures of the tibia may occur from a direct impact to the bone, or by a medial or lateral rocking motion. A fracture may occur to the shaft through a direct force, such as that from a motor vehicle striking the leg, or by a twisting force that leads to a stress fracture.

Injuries to the ankle in older patients often result from the foot rolling under the leg, causing a fracture of the bone. This type of injury is commonly seen as an older person attempts to step down from a curb or step and misjudges the height. Another common cause for this pattern of injury is depressing the brake pedal of a vehicle with great force in anticipation of or during a collision.

Upper Extremity Injuries

Injuries to the upper extremities typically pose a low risk of death, but loss of function of the extremity can greatly reduce the older person's independence and can lead to a permanent reduction in function, even after healing. The effective use of the upper extremities depends on an intact shoulder, elbow, and wrist site, which are often injured by older patients.

The **rotator cuff** is composed of four muscles that attach to the humerus to allow motion and provide stability to the arm and shoulder. With time, the rotator cuff undergoes progressive degeneration, making it highly susceptible to tears and injury. Older patients who sustain a traumatic injury to the shoulder region are at risk for further damage to the rotator cuff, leading to pain, instability about the shoulder, and decreased upper extremity function.

Fractures, dislocations, sprains, and strains are all injuries that can occur about the shoulder in older patients. Osteoporosis predisposes older people to fracture of the proximal humerus. Common mechanisms of injury include falling onto an outstretched arm or falling onto an arm while carrying something in it. Distal forearm and wrist fractures are also common injuries that occur in older patients because of osteoporosis. Again, falls are a frequent cause of these injuries, with fractures occurring as the patient extends the arm and lands on the outstretched wrist.

Injuries Associated with Prosthetic Joint Replacement

Prosthetic joint replacements are used commonly in the hip, knee, and shoulder (**Figure 7-6**). The primary reason for the use of prosthetic joints is the treatment of underlying arthritis. The devices are implanted to replace joints; however, they rely on the remaining bone for support and stabilization. Fractures that occur in close proximity to implanted devices may compromise

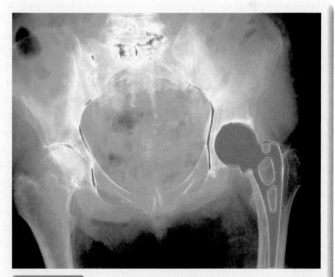

Figure 7-6 Prosthetic joints replace joints, but rely on the remaining bone for support and stabilization.
© Mediscan/Corbis

CASE STUDY 2

© 123dartist/Thinkstock

You are dispatched for a female who has fallen. Ethel is an 85-year-old woman who lives alone. Upon arrival to the scene, you find her in her living room, lying on her left side. The patient is conscious, but confused. She tells you she thinks she fell yesterday but does not remember the time. She also tells you that she has discomfort in her hip. The neighbor who found Ethel is present and states she last saw the patient outside 2 days ago.

- What are your thoughts?
- What information should you gather?

stability of the prosthesis. Common causes of this type of fracture are falls, motor vehicle crashes, reduced bone strength from osteoporosis, stress associated with poor prosthesis fit, or loosening of the prosthesis from infection. Dislocation of hip replacements can occur if there is excessive motion of the hip joint. The risk of this is highest within the first 6 weeks after prosthesis implantation.

Assessment of Geriatric Trauma

As in all other situations, scene size-up should be established. Although it may be easy to assume that an older patient found in a damaged vehicle was in a car crash and is therefore purely a trauma patient, medical conditions such as syncope secondary to cardiac arrhythmia need to be ruled out as a potential cause of the crash. Information from bystanders, such as the patient's level of consciousness before the crash, is useful in making a determination about the entire scope of the emergency.

In evaluating disability, do not assume that a decreased level of consciousness is the baseline mental status of an older patient. Obtain assistance with determining level of consciousness from people familiar with the patient, if available. It is helpful to ask questions such as, "What was he like an hour ago? What was he like yesterday? Does he usually talk like this? Can he usually move his arms and legs?" If medical history is not immediately available, observe for clues during the physical exam. For example, does the patient have a midline scar to the chest indicating heart surgery? Is there indication of a pacemaker? Does the patient have a dialysis shunt?

Evaluating the range of motion should be performed in older patients who have specific complaints in a particular limb. Evaluate range of motion by asking the patient to move the joints in question. It is important to ask patients who have a history of arthritis or previous joint replacement about their normal range of motion. Avoid excessive flexion or extension of replaced joints, as this may lead to injury or damage of the limb.

Communication Tip

When evaluating range of motion, it is important to ask patients who have arthritis or joint replacements about their normal range of motion.

Investigating the cause of a fall is as important as treating the sustained injury, yet this process is often overlooked. Indeed, the causes of a fall are often multiple, resulting from a combination of age-related changes in balance and strength, diseases that affect balance (such as cataracts or strokes), environmental factors (such as a loose rug or wet floor), and acute medical problems (such as a urinary tract infection [UTI] or hypoglycemia). Although many falls in older individuals are related to mobility problems, it is often useful to ask the patient, "But why did you fall today?" It is particularly important to seek out medical causes, since falling is frequently a nonspecific presentation of an acute medical disease and can be the only symptom of a serious illness. Therefore, evaluate the scene for trip hazards, walkers, and canes to determine the nature of the fall, and ask bystanders and the patient about the fall and the events immediately preceding it. The key components of a fall history can be remembered by the SPLATT acronym (**Table 7-2**). Assume the presence of a medical complication leading to trauma until proven otherwise.

Inquire as to exactly what the patient was doing and feeling at the time of the fall. Does he or she know what caused the fall? Were there any warning symptoms? It is important to ask specifically if the fall was caused by the patient "passing out" or losing consciousness, or if the patient struck his or her head or lost consciousness when hitting the ground. The older patient who has fallen may not recall when the fall occurred; therefore, the provider should inspect the scene for indications as to where and when the patient may have fallen. Clues as to when the patient fell include newspapers, meals found sitting out, appliances left on, and the patient's attire. It is also important to interview neighbors who may watch out for the

Table 7-2   Essential Components of a Fall Assessment: SPLATT
Symptoms
Previous falls
Location of fall
Activity at time of fall
Time of fall
Trauma, both physical and psychological

Data from: Tideiksaar R. Preventing falls: How to identify risk factors and reduce complications. *Geriatrics* 1996:51:43–53.

well-being of the patient to find out when he or she was last contacted or seen.

Next, ask about and examine the patient for any injuries requiring treatment. While examining the patient in search of injuries, it is also important to evaluate the patient for the presence of fall and injury risk factors and to determine the contributing factors to each fall, since many factors and contributors are subject to interventions that could reduce the chance of a subsequent fall (**Table 7-3**). For example, does the patient smell of alcohol? Are there pill bottles nearby? Are there signs of mobility problems, such as a walker? Is the patient having a hard time seeing or hearing you? Providers also need to gather information about the environment in which the incident occurred. Is the environment well lit? Are there loose throw rugs? A study of falls in community-dwelling older individuals showed that for each risk factor that was identified and modified, the chances of falling in the next year were reduced by 11%. Thus, EMS providers are in a unique position to make an enormous impact on the quality of life of the older patients they serve.

The physical exam focuses on evaluation of the patient's complaints, such as examining a painful extremity to determine if a fracture may be present, but remember that older patients are very prone to injury even from minor trauma. A thorough exam may be required to determine the full extent of injuries; the older patient presenting to an emergency department with one complaint from a trauma event may be found to have a second injury they were not initially aware of. The management of the older patient who has fallen begins with investigating the cause of the fall. If there is a medical condition that caused the fall, treat as appropriate. Patients who fall and strike their head and are taking anticoagulants, aspirin, or newer antiplatelet agents should be considered for evaluation in a trauma center, as the risk of bleeding is increased.

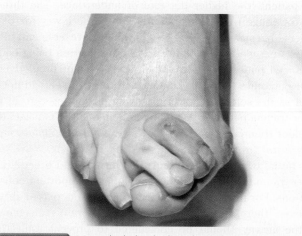

Figure 7-7 Musculoskeletal disorders that cause bone deformity or leg or foot weakness are a risk factor for falls in older people.
© Mike Devlin/Science Source

Management of Geriatric Trauma

Adequate management of the older trauma patient begins with triage. Studies reveal that older trauma patients are often undertriaged and transferred to facilities that do not have the essential resources required for definitive care because their underlying comorbidities and decreased physiologic reserves are not appreciated. One study showed that patients older than 80 years who were transferred to an acute care hospital had a mortality rate of over 50%, compared to 8% when transferred to a trauma center. [10] Other studies concluded that the older

Table 7-3 Intrinsic Risk Factors for Falls and Injuries in Older Adults
• *Sensory impairment*, particularly vision, hearing, and **proprioception** (perception of movement and body's position)
• *Brain diseases* that affect balance (stroke and Parkinson's disease are major conditions)
• *Dementia*, which influences balance, judgment, and problem-solving ability
• *Musculoskeletal disorders*, especially those that cause leg or foot weakness or boney deformity (**Figure 7-7**)
• *Medications*, particularly those with sedative effects such as sleep aids and anxiety medications; also, simultaneous use of many medications (polypharmacy)
• *Depression* and the use of antidepressant medications
• Use of *alcohol*
• *Advanced age*: the older the patient, the more likely are falls and injuries
• *Poor energy-absorbing capacity* of tissues ("onion skin") or bone (osteoporosis)

the patient, the higher the rate of undertriage. The threshold for triage to a trauma center should be lower for older patients because they have less physiologic reserve and more preexisting medical conditions. All other factors being equal, advanced patient age—in and of itself—is not predictive of poor outcomes following trauma, and therefore should not be used as the sole criterion for denying or limiting care in the older trauma patient.[12] A guiding principle in the management of older trauma patients is that *less mechanism equals more significant trauma*.

Initial evaluation of circulation, airway, and breathing in older trauma patients includes a number of important considerations. For example, the older patient has decreased airway reflexes; therefore, expeditious and deliberate management of the airway should be considered to prevent aspiration. Because the ventilatory response to hypoxia and hypercarbia are blunted in the older patient, occult respiratory insufficiency is common. Anatomically, the older person's airway can be difficult to manage. Mouth opening may be impaired. Laryngosopy may be particularly difficult when coupled with the need to maintain in-line stabilization of the spine, kyphosis, or impaired mobility in an uncleared cervical spine. Pharmacologic therapy for rapid sequence intubation in the older patient also merits special consideration. Doses of nearly all sedatives, including barbiturates, benzodiazepines, and etomidate, should be reduced in the older patient to avoid hypotension (**Table 7-4**). Doses of lidocaine and opiates, frequently used as premedication before intubation of patients suffering head injury, should also be reduced.[13]

The establishment of intravenous therapy should be accomplished early. However, no more than several minutes should be spent on-scene attempting to establish an IV, as additional attempts can be made while enroute to definitive care. Provided that lung sounds are clear, fluids should be administered liberally in an attempt to maintain a systolic blood pressure of 100 mm Hg. If a hypotensive patient presents with rales or other evidence of congestive heart failure, prompt medical direction should be obtained to determine how aggressively fluids should be administered. Lung sounds must also be reassessed periodically, and cardiac monitoring and glucose evaluation should be standard for older trauma patients. Acute and chronic medical conditions predispose the older person to hypothermia, especially when ambient temperatures are low, so patients need to be protected. Considerations for cervical and spinal immobilization are discussed later in the chapter.

One challenge while managing older trauma patients is determining whether pain being experienced following a traumatic event is acute or chronic. **Acute pain** represents the body's means of indicating the presence of a new injury; **chronic pain** is experienced consistently and includes behavioral as well as physical factors. It is always important to question patients in detail about the nature of the pain they are describing and how it compares to any level of discomfort they may normally experience. Providers should always assume that pain is real. The goal of evaluating a patient's complaint of pain is to determine whether the pain being experienced indicates a new injury or represents an aggravation of a preexisting condition (**Figure 7-8**).

Immobilizing an Older Trauma Patient

There are several circumstances in which immobilization of an older trauma patient is warranted, such as cervical/spinal injury management, hip fracture stabilization, and facilitating extrication and movement. Older patients present several unique challenges to EMS providers with regard to managing spinal injuries (**Figure 7-9**). For example, to immobilize kyphotic patients, several blankets and pillows may be required to provide support to the head and upper back. **Skill Drill 7-1** discusses the technique for immobilizing kyphotic patients. To provide extra padding and prevent pressure sores, place a blanket on the backboard prior to placing the patient onto the board. Void spaces should also be padded. Do not attempt to force the kyphotic patient to lay flat on the backboard, as this will cause considerable pain to the

Table 7-4	Rapid Sequence Induction Medications and Suggested Dose Adjustments
Medication	**Adjustment**
Succinylcholine 1.5 mg/kg IV	No change
Etomidate 0.1 mg/kg to 0.2 mg/kg IV	Decreased from 0.3 mg/kg IV
Versed	Decrease 20% to 40%
Fentanyl	Decrease 20% to 40%
Ketamine	Should be avoided secondary to cardiac effects

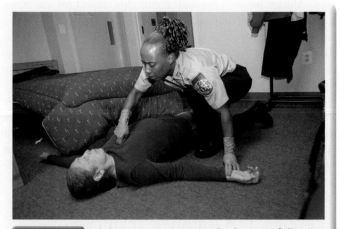
Figure 7-8 It is important to assess whether pain following a traumatic event is acute or chronic.
© Jones & Bartlett Learning. Courtesy of MIEMSS.

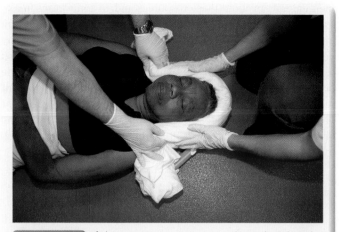
Figure 7-10 If the attempt to move a patient's head to the midline results in changes in neurological status or complaints of increasing pain, secure the head in the position in which it was found by using blankets and tape.
© Jones & Bartlett Learning. Courtesy of MIEMSS.

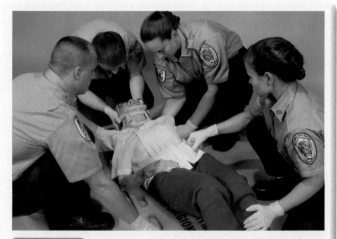
Figure 7-9 Kyphotic patients may require additional personnel to log-roll effectively.
© Jones & Bartlett Learning

Controversy

Many discussions have taken place regarding the use of backboards. It is beyond the scope of this text to cover the subject definitively. Providers should be guided by the patient's presentation, need for spinal immobilization, and local protocol.

continually monitored for distal neurovascular status, as well as signs and symptoms of shock. **Skill Drill 7-2** discusses immobilization of a patient with a hip fracture.

Preventing Falls and Injuries in Older People

EMS providers are in a strategic position to be proactive in the prevention of falls and injuries in the older adult population. Research has demonstrated that a number of risk factors contribute to a person's risk of falling. In addition, many older adults who fall do so repeatedly. One of the best predictors of falls among older persons is having a history of a previous fall; therefore, it is important to identify such a history. The identification of risk factors and the prevention of subsequent falls should include a review of medications, improvement of sensory function to the extent possible, elimination of environmental obstacles, and promotion of an exercise program that can help an older adult regain and maintain strength and balance. EMS providers should also be knowledgeable about community resources and the appropriate recommendations to make to older adults and families regarding fall prevention. Knowing the resources that local departments of aging and social services can provide to older adults in the community will allow an EMS provider to educate older people and

patient and could fracture or displace already fragile vertebrae. In addition, it may not be possible to apply a standard cervical collar to some older patients, as the patient's head may not move to a midline position. If this is the case, simply wrap a blanket around the patient's head (**Figure 7-10**). Prior to securing the patient's head to the board, place a piece of gauze over the forehead, so that the skin will be protected from the tape.

Hip fractures should be treated by splinting the injured extremity with a blanket roll or long board splint. Fractures of the hip do not necessarily require the use of traction splints. The purpose of the blanket roll is to maintain the leg in a static position so that further injury does not occur and pain is controlled. The blanket roll should be placed between the patient's legs and the injured extremity secured in the position in which it was found by using blankets and pillows. A long backboard or scoop stretcher should be used, so that the patient and splinting material may be secured in position. These patients should be their caregivers about these resources and, in some cases, make a referral. For example, many senior centers offer aerobic training and other health-related programs that an older adult may not be aware of. Some communities even offer transportation to these centers. Not only can an older person benefit from the programs that are offered, but there is also the added benefit of socialization. Establishing relationships with local agencies that provide services to older people will streamline the reporting process, establish a better feedback loop, and enhance the quality of the lives of the older people in the community.

Reducing Medications

Persons who have fallen should have their medications reviewed and perhaps changed or discontinued. Medical research consistently demonstrates a strong relationship between falls and the use of **psychotropic** and **psychoactive** medications that cause sedation, dizziness, or loss of balance. Examples of these medications include benzodiazepines, sedative–hypnotics, antidepressants, and antipsychotics.

Cardiovascular drugs and antihypertensives can also place an older adult at risk for falls by causing low blood pressure. Orthostatic hypotension can be triggered by certain types of cardiac drugs such as digoxin, antiarrhythmics, and diuretics. Also, alcohol—even in very small doses—affects gait and balance and places an older adult at risk for falls.

Not only does the type of medication contribute to falls, but also the number of medications taken. The American Geriatric Society's "Guideline for the Prevention of Falls in Older Persons" recommends medication reduction in older persons who are taking four or more medications. It is vital that EMS providers gather a thorough medication history for every older patient. With this information, the emergency department physician can evaluate the older patient's medication use and potentially make recommendations to the patient or to his or her primary care physician.

Medication Tip

The American Geriatrics Society recommends paying particular attention to medication reduction in older persons who are taking multiple medications.

Improving Sensory Function

Poor visual acuity has been identified as a contributor to falls. Lighting is the environmental factor most easily modified in order to improve vision and reduce the risk of falling. Lighting should be bright and kept at consistent levels throughout the home, with glare and reflection minimized. When possible, a nightlight in the bedroom, bathroom, hallways, and kitchen will ease the transition from darkness to brighter

light. Motion-sensor-operated nightlights that turn on when someone enters a room and turn off when the room is unoccupied are inexpensive and easily obtained at local hardware stores. While in the older patient's home, the EMS provider can observe the lighting conditions and make recommendations for improvement.

In addition, older people should have yearly eye exams. After a fall or if an older person has risk factors for falling, he or she should be asked about any difficulties related to vision and should visit a physician promptly for a thorough ophthalmologic evaluation. Many local health departments also offer eye screening. This is another opportunity to make a referral for improved health.

Exercise and Balance Training

Perhaps the most important indications of an older person's risk of falling are difficulties with balance, mobility, and performing activities of daily living (ADLs). Lower extremity weakness is also a major risk factor. An easy test to evaluate gait, balance, and strength is the "get up and go" test (**Figure 7-11**). This test can be

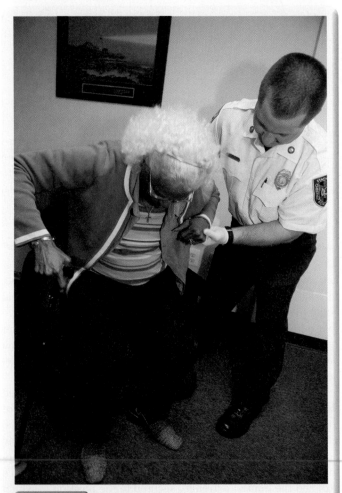

Figure 7-11 The "get up and go" test is an easy way to evaluate gait, balance, and strength, and thus the overall risk of falling.
© Jones & Bartlett Learning. Courtesy of MIEMSS.

SKILL DRILL 7-1

Immobilizing a Kyphotic Patient to a Long Backboard

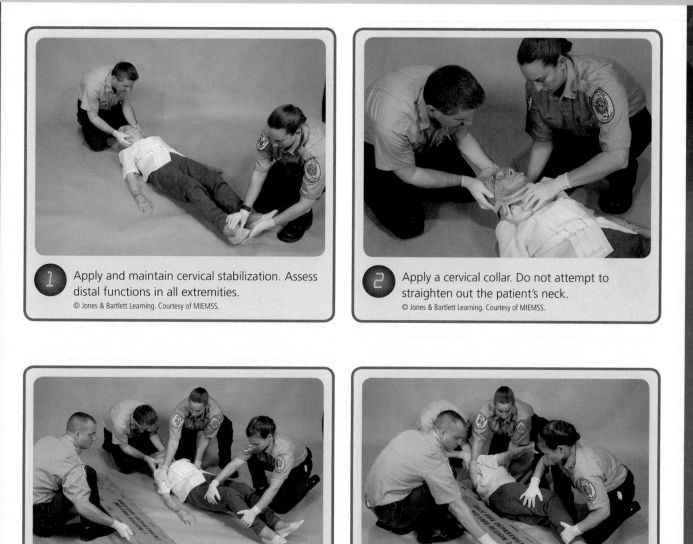

1 Apply and maintain cervical stabilization. Assess distal functions in all extremities.
© Jones & Bartlett Learning. Courtesy of MIEMSS.

2 Apply a cervical collar. Do not attempt to straighten out the patient's neck.
© Jones & Bartlett Learning. Courtesy of MIEMSS.

3 Rescuers kneel on one side of the patient and place hands on the far side of the patient.
© Jones & Bartlett Learning. Courtesy of MIEMSS.

4 On command, rescuers roll the patient toward themselves.
© Jones & Bartlett Learning. Courtesy of MIEMSS.

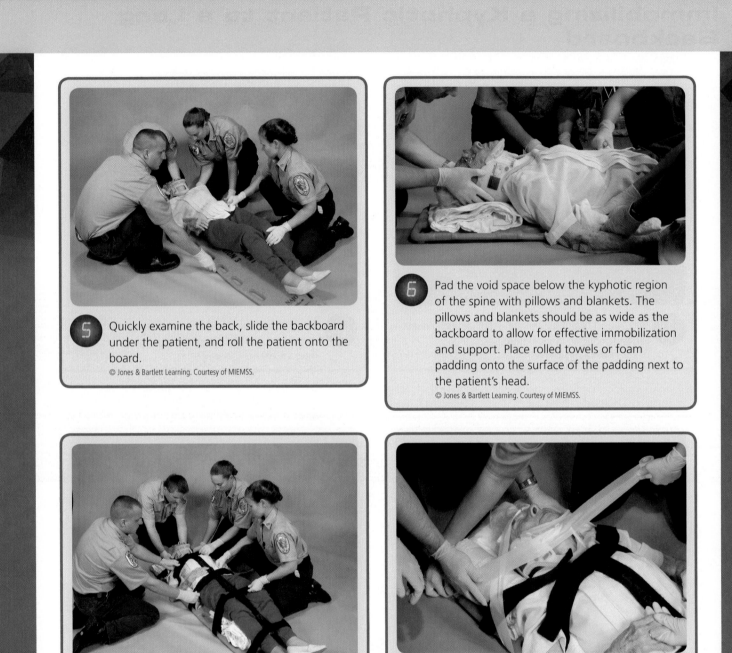

5 Quickly examine the back, slide the backboard under the patient, and roll the patient onto the board.
© Jones & Bartlett Learning. Courtesy of MIEMSS.

6 Pad the void space below the kyphotic region of the spine with pillows and blankets. The pillows and blankets should be as wide as the backboard to allow for effective immobilization and support. Place rolled towels or foam padding onto the surface of the padding next to the patient's head.
© Jones & Bartlett Learning. Courtesy of MIEMSS.

7 Secure the torso to the backboard with straps.
© Jones & Bartlett Learning. Courtesy of MIEMSS.

8 Secure the patient's head and padding to the backboard with 2-inch medical tape. The tape should be applied across the forehead and cervical collar and should prevent the padding from becoming dislodged. Immobilize the remainder of the body as normal.
© Jones & Bartlett Learning. Courtesy of MIEMSS.

SKILL DRILL 7-2

Splinting a Hip Fracture

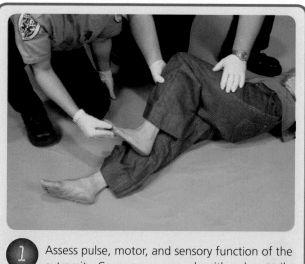

1 Assess pulse, motor, and sensory function of the extremity. Cover open wounds with a dry, sterile dressing and apply direct pressure, if necessary.
© Jones & Bartlett Learning. Courtesy of MIEMSS.

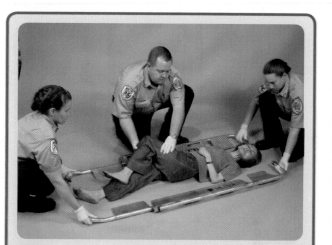

2 Place the patient onto an orthopedic stretcher or long backboard by logrolling the patient onto the uninjured leg while having a provider support the injured extremity.
© Jones & Bartlett Learning. Courtesy of MIEMSS.

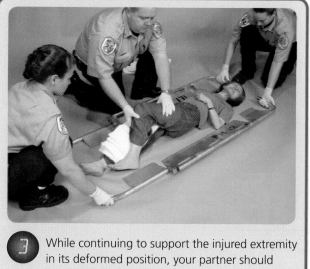

3 While continuing to support the injured extremity in its deformed position, your partner should place a blanket roll between the patient's legs.
© Jones & Bartlett Learning. Courtesy of MIEMSS.

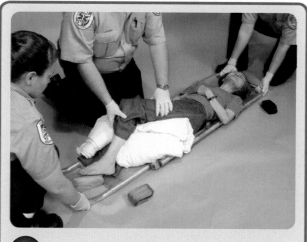

4 Place blankets and pillows under the injured extremity to provide support to fracture site in the deformed position.
© Jones & Bartlett Learning. Courtesy of MIEMSS.

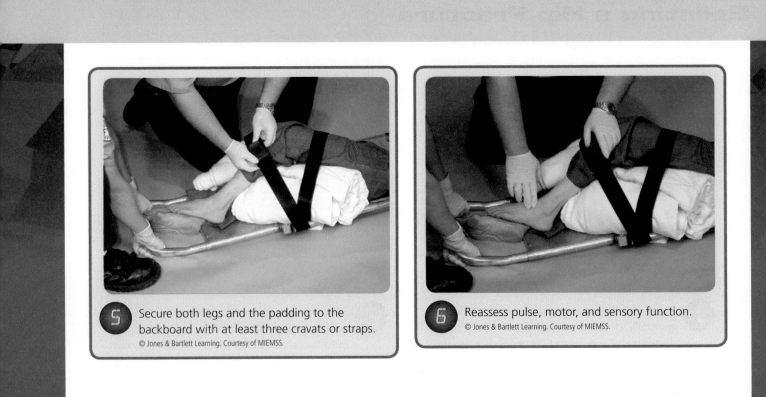

5 Secure both legs and the padding to the backboard with at least three cravats or straps.
© Jones & Bartlett Learning. Courtesy of MIEMSS.

6 Reassess pulse, motor, and sensory function.
© Jones & Bartlett Learning. Courtesy of MIEMSS.

performed in the home setting by asking a patient to rise from a chair that has been placed 10 feet from the wall, stand in place for a few seconds, walk to the wall, turn around and walk back to the chair, and then sit down. Observe whether or not the patient needs to use his or her hands to rise from the chair and how steady he or she is while walking and turning. This test requires little time and provides an excellent assessment of an older person's overall mobility and risk of falling. If an older person is being transferred to the emergency department, the test can be modified by having the person rise from his or her seated position and walk 10 feet to the stretcher. While performing this test, EMS providers should be on either side of the patient in case the patient develops difficulty. The results of the test should be reported to the emergency department physician. Never perform this test on a patient for whom walking is contraindicated, such as someone with cardiac or neurologic complaints or someone with a lower extremity injury.

One of the major contributors to muscle weakness, as well as gait and balance instability, among older adults is a lack of physical activity. Although muscle bulk and strength decrease with age, the decrease can be partially offset with exercise. Exercise also improves bone strength and balance, and reduces the risk of falls. A reasonable exercise goal for the older patient is to increase activity levels with an eventual target of a total of 30 minutes—either in one session or divided into multiple small sessions throughout the day—on most days of the week.

> ### Attitude Tip
>
> More aggressive assessment, field management, and communication of important observations made at the home can result in decreased morbidity and mortality, and an improved outcome for the injured patient.

Walking and dancing are weight-bearing exercises that may improve balance and bone density and are very inexpensive. Balance training, particularly Tai Chi, has proven to reduce falls in frail individuals. Most importantly, the patient should pick exercises that he or she is likely to continue to perform in a setting that encourages adherence to the program. An EMS provider's familiarity with local resources available through senior centers and community colleges will be helpful. Often the local chapter of the Arthritis Association can provide a list of exercise facilities for seniors. Preferences will differ regarding structured classes, exercising with a spouse, or exercising alone. Some patients may need to be evaluated by a physician or physical therapist to help them determine a safe and optimal exercise regime for their individual needs.

Use of Assistive Devices

An older person's gait and balance may improve with the use of an assistive device (**Figure 7-12**). However, while canes and walkers increase the base of support, an older person will need instruction on how to use these devices, as they can be

hazardous if used improperly. A knowledgeable healthcare provider can share this instruction with the patient. Ambulation devices should be assessed regularly for problems such as loose hardware on walkers or worn rubber tips on canes. When these types of problems are present, the assistive device will not provide adequate support.

It is also important to evaluate the older adult's use of the device in the home setting. A cane is properly held on the side opposite the affected extremity, and the cane and the affected extremity are advanced together. For a walker, it is important to evaluate its use in relation to the space availability in narrow hallway passages, doorways, bathrooms, and other rooms of the house; it is also important to evaluate the type of flooring the walker is being used on. Even a standard walker can tip over, so advise the patient to keep the walker ahead and step into it. The bathtub tends to be a particularly hazardous area of the home. To reduce the risk of falling in the bathtub, many people will use a tub bench, a secure seat that allows them to sit rather than stand in the shower. Proper use of assistive devices such as these will decrease the risk of falling and serve as an aid to improved gait and balance.

Making the Home Safe

Approximately 70% of falls occur in the home; this statistic suggests that a careful assessment of the safety of the home may yield dramatic reductions in fall risk. Again, this is a golden opportunity for an EMS provider to dramatically improve the quality of life for an older individual—an opportunity not available to all healthcare providers. A checklist of common hazards associated with falls in the home, such as that proposed by the U.S. Consumer Product Safety Commission, can be given to the patient and family.

Modifications can then be made in the home to improve its safety. For example, removing loose throw rugs, moving frequently used items to easy-to-reach shelves, and installing necessary durable equipment (i.e., toilet risers and grab bars, bathtub/shower chairs or benches and grab bars) can maintain safety in ADLs (**Figure 7-13**). Although cost may be a concern to some patients, the necessary supportive equipment to improve safety can be found in medical device catalogues obtained from local pharmacy stores, mail order companies, or the Internet.

> ### Attitude Tip
>
> Identifying home hazards that may cause falls is an opportunity for an EMS provider to dramatically improve the quality of life for older patients—an opportunity not available to all healthcare providers.

Stairs in particular can be hazardous to an older person. It has been estimated that at least 10% of falls occur on stairs, usually while the patient is descending; this may be due to misjudgment about the next or last step. Recommendations to correct

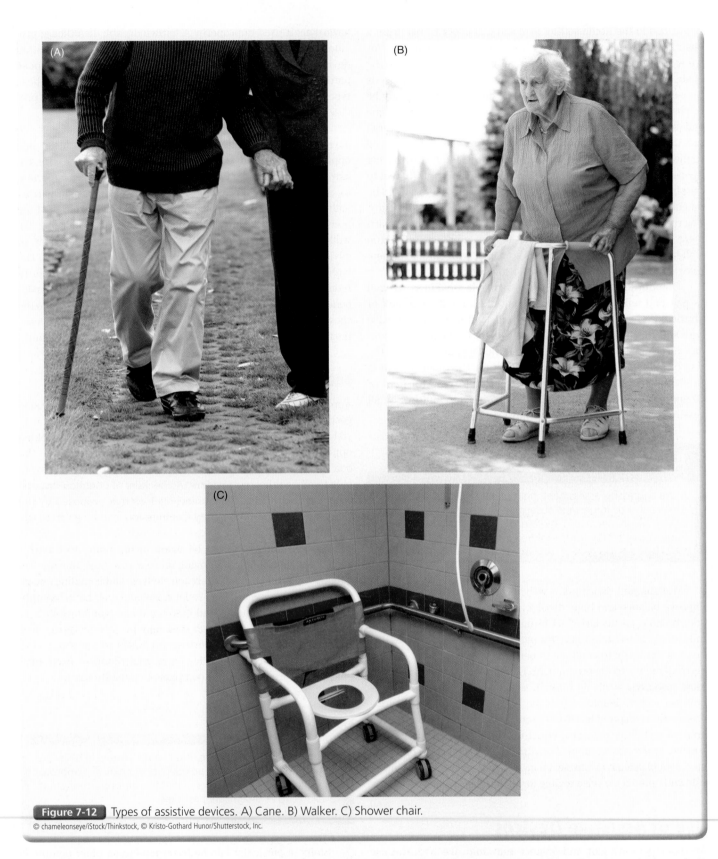

Figure 7-12 Types of assistive devices. A) Cane. B) Walker. C) Shower chair.
© chameleonseye/iStock/Thinkstock, © Kristo-Gothard Hunor/Shutterstock, Inc.

this problem include placing a contrasting marker, such as tape, at the end of each step and securely installing handrails on each side of the staircase. For patients who are unable to use the home safety checklist themselves, a social worker or healthcare provider such as an occupational therapist may assist in evaluating home safety and making recommendations for improvement. An EMS provider is often in an ideal position to refer the patient for this help.

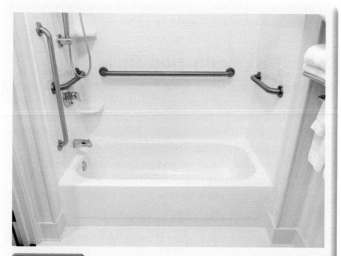

Figure 7-13 Installing equipment such as grab bars and shower chairs helps maintain safe activities of daily living for older adults at risk for falls.
© nazdravie/iStockphoto

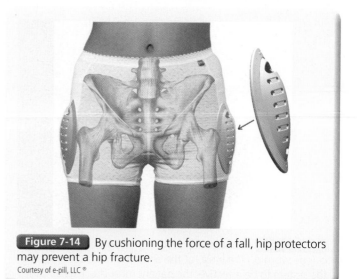

Figure 7-14 By cushioning the force of a fall, hip protectors may prevent a hip fracture.
Courtesy of e-pill, LLC ®

Proper Footwear

Fall risk may increase if an older person has any type of foot problem. Abnormalities of the feet, such as corns, bunions, and hammertoes, can affect safe mobility. Long toenails or painful bunions usually require correction, which may mean a visit to the podiatrist. In addition to problems related directly to the feet themselves, improperly fitted shoes can lead to walking difficulties that place the older adult at risk of falling. Older patients frequently wear larger shoes or slippers for comfort and convenience when they have foot problems or foot swelling; however, this does not provide for proper fit and support. Additionally, in order to keep larger shoes on the feet, an older person may develop a shuffle walk that can lead to tripping. On the other hand, shoes that are narrow and squeeze the foot can contribute to foot pain when walking. The best recommendation for the older patient is to wear a shoe that fits the entire foot, such as a walking shoe with a low heel and nonskid bottom. Rubber- or crepe-soled footwear is also recommended. Instruct older adults to avoid walking in stocking feet and to eliminate the use of loose slippers.

Hip Protectors

The majority of hip fractures result from a fall during which there is impact to the **greater trochanter** of the proximal femur (the bony prominence on the proximal lateral side of the thigh, just below the hip joint). Padding this area cushions the force of the fall, and therefore may prevent a fracture. Any older adult who is at high risk of falling, or who may have osteoporosis, muscle weakness, or difficulty with gait and balance, should consider wearing hip protectors to reduce the chance of a hip fracture. Hip protectors are anatomically designed external hip pads that fit over the side of each hip in the pockets of a stretchy undergarment (**Figure 7-14**). They can be worn under a skirt or pants, and there are currently about 10 different brands on the market.

In one study of ambulatory older adults who were at increased risk for hip fracture, the risk of a fracture was reduced by 60% if they were wearing a hip protector at the time of the fall. However, some older persons find wearing the hip pads to be uncomfortable or are unwilling to wear them as part of their daily clothing; therefore, they may not be suitable for everyone.

Personal Alarms

A personal emergency response system (PERS) consists of a small battery-powered transmitter or portable help button that the user usually wears on a wristband or a chain around the neck (**Figure 7-15**). It can also be carried on a belt or in a pocket. The receiving unit is connected to the user's telephone and acts as an automatic dialing machine that connects to an emergency response center for assistance. For this type of system to work well, an older adult needs to accept the concept and be compliant with wearing the transmitter. Additionally, the batteries of the transmitter must be checked periodically to ensure they work.

There are several psychological benefits to an older adult using the PERS. These include an increased sense of security, reduced fear of falling, and increased sense of autonomy and independence. A PERS can be purchased, though Medicare, Medicaid, and other insurance companies do not pay for the purchase of the equipment. Rental may be available through national manufacturers, local distributors, hospitals, and social service agencies. The installation fee and subsequent monthly

Attitude Tip

As an advocate for the older population, and in order to prevent fall injuries, you and your EMS agency can become proactive in injury prevention and home safety evaluation programs for older members of your community's service area.

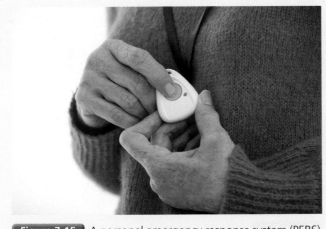

Figure 7-15 A personal emergency response system (PERS) can be worn on the wrist, at the belt, or around the neck. For the system to be effective, the patient must check its batteries regularly and wear the device consistently.
© Image Point Fr/Shutterstock, Inc.

fees are relatively inexpensive. The Federal Trade Commission provides information on personal emergency response systems.

Teaching the Older Adult to Get Up Safely After a Fall

In order to prevent long "down times" after a fall, and to build the confidence of a person who has fallen in the past, older adults need to be taught what to do if a fall occurs. The first lesson is, "Don't panic!" If the patient has a way of giving an alert that he or she has fallen, the patient should not get up until he or she has been checked. If injury makes it impossible to get up, the patient should attempt to stay warm by covering up with a coat, rug, blanket, or other available material. Instructions for getting up safely include:

- Roll onto the stomach, get up on all fours, and crawl to a nearby piece of sturdy furniture.
- Shuffle on the bottom or side of the body to a telephone or piece of sturdy furniture.
- Scoot up the stairs and, when able, stand.

In addition, it is wise for patients with mobility problems to keep a cellular telephone nearby at all times.

Other Risk Reduction Tips

To reduce the risk of being involved in a motor vehicle incident or being struck by a car, older people and their families should:

- Not drive if medications are being used that may impair judgment or cause drowsiness
- Periodically have vision and hearing checkups
- Monitor driving ability on a regular basis
- Avoid attempting to cross busy intersections or intersections that do not have crosswalks and signals

To reduce the risk of being burned, older people and their families should:

- Check the batteries on smoke detectors semiannually
- Have an escape plan
- Provide information to the fire department about the location of disabled family members in the house
- Exit the house if there is a fire
- Lower the temperature of the water heater to 120° F to reduce the frequency and severity of burns while still providing warm water to wash

Injuries that occur as a result of violence and elder abuse may also be preventable. To reduce the risk of these injuries, older people and/or their family members and friends can take the following measures:

- Accompany older people on trips outside the home, particularly at night.
- Ensure that doors and windows are secured.
- Answer the door only if the person who is knocking is known by the older person.
- Remove weapons from the home, particularly if an older person suffers from depression or mental status alterations.
- Constantly monitor older patients in both the in-home and long-term-care facility settings for signs of neglect and abuse, such as bruises, an unkempt environment, and injuries.

CASE STUDY 3

© 123dartist/Thinkstock

You are called to the scene of a motor vehicle crash. Upon arrival, you find a mid-sized car that has collided head-on with a large tree. There is significant front-end damage to the car and a starburst on the windshield. Additionally, you note that the road on which the crash occurred is dry, does not consist of any curves or bends, and there is minimal traffic.

As you approach the vehicle you see a male who appears to be about 75 years old in the driver's seat. He is not wearing a seat-belt, and the airbag has not deployed. The patient is semiconscious with a laceration of the forehead and signs of respiratory difficulty. He moans when stimulated. On physical exam, you find deformity and crepitus of the right rib cage, as well as bruising of the right ribs and upper abdomen.

- How should you manage this patient?
- What are your concerns?

Summary

Older trauma patients present unique challenges and face more significant obstacles to recovery than younger patients. There are also several pitfalls in the management of older trauma patients, including:

- Failure to recognize low mechanism of injury
- Lack of classic exam findings
- Lack of changes in vital signs
- Failure to appreciate comorbidities
- Failure to appreciate medication effects
- Failure to appreciate the risks presented by age alone

Despite overall higher mortality rates, most older trauma patients return to independent or pre-injury functional status. Critical to improving these outcomes is an understanding that although similar trauma principles apply to older people, they require more aggressive evaluation and resuscitation. Knowledge of the physiologic changes associated with aging, the impact of coexistent acute and chronic medical conditions, and an understanding of the unique patterns of injury in geriatric trauma patients is critical to optimizing outcome.

References

1. Centers for Disease Control and Prevention, National Center for Health Statistics, Ten Leading Causes of Death and Injury, Causes of Death by Age Group, 2011.
2. Summary Health Statistics for the U.S. Population: National Health Interview Survey, 2012, Table 7.
3. Centers for Disease Control and Prevention, National Center for Health Statistics, National Vital Statistics.
4. Aschkenasy & Rothenhaus, p.419.
5. Ibid, p. 420.
6. Aresco C, Stein DM. Cervical spine injuries in the geriatric patient. *Clin Geriatr* 2010:18(2)
7. Ibid.
8. Ibid.
9. Bala M, Menaker J. Torso trauma in the elderly. *Clin Geriatr* 2010:18(3).
10. Anderson D, Osei-Boamah E, Gambert SR. Impact of trauma-related hip fractures on the older adult. *Clin Geriatr* 2010:18(6).
11. Ibid.
12. Rushing AM. Scalea TM. Trauma resuscitation of the elderly patient. *Clin Geriatr* 2010:18(5).
13. Aschkenasy & Rothenhaus, p. 423.

CASE STUDY SUMMARIES

© 123dartist/Shutterstock, Inc.

Case Study 1 Summary

In evaluating older trauma, the provider must always consider that a medical reason may have caused the traumatic event. Knowledge of the physiologic changes associated with aging, the impact of coexistent acute and chronic medical conditions, and the unique patterns of injury in older trauma patients is essential in achieving a successful outcome. In this case, the patient presents with a fall from a bicycle accident, and there is an obvious injury to the patient's left humerus. Perhaps more critically, the patient presents with confusion and left-sided facial droop and slurring of speech.

Both the patient's medical and trauma conditions must be managed concurrently. Immobilization of the humerus, and cervical and spinal immobilization should occur. The patient must also be evaluated for the occurrence of a stroke. Based upon the symptoms, the patient should be considered for transport to a hospital that can manage both the patient's trauma and the possibility of a stroke. It may be logical for the provider to assume that the onset of the patient's symptoms places him in the critical time for stroke therapy since the patient was riding his bicycle. Since *time is brain*, the patient must be given the benefit of aggressive care. Although similar trauma principles apply to older people, they require more aggressive evaluation and resuscitation.

Case Study 2 Summary

A thorough patient assessment must be performed. Upon evaluation, you note that the patient is confused. You will want to determine if this is the patient's baseline or a new presentation. The neighbor may be able to assist in making this determination. Your assessment also reveals a lateral rotation of the left foot and the left leg appears shorter than right. The leg and hip must be stabilized. Additional information that should be gathered includes the following:

- Is the patient's confusion new?
- How long has the patient been lying on the floor?
- Is the home well kept?
- Is the patient able to care for herself?

This patient has suffered a fall, presents with a possible hip fracture, is confused, and takes Coumadin. Given this information, medical direction with—and transport to—a trauma center should be considered. During transport, the patient's vital signs should be evaluated frequently. In addition, glucose should be evaluated, intravenous access should be established, and the patient's cardiac rhythm should be monitored. It is important to monitor glucose in this patient as the patient's actual downtime is unknown. Additionally, the patient takes Lanoxin for her atrial fibrillation; depending on her downtime, the patient may have missed doses and the likelihood of decreased functional reserve must be anticipated.

Case Study 3 Summary

Based on the mechanism of the crash, you should have high suspicion for significant injury. The risk of a head and brain injury (including bleeding in the brain) are high in this case. A complete head-to-toe exam is needed, keeping in mind that the bones of older persons are more fragile and easily fractured. Palpate the neck and be sure to take precautions with the spine. The patient may or may not have a neck injury but, due to his decreased level of awareness, he is unable to tell you if he has pain, weakness, or numbness. The starburst on the windshield and head laceration leads you to be concerned about a coup-contre coup head injury as well as a neck injury. Atrophy of the brain in the older person places this patient at a higher risk of a subdural hematoma. Further concern should include upper abdominal injury from the steering wheel. Additionally, the lack of a seat belt and airbag deployment place this patient at high risk of multiple rib fractures, a flail chest, and underlying pulmonary and upper abdominal organ damage. Flail chests often are not immediately apparent, and the patient may not exhibit significant work of breathing due to the decreased muscle strength of the rib cage and diaphragm seen in older adults.

Additional consideration in this case is the reason for which the patient crashed. Did he have a stroke/transient ischemic attack, cardiac arrhythmia, syncopal episode, drop in blood sugar, or some other medical event? You may gain more insight to this matter by obtaining readings from a 12-lead ECG, rhythm monitoring, oximetry, and finger-stick blood glucose test. You should also look for signs of facial droop or lack of response to pain with one extremity.

Older patients do not tolerate shock or hypoxia, and it is likely this patient will have both. Therefore, rapid extrication, assessment of injuries and vital signs, and transport to a trauma facility is necessary.

CHAPTER 8

Respiratory Emergencies

LEARNING OBJECTIVES

1. Discuss assessment of the older patient with pulmonary complaints.

2. Differentiate the lung sounds associated with various respiratory problems and conditions.

3. Describe the epidemiology of pulmonary diseases in the older population, including chronic obstructive pulmonary disease (COPD), influenza, pneumonia, pulmonary embolism, lung cancer, tuberculosis, acute respiratory distress syndrome (ARDS), pulmonary fibrosis, congestive heart failure, and pulmonary edema.

4. Identify the need for intervention and transport, and develop a treatment plan for the older patient with pulmonary complaints.

Introduction

Most older adults are generally healthy and mentally sharp. However, due to a decrease in physiologic reserves, the older age group is disproportionately affected by acute illness. Combined with declines in lung function, lifelong risk factors, and medication side effects, certain age-related changes can be devastating. This is especially true with respect to heart and lung function. Respiratory symptoms—both acute and chronic—are very common in older adults, but are often nonspecific. In order to prevent exacerbation, the EMS provider often must make decisions rapidly and initiate treatment without a specific diagnosis.

In general, respiratory assessment of older patients can be challenging. In addition to having nonspecific symptoms, this age group commonly has atypical presentations and many respiratory diseases overlap in their presenting symptoms. For example, **pneumonia** may occur without fever or cough, and **pulmonary edema** can be present without the need to sit up to improve breathing. A patient's outcome will be positively affected by a thorough initial assessment that includes recognition and treatment of potentially life-threatening problems and continues through identification of likely disease processes.

It is important to note that age itself is not a major factor in the outcome of the older adult: It is the patient's physiologic function and disease status that has the greatest impact. In terms of morbidity and mortality, older adults in the intensive care unit—even those requiring mechanical ventilation—have the same outcomes as younger patients in similar clinical situations *if* both have equal functional status.

Approach to the Older Patient with Respiratory Signs and Symptoms

Recall that the purpose of the respiratory system is to bring oxygen to the alveoli and to clear carbon dioxide that is produced from metabolic processes. Once the oxygen is brought to the alveoli, it then crosses the alveolar membrane into the circulatory system, where it is transported to the tissues to support **aerobic metabolism** at the cellular level. Because the respiratory and cardiovascular systems are so inextricably linked, recognition of problems during your initial assessment is crucial. It is also important to remember that the brain cannot store oxygen, so as a result it needs a constant supply, which comes from properly functioning respiratory and cardiovascular systems.

Normal cardiopulmonary changes that occur with age are usually benign and include: (1) a slight reduction in tidal volume and airflow speed, (2) gradual reduction in arterial oxygen levels, (3) a decreased sensitivity to low oxygen and high carbon dioxide levels, (4) a decreased cough response, and (5) loss of **reserve capacity**—the body's ability to respond to increased demands under stress, such as illness or exercise. Most other significant declines in lung function result from disease or risk factors such as cigarette use and obesity. In addition, drug side effects can cause major complications for older people. For example, beta-blocker eye drops, such as timolol, can precipitate asthma, and antihistamines, such as diphenhydramine (Benadryl), can cause confusion and drying of lung secretions.

Signs and Symptoms

Signs and symptoms of respiratory problems in older people can by atypical and subtle. Mental status changes are often the first sign of respiratory trouble. Because many heart conditions present similar to lung conditions, EMS providers must pay close attention to the older person's presentation and gather a thorough history from the patient. General signs and symptoms that may present during respiratory emergencies are covered below; detailed signs and symptoms of specific respiratory problems are discussed later in the chapter.

Dyspnea, or shortness of breath, is a presenting symptom in older people with respiratory problems. It is sometimes difficult to decipher between a subjective shortness of breath and chest pain in an older patient, and it is also possible for both of these symptoms to be present at the same time. A history of

CASE STUDY 1

You are called to the home of a 78-year-old man with difficulty breathing. Upon entering the home, you find the patient, Mr. Henry, sitting in a tripod position in obvious distress. He has placed a fan in front of himself in order to try to get more air. Mr. Henry is tachypneic, diaphoretic, and slightly cyanotic in the lips and fingers. He can only speak in one-word sentences and must take several breaths between each word. You learn from Mr. Henry's wife that he has been a smoker for more than 35 years, has a history of emphysema, always has some degree of breathing difficulty, and has a cough that produces clear sputum every morning. The patient takes inhalers and Prednisone; however, over the past 3 days, his breathing has gotten worse.

There is no report of any history of heart problems. The patient's vital signs are: BP: 186/94; P: 120; R: 32 and labored with an oxygen saturation of 89% on room air. He has diminished lung sounds throughout, but some expiratory wheezing can be heard.

- What is your impression of this patient?
- What should your treatment be?

past illness and a list of current medications are often helpful in determining whether the symptoms are indicative of heart disease or lung disease. Generally speaking, cough, sputum, fever, and signs of emphysema suggest lung disease, whereas chest tightness, sweating, leg swelling, or a history of high blood pressure or heart disease suggests the heart is the source of the problem.

Attitude Tip

Patients over the age of 85 years are more likely to initially present with shortness of breath than with chest pain when suffering an acute myocardial infarction.

Coughing is another symptom of respiratory problems in older patients. A cough may produce sputum or may be nonproductive. A cough productive of thick sputum can be the result of acute infection, such as pneumonia or bronchitis. Sputum that is colored yellow or green is a sign that it contains white blood cells (neutrophils), which is indicative of an infection. Watery or bubbly pink sputum is characteristic of pulmonary edema. A cough caused by pulmonary edema or postnasal drip will worsen when the patient lays flat. Nonproductive coughing, on the other hand, is most often caused by an infection or asthma. Coughing associated with eating may indicate **dysphagia** (inability to swallow or difficulty swallowing) with aspiration of food or liquid or **esophageal reflux** (regurgitation of food or acid from the stomach into the esophagus). Using these clues while taking a careful patient history can often help to determine the cause of the cough.

Hemoptysis (coughing up blood) most often presents as streaks of blood in the sputum. Although this symptom is usually not life threatening, it is never normal. Patients with even minor hemoptysis will often have anxiety; these patients need to be reassured and referred expediently into the healthcare system for a firm diagnosis. Massive welling up of blood may be related to a ruptured blood vessel, which can be a life-threatening situation and will require immediate and ongoing suctioning to prevent aspiration and **hypoxia**. Infections, foreign bodies, **bronchiectasis**, and cancer are the most common pulmonary causes of hemoptysis in the older age group.

The presence of chest pain may be acute or chronic and may be related to breathing. Chest pain, combined with a history of a myocardial infarction, abnormal heart sounds (murmurs), and **orthopnea** (dyspnea while lying flat), is indicative of heart disease. Continuous, dull substernal chest pain also suggests cardiac or esophageal causes. On the other hand, chest pain that is associated with breathing, known as **pleuritic chest pain**, strongly suggests problems with the lungs or chest wall, or other noncardiac problems such as rib fracture. Chest pain related to breathing may also be known as pleurisy, an irritation of the membranes (pleura) that cover the lungs and internal chest wall (**Figure 8-1**). Pneumonia, pulmonary embolism,

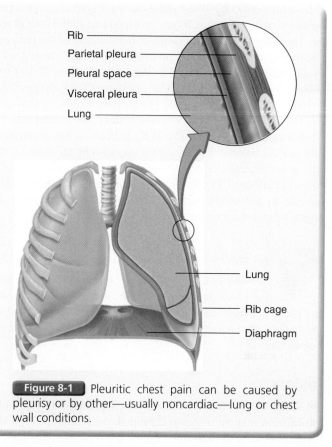

Figure 8-1 Pleuritic chest pain can be caused by pleurisy or by other—usually noncardiac—lung or chest wall conditions.

and pneumothorax are all causes of pleuritic pain. For example, shingles (herpes zoster infection), which shows up as a rash with blisters in a line over nerve pathways, can result in chest pain of a steady nature, though the pain associated with shingles may present 2 to 3 days prior to the appearance of the rash.

Unless it is severe, hypoxia does not usually cause dyspnea (although many of the causes of acute dyspnea also cause hypoxia). Assess the patient's presentation, symptoms, and history of heart or lung disease. The most common lung problems in older people are chronic obstructive pulmonary disease (COPD), **acute pulmonary edema** (fluid accumulation in the lungs), and aspiration. Normal oxygen saturation in a healthy adult is usually greater than 95%, though in patients with COPD, oxygen saturation (as a result of the disease) can be 89% to 92% at rest. These numbers should be compared against the patient's baseline and current level of distress when considering treatment. Other causes of low blood oxygen are pneumonia, pulmonary embolism, and cardiac disease. Although rare, drug overdose and brain disorders can also slow breathing so much that blood oxygen is lowered. Unless it is severe, hypoxia is treated by administration of oxygen via nasal cannula or non-rebreather face mask. In severe cases of hypoxia, the use of continuous positive airway pressure (CPAP) or bag-valve mask (BVM) ventilation must be used.

Oxygen administration should be monitored by pulse oximetry, capnography, and continued assessment of the patient's level of breathing difficulty. While pulse oximetry is an accurate representation of oxygenation, it only provides part of the overall picture. In order to have a thorough understanding of the patient's respiratory compliance, the provider should use capnography to evaluate the patient's end-tidal carbon dioxide ($ETCO_2$) to ensure appropriate gas exchange. Normal $ETCO_2$ ranges from 35 mm Hg to 45 mm Hg. A value lower than 35 mm Hg indicates that the patient has an increased respiratory rate or tidal volume, while a value greater than 45 mm Hg indicates a low respiratory rate or tidal volume. $ETCO_2$ values may also be increased if the patient is retaining CO_2 because of poor gas exchange, such as in cases of CHF or COPD. While pulse oximetry may take a couple minutes to accurately portray an issue with oxygenation, capnography can show changes within seconds.

Assessment

Respiratory assessment of older patients proceeds best with simple and traditional history and physical examination techniques (see the *Assessment of the Older Patient* chapter for a more general discussion of patient assessment).

History

Often, the chief complaint clearly indicates the problem. Useful information may be revealed if you ask the patient if he or she has experienced the same problem in the past and what kind of chronic medical problems he or she has. For example, the patient may say, "My asthma is acting up," or "This pain is just like my last heart attack." A medication review will also often help clarify the situation, and is especially important if there have been any recent changes in medications. Of additional importance to note during the history of the present illness are allergies to medications and any events that have occurred in conjunction with the onset of symptoms. Questioning family members or a care provider in addition to the patient may turn up important information that the patient is too distressed, confused, or anxious to provide.

Communication Tip

The patient's chief complaint can be very accurate in identifying the problem, even if the patient is confused or anxious.

Examination

The physical examination focuses on determining the extent of the acute illness. Initial assessment of the respiratory system involves inspection, palpation, and auscultation. Inspection begins with the upper airway to determine patency. Anything that impedes the movement of air (food, secretions, foreign body obstruction, etc.) must be immediately cleared. For some older

adults—such as those suffering from dysphagia—food must be cut into small pieces or puréed in order to avoid a choking or aspiration event. Loose-fitting dentures can also cause an airway obstruction; if placing an older person who has dentures in a supine position, carefully observe that the dentures do not come loose and become an airway obstruction. Pay close attention to the pattern of breathing and to the movement and symmetry of the chest wall on both inspiration and expiration. Check for the use of accessory muscles, such as the intercostal muscles and the sternocleidomastoid muscles.

Palpation includes checking the trachea to see if it is displaced from the midline and feeling the chest wall for vibrations (caused by retained secretions) arising in the airway when the patient breathes. You should also confirm any asymmetrical movements that were seen on inspection and note any chest wall tenderness or crepitus. Next, auscultate all lung fields for any sounds other than movement of air. **Crackles** are high-pitched popping sounds that occur during inspiration; these sounds are similar to the sounds heard when you rub hair near your ear, and their presence indicates fluid in the alveoli. **Rhonchi** are sounds of bubbling of a thicker, more viscous material as opposed to the fluid indicated by crackles. These sounds are caused by the aeration of mucous often associated with pneumonia. **Wheezes** are musical, continuous sounds caused by the narrowing of the lower airways due to constriction or secretions in the bronchioles. Such sounds may change after deep breathing or coughing. Absent breath sounds on one side of the lung (compared to the other) can indicate a pneumothorax or a large **pleural effusion**.

If breathing is adequate, oxygen may be administered by nasal cannula. Many older people with chronic lung conditions receive home oxygen therapy. The flow rate should be continued to ensure adequate oxygenation and work of breathing. A determination of inadequate oxygenation requires intervention using a non-rebreather mask (which is capable of delivering 90% to 100% oxygen), a BVM device, or CPAP. Once airway problems are addressed, an assessment of the cardiovascular system must be accomplished.

Initial assessment of the cardiovascular system focuses on determination of the presence, rate, rhythm, and quality of the pulse, and inspection of the color, temperature, and condition of the skin. Central cyanosis, seen around the mouth and on the trunk, indicates significant hypoxia that requires immediate care, including oxygen administration or ventilation with a BVM. Peripheral cyanosis of nail beds or ear lobes may also indicate circulatory problems. See the *Cardiovascular Emergencies* chapter for a detailed description of cardiovascular assessment.

Attitude Tip

Always let the patient and the patient's family know how much you care, not how much you know.

Specific Lung Conditions

Chronic Obstructive Pulmonary Disease

Chronic obstructive pulmonary disease (COPD) is a term used to describe a group of diseases that are characterized by chronic airflow obstructions of the lower airway, including emphysema, chronic bronchitis, and asthma. It is the third leading cause of death in the United States, behind cancer and heart disease.[1]

Emphysema and Chronic Bronchitis

Emphysema and chronic bronchitis frequently present together and are almost always the result of prolonged tobacco use (though nonsmoking COPD is common in older persons). In 2012, the prevalence of these diseases was 11.3 million adults. Two years prior, COPD was responsible for 1.2 million physician office visits; 1.8 million emergency department visits; 700,480 hospitalizations; and 133,660 deaths.[2]

The bronchitis component of COPD is manifested by cough (especially in the morning) and sputum associated with inflammation of the airways. With emphysema, the alveolar membrane becomes damaged and does not allow diffusion of oxygen and carbon dioxide into and out of the bloodstream; therefore, this condition produces lung destruction that leads to progressive dyspnea.

Acute COPD attacks are most often due to infection or nonadherence to prescribed COPD medications. Dehydration, exposure to irritating pollutants, heart failure, and fever from any cause may also precipitate a decline in lung function in these patients. Symptoms are usually gradual, even subtle: progressive breathlessness, cough with a change in sputum color, and increased volume of sputum. Use of the accessory muscles of respiration is common, and the patient may feel and look desperate. The expiratory phase of breathing is often prolonged and breath sounds are distant. Wheezes and rhonchi may still be evident, even when the breath sounds are so soft that they are difficult to hear. Patients with emphysema will often breathe with their lips pursed, as this causes increased airway pressures and slower exhalations which ultimately improve expiratory flow rates. Medications such as sedatives, antihistamines, and beta-blockers can cause or contribute to the worsening of symptoms.

Medication Tip

Medications such as sedatives, antihistamines, and beta-blockers may cause symptoms or contribute to their worsening in an attack of emphysema or chronic bronchitis.

Asthma

Asthma in older adults causes bronchospasm, edema of the lining of the bronchioles, and an accumulation of secretions in the airways. It is a recurrent, chronic disorder, and between attacks, the patient may feel relatively well and have near-normal pulmonary function. The prevalence of asthma in adults in 2012 was 18.7 million. In 2010, the disorder was responsible for 14.2 million physician office visits; 1.8 million emergency department visits; 439,000 hospitalizations; and 3,404 deaths.[3] While outpatient visits for asthma are less common in the older population, hospitalizations are more common.

CASE STUDY 2

You are called to a local assisted-living facility for a patient with a reported change in mental status. Upon your arrival, the nurse on duty reports that a resident by the name of Mr. Fisher has not been acting right for several days. She reports that the patient is 80 years old, independent with most activities of daily living, and mentally cognizant. Over the past 2 days, however, the patient's mental status has declined. The nurse reports the patient's vital signs to be: BP: 140/90; P: 110; R: 26; and temperature: 99.3° F. She also informs you that the patient's only medical history is hypertension and a right hip replacement, and that Mr. Fisher has resided in the assisted-living facility for 2 years since his wife passed away. His children reside in state but live several hours away from the facility. The oldest son, who has power of attorney, has been notified by the facility that his father is being transported to the hospital.

Upon entering Mr. Fisher's room, you find him in bed. You introduce yourself and explain that you will be taking him to the hospital. The patient states that he does not understand why. The nurse explains to Mr. Fisher that he has not been feeling well over the past several days and is "not himself." Before transferring the patient to the stretcher, you conduct a brief patient assessment. Mr. Fisher is alert but does not know the day of the week or understand what is happening. You notice that he feels warm to the touch, and is slightly diaphoretic and tachypneic. You ask him to take a deep breath in order to listen to lung sounds. When attempting to do so, Mr. Fisher begins to cough and states it "hurts" his chest to do so. You auscultate lungs sounds and hear fine crackles. Pulse oximetry reveals an oxygen saturation of 93% and capnography reveals an $ETCO_2$ of 50 mm Hg on room air.

- What is your initial impression of this patient?
- How should the patient be treated?

Asthma attacks may be triggered by viral infections, air pollutants, cold air, allergens such as pollen, and medications, and are made worse by anxiety and dehydration. The patient often complains of breathlessness, has diffuse wheezing and a cough, is sitting bolt upright, and is anxious. Waveform capnography often will have a prolonged phase II and phase III with a shark-fin–like appearance. On exam, there may be both inspiratory and prolonged expiratory wheezes. Distant breath sounds may indicate impending respiratory failure. Signs of life-threatening asthma also include changes in mental status, inability to speak more than a few words at a time, cyanosis, diaphoresis, retractions of the sterno-mastoid and intercostal spaces, and **pulsus paradoxus**.

Management of COPD and Asthma

Assessment of patients with acute exacerbation of COPD or asthma should be rapid, with special attention paid to the time, course, and onset of the attack. It may be difficult to differentiate asthma from bronchitis or emphysema, but management is quite similar.

Administer oxygen if the patient feels short of breath or has hypoxia or tachypnea, but closely monitor for a lowered level of consciousness caused by a buildup of carbon dioxide that occurs in certain patients with COPD prior to receiving oxygen. Basic life support providers can assist the patient who has his or her own short-acting bronchodilator medication, such as albuterol (**Figure 8-2**). Advanced life support providers should consider the administration of albuterol (2.5 mg)/Atrovent (500 mcg) via nebulizer. If further treatment is indicated, additional albuterol-only nebulizers can be administered. For patients with severe asthma or COPD, consider the administration of epinephrine (1:1000 0.5 mg intramuscular [IM]). For moderate to severe exacerbations, consider the administration of magnesium sulfate (2 g IV infusion over 20 minutes).

Depending on transport time and local protocols, the EMS provider may also consider reducing inflammation by administering steroids, such as methylprednisone (125 mg IV), prednisone (60 mg PO), or dexamethasone (10 mg IV/PO). While the EMS provider will most likely not see the effects of the steroid, the earlier it is administered, the sooner the patient will experience the anti-inflammatory benefits.

> ### Medication Tip
>
> If covered in your protocols, help administer the COPD patient's inhaled bronchodilator medicine. Administration of the medicine may considerably improve the patient's clinical condition, and you do not have to be sure what type of COPD is present to do it.

Patients with moderate to severe respiratory distress may also require high-flow oxygen via non-rebreather mask, CPAP with inline nebulization, or BVM while receiving medication via nebulizer. The patient's work of breathing, oxygen saturation, $ETCO_2$, and electrocardiogram (ECG) must be continuously monitored. Patients who are eligible for CPAP should be conscious and cooperative, and have a systolic blood pressure over 90 mm Hg. The EMS provider may need to coach the patient on the proper use of CPAP and ensure that a good seal is present. In addition to patients who have a decreased level of consciousness or who cannot tolerate the system, CPAP should not be used in patients who have acute abdominal problems; have had recent surgery of the face, ENT (ear, nose, and throat), or esophagus; or have facial trauma. If the patient shows signs of decreasing mental status, becomes hemodynamically unstable, or is suspected of developing pneumothorax, immediately discontinue the treatment and be prepared for advanced airway management (**Figure 8-3**).

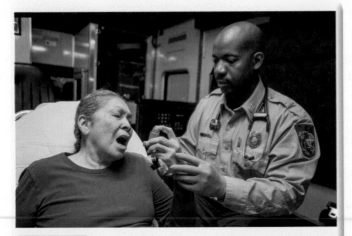

Figure 8-2 The patient having an asthma attack may have a bronchodilator medication in a metered-dose inhaler. If your protocols allow, assist the patient in administering the medication.
© Jones & Bartlett Learning. Courtesy of MIEMSS.

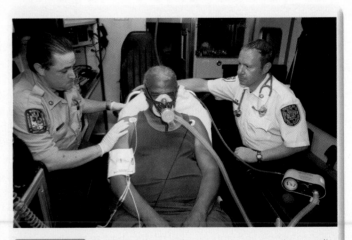

Figure 8-3 Patients with moderate to severe respiratory distress may require continuous positive airway pressure with inline nebulizations.
© Jones & Bartlett Learning. Courtesy of MIEMSS.

Influenza

Flu, or **influenza**, is a contagious respiratory infection caused by a variety of viruses. Human influenza A and B viruses cause seasonal epidemics of disease almost every winter in the United States, and the emergence of a new human influenza virus can cause an influenza pandemic. Influenza type C infections, on the other hand, cause a mild respiratory illness and are not thought to cause epidemics.

Influenza-like illness in older people may be atypical. Older patients generally present with a new onset of cough, sore throat, nasal congestion or rhinorrhea, or a temperature of 100° F or greater; however, fever may be absent. In addition, atypical complaints may include loss of appetite, mental status changes, or unexplained fever as the only presenting symptoms.

Adults aged 65 years and older are at greater risk of serious complications from influenza compared to young, healthy adults. Examples of these complications include primary viral pneumonia and bacterial superinfection leading to tracheobronchitis or pneumonia, and dehydration. An unrecognized complication may be worsening respiratory status in older patients with underlying chronic obstructive lung disease or congestive heart failure.

Each year, the older population accounts for an estimated 90% of seasonal influenza-related deaths and more than 60% of seasonal influenza-related hospitalizations in the United States.[4] Because hospitalization in this age group often precipitates disability and has the potential to result in loss of the ability to live independently, prevention and prompt treatment of influenza may reduce the risk of associated complications, including hospitalization and death. Prehospital treatment for influenza in older people includes supportive oxygen therapy and fluids for dehydration.

Pneumonia

Pneumonia is a condition of the lung primarily affecting microscopic air sacs known as alveoli. The condition is usually caused by viral or bacterial infection. Approximately 90% of pneumonia deaths occur in persons 65 years or older.[5] It is the second-most-common nursing home-acquired infection. Additionally, community-acquired pneumonia—that is, pneumonia acquired in the community setting, not in a hospital or other care facility—is responsible for 350,000 to 620,000 hospitalizations of older people every year.[6]

Pneumonia in older people is a serious problem and has a different clinical presentation than in younger patients. Older patients with pneumonia complain of significantly fewer symptoms and signs. Delirium, worsening of chronic confusion, or falls may be the only manifestation of the condition in older patients. Additional signs and symptoms may include:

- New or worsening cough
- Newly **purulent sputum**

- Respiratory rate greater than 25 breaths per minute
- Tachycardia
- New or worsening hypoxia
- Pleuritic chest pain
- Cognitive or functional decline
- Change in respiratory exam (e.g. crackles or rhonchi)
- Fever or temperature instability (such as a temperature higher than 100.5° F or lower than 96° F, or a temperature that is higher than 2° F over baseline)

Additional complications may arise from pneumonia. These include:

- Bacteremia/sepsis
- Pleurisy and **empyema**
- Lung abscess
- Acute respiratory distress syndrome (ARDS)

Prehospital treatment of older patients with pneumonia includes ensuring adequate oxygen saturation and administering intravenous fluids as necessary for hypotension.

Pulmonary Embolism

A **pulmonary embolism (PE)** is an obstruction of the pulmonary arteries caused by a blood clot (embolus) that is carried to the pulmonary vasculature by the circulatory system. Any obstruction in blood flow to the lung can result in damage or infarction to the lung tissue. In most cases, a PE is caused by a **deep vein thrombosis (DVT)**. A DVT occurs when an abnormal blood clot forms in a large vein, usually in the lower leg, thigh, or pelvis, (though it can also occur in other large veins in the body).

With or without death of lung tissue, a PE is a life-threatening emergency that may present similar to other diseases such as pneumonia, heart failure, and COPD. Predisposing factors include recent surgery (especially an orthopaedic procedure such as that used to treat a lower extremity injury, or a knee or hip replacement), cancer, prior history of blood clots, obesity, and recent sedentary behavior such as sitting in a car for a long trip. Additional risk factors include medical disorders that lead to immobility, as well as genetic defects known as inherited thrombophilias.

Approximately 300,000 to 600,000 people are affected by DVT/PE each year in the United States. For those over 80 years of age, cases are as high as 1 in 100. Estimates suggest that 60,000 to 100,000 Americans die of DVT/PE every year, with sudden death being the first symptom of PE in about 25% of cases. Among people who have had a DVT, 50% will have postthrombotic syndrome, which includes long-term complications such as swelling, pain, discoloration, and scaling in the affected limb, and about 33% of patients will have a recurrence within 10 years.[7] Nursing home residents are often overlooked as a risk group for DVT/PE, even though they are more than twice as likely as nonresidents to develop these conditions and they account for over 13% of incidents that occur outside the hospital.[8]

The classic symptom of DVT/PE is a triad of pain, dyspnea, and hemoptysis; however, this group of symptoms is less commonly seen in older people. Instead, common presentations include brief paroxysm(s) of breathlessness or tachypnea; collapse, cardiac arrest, syncope, presyncope, or hypotension; pulmonary hypertension and right heart failure, presenting as chronic, unexplained breathlessness; and nonspecific clinical signs such as fever, wheezing, pulmonary edema, arrhythmia, confusion, or functional decline. Pleuritic chest pain may also be present as a result of a lung infarct (**Figure 8-4**). Treatment should include oxygen administration (as hypoxia is likely), a 12-lead ECG (if available), and symptom-based care.

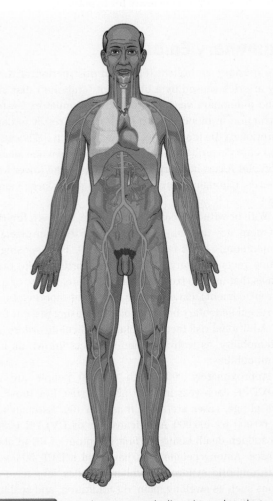

Figure 8-4 A pulmonary embolism is a clot that develops in a leg or pelvic vein, breaks loose, and travels through the venous system to lodge in the lungs.

Lung Cancer

The American Cancer Society (ACS) estimates that in 2014 there will be about 224,210 new cases of lung cancer in the United States, with, 159,260 people dying of the disease.[9] This type of cancer is by far the leading cause of cancer death among both men and women: Each year, more people die of lung cancer than of colon, breast, and prostate cancers combined. Almost 70% of people diagnosed with lung cancer are older than 65 years of age.

Most lung cancer statistics include both small cell and non-small cell lung cancers. About 85% to 90% of lung cancers are non-small cell lung cancer (NSCLC). The other 10% to 15% of lung cancers are small cell lung cancer (SCLC), named for the size of the cancer cells when seen under a microscope. It is very rare for someone who has never smoked to have SCLC. Starting in the bronchi near the center of the chest, SCLC tends to widely spread through the body early in the course of the disease.

Cigarette smoking is the leading cause of lung cancer; however, the following factors may also increase a person's risk:

- Exposure to asbestos
- Exposure to cancer-causing chemicals such as uranium, beryllium, vinyl chloride, nickel chromates, coal products, mustard gas, chloromethyl ethers, gasoline, and diesel exhaust
- Family history of lung cancer
- High levels of air pollution
- High levels of arsenic in drinking water
- Radiation therapy to the lungs
- Exposure to radon gas

Treatments for lung cancer include chemotherapy, radiation, and surgery. Older adults usually handle radiation therapy well, with side effects dependent on the type and dose of radiation and the location of the cancer being treated. For lung cancer patients, radiation therapy often causes fatigue and loss of appetite.

Unlike radiation therapy, chemotherapy affects the entire body; therefore, the risk of side effects is increased with this type of treatment. Although the types of side effects experienced by older and younger patients are similar, they occur more often in older adults. A prime reason for this is that as a person ages, kidney function decreases, making the kidneys less able to cleanse the toxic chemotherapy drugs from the body. Drug build-up results in more side effects; however, harmful reactions to chemotherapy only account for about 10% of all hospital admissions for older people with cancer. Side effects may include:

- Lowered white blood cell, red blood cell, and platelet counts, which can increase the risk of infection, **anemia**, bleeding, and bruising
- Stomach and intestinal problems, such as nausea, vomiting, diarrhea, and dehydration

- Damage to the nervous system that may further weaken the person's mental capacity (such as thinking or judgment abilities), increase memory loss, and cause fatigue and nerve damage (peripheral neuropathy)

Many lung cancer patients are on supplemental oxygen therapy. Prehospital treatment includes continuation of oxygen therapy to support adequate oxygenation and the provision of supportive care.

Tuberculosis

Tuberculosis is an airborne infectious disease caused by a bacterium called *Mycobacterium tuberculosis*. While tuberculosis appears to have peaked in the United States during the early 1990s, it continues to be a problem in certain populations, including the older population. Older individuals considered to have an increased risk of tuberculosis infection include, among others, those who reside in long-term care facilities.

Reactivation of old disease is a major concern with tuberculosis, particularly among the older population. With age, the T-cell-mediated immune response wanes, allowing for latent tuberculosis to become active. Certain conditions have been associated with an increased likelihood of tuberculosis reactivation, including HIV infection, diabetes mellitus, chronic steroid use, immunosuppressive treatments, silicosis, end-stage renal disease, prior gastrectomy or intestinal bypass, oropharyngeal or upper gastrointestinal cancers, leukemia or lymphoma, chronic malabsorption, and malnutrition.[10] Other factors contributing to reactivation of tuberculosis include:

- Age-associated diseases such as cardiovascular disease and COPD
- Poor nutrition
- Chronic renal failure
- Chronic institutionalization, with incidence among nursing home residents two to three times more likely

Tuberculosis in older adults may be difficult to diagnose, as this population often does not have the classic presentation of the disease. For example, older adults are less likely than younger patients to have hemoptysis, fever, and night sweats. Instead, nonspecific symptoms are common among the older population and may include:

- Changes in activities of daily living
- Chronic fatigue or weakness
- Cognitive impairment
- Anorexia or weight loss
- Persistent low-grade fever

The duration of these symptoms may be greater in the older person, and may be confused with age-related illnesses such as

malignancy, diabetes mellitus, and malnutrition. In cases such as these, diagnosis often only occurs postmortem.

The most common drugs used to fight tuberculosis are isoniazid (INH), rifampin, pyrazinamide, ethambutol, and streptomycin. Prehospital treatment includes administering oxygen as needed and providing symptomatic care. When caring for tuberculosis patients, EMS providers should place an N95 respirator on themselves and a surgical mask on the patient. Providers should also receive a yearly tuberculosis skin test or X-ray along with an annual respirator fit test.

Acute Respiratory Distress Syndrome (ARDS)

Acute respiratory distress syndrome (ARDS) is the end-stage of acute lung injury. It results from pulmonary inflammation, which causes the alveolar-capillary membrane to have an increased permeability to water, solutes, and plasma proteins. The condition is characterized by an acute onset of respiratory failure associated with diffuse alveolar damage and **hypoxemia** (resistant to oxygen therapy), which result from a variety of systemic and pulmonary insults. Common causes include:

- Sepsis (the most common cause)
- Inhalation of harmful substances (such as high concentrations of smoke or chemical fumes)
- Aspiration of vomit
- Severe pneumonia
- Head or chest injury (accidents, such as falls or car crashes, can directly damage the lungs or the portion of the brain that controls breathing)

The incidence of ARDS has been difficult to determine partly because of the variety of causes, clinical manifestations, and criteria used to define it, though estimates have ranged from 1.5 to 75 cases per 100,000 persons. In 2007, the National Heart, Lung and Blood Institute estimated that approximately 190,000 persons living in the United States are affected by ARDS annually.[11] ARDS continues to have a high mortality rate (30% to 40%), particularly among older people.

The diagnosis of ARDS is made clinically. Cardinal features of the condition include:[12]

- Dyspnea with an increase in respiratory rate and involvement of accessory musculature
- Hypoxemia (oxygen saturation less than 90% by pulse oximetry, on at least 40% oxygen) caused by deoxygenated blood bypassing gas exchange owing to the perfusion of fluid-filled alveoli
- Large pulmonary shunt (little or no improvement in oxygen saturation with 100% oxygen)
- History of a precipitating condition

- Increased work of breathing due to a reduced volume availability for ventilation and a "stiffening" of lung tissue (decreased lung compliance), accounting for up to 50% of the body's oxygen requirements
- Diffuse infiltrates on radiographic studies
- Complications resulting from multiple organ dysfunction

If ARDS is suspected, oxygen should be administered by mask at the highest concentration. These patients may need assistance with ventilations by BVM and possible intubation. Providers should be aware that due to decreased lung compliance, ventilations may require an increased amount of pressure. If possible, add a positive end expiratory pressure (PEEP) valve to the BVM to increase airway pressure. Aggressive ventilations may cause a tension pneumothorax requiring needle decompression.

Pulmonary Fibrosis

Pulmonary fibrosis is a disease in which tissue deep in the lungs becomes thick and stiff, or scarred, over time (**Figure 8-5**). As

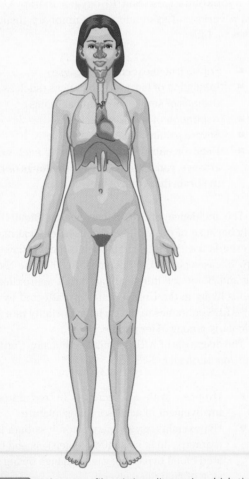

Figure 8-5 Pulmonary fibrosis is a disease in which tissue deep in the lungs becomes thick and stiff, or scarred, over time.

the tissue thickens, the lungs cannot properly move oxygen into the bloodstream. As a result, the brain and other organs do not get the oxygen they need.

When a cause cannot be found for the fibrosis, the disease is referred to as idiopathic pulmonary fibrosis (IPF), a serious disease that usually affects middle-aged and older adults. The progression of IPF varies from person to person: In some people, fibrosis happens quickly, while in others, the process is much slower, and the disease stays the same for years.

There is no cure for IPF, and many patients only live an additional 3 to 5 years after diagnosis. An estimated 40,000 people die of the disease each year, with respiratory failure being the most common cause of death. Other causes of death include pulmonary hypertension, heart failure, PE, pneumonia, and lung cancer.

Potential risk factors of IPF may include exposure to environmental pollutants such as inorganic dust (silica and hard metal) and organic dust (bacteria), as well as certain medications, including nitrofurantoin (an antibiotic), amiodarone (a heart medication), methotrexate and bleomycin (both chemotherapy medications), and many others. Additional IPF risk factors include cigarette smoking and viral infections, including infections caused by the Epstein–Barr virus (which causes mononucleosis), influenza A virus, hepatitis C virus, HIV, and herpes virus 6. A significant number of people with gastroesophageal reflux disease (GERD) also develop IPF.

The signs and symptoms of IPF develop over time. They may not even begin to appear until the disease has seriously damaged the lungs. The most common signs and symptoms are shortness of breath, which is usually the main symptom, and a dry, hacking cough that does not improve. Shortness of breath may initially occur only during exercise; however, after time, it will also occur while the patient is at rest. Additional signs and symptoms of IPF that may develop over time include:

- Rapid, shallow breathing
- Gradual, unintended weight loss
- Fatigue or malaise
- Aching muscles and joints
- Clubbing of the fingers or toes
- Crackles on auscultation

Treatment for symptoms related to pulmonary fibrosis includes administering oxygen therapy for shortness of breath and providing supportive care.

Congestive Heart Failure and Pulmonary Edema

Congestive heart failure (CHF), a condition in which the heart is unable to maintain adequate output to meet the metabolic needs of the body, and acute pulmonary edema (APE), the buildup of fluid in the alveoli, can be difficult to accurately diagnose as the cause of respiratory distress. (These conditions are discussed in depth in the *Cardiovascular Emergencies* chapter.) Both of these conditions are most accurately identified through the review of a patient's medical history, risk factors, medications, and physical exam, along with interpretation of blood pressure. Factors that help distinguish CHF from other respiratory causes include a history of CHF, exam features of jugular venous distension, and ECG evidence of atrial fibrillation. Patients with CHF are commonly on antihypertensive medications, diuretics, and other cardiac medications. These patients frequently have an elevated blood pressure, which is usually greater than 160/100 mm Hg but not uncommonly greater than 180/120 mm Hg. Additional symptoms associated with CHF or APE include orthopnea, dyspnea on exertion, and paroxysmal nocturnal dyspnea (PND).

CHF or APE should be strongly considered in patients possessing the previously mentioned characteristics and presenting with acute respiratory distress, tachypnea, hypoxia, or wheezing and marked hypertension, even in the absence of peripheral edema. Acute respiratory distress resulting from CHF may range from asymptomatic or mild to severe, life-threatening cases of APE. The New York Heart Association places patients with heart failure in one of the following classes:

- Class I: Patients with cardiac conditions that are generally asymptomatic regardless of physical exertion
- Class II: Patients with cardiac conditions who exhibit complications, such as dyspnea or other symptoms of heart failure, during normal physical exertion
- Class III: Patients with cardiac conditions who exhibit complications, such as dyspnea or other symptoms of heart failure, during mild physical exertion
- Class IV: Patients with cardiac conditions that cause complications during any physical activity

The goals of treatment are to reduce the pressure of blood returning to the heart (preload) and to reduce the resistance that the left ventricle must pump against (afterload). Treatment may vary according to local protocol but typically involve the following steps:

1. Position the patient in high Fowler's position.
2. If the patient is able, ask him or her to rate their breathing difficulty on a scale of 0 (no trouble breathing) to 10 (the worst trouble breathing).
3. CPAP should be considered for moderate dyspnea and must be implemented in severe dyspnea. (Use early; attempt to administer 3 doses of nitroglycerin [NTG] while setting up, acclimatizing the patient, and applying CPAP.)

A 12-lead ECG should be performed (if available). Withhold NTG in the face of an inferior wall myocardial infarction (MI)

with posterior wall extension MI. Use medical control for further administration.

1. Initiate an intravenous line.
2. Identify the cardiac rhythm and treat according to local, regional, or state medical protocol.
3. For patients with hypertension and moderate to severe symptoms, administer NTG. If systolic blood pressure drops below 90 mm Hg, treat with a medical fluid bolus.

- Asymptomatic: apply oxygen to maintain oxygen saturation greater than 93%.
- Mild: administer low-dose NTG (0.4 mg SL) at 3 to 5 minute intervals, to a maximum dose of 1.2 mg.
- Moderate and severe: CPAP is the preferred therapy. Until CPAP is applied, administer high-dose NTG. Assess blood pressure before each administration.

CPAP is the preferred therapy. Do not remove CPAP to continue administering NTG. Administer high-dose NTG (at 3 to 5 minute intervals) until CPAP is applied or if CPAP is not tolerated.

1. Administer 1 dose of 0.4 mg NTG and apply 1 inch of NTG paste.
2. Administer 1 dose of 0.8 mg NTG.
3. Continue 0.8 mg NTG dosing to achieve a 20% reduction in systolic blood pressure.

If blood pressure is low, consider administering medical fluid bolus(es) followed by dopamine (2 mcg/kg/min to 20 mcg/kg/min). Titrate to systolic blood pressure of 100 mm Hg or as directed by medical consultation. IV infusion pump is preferred.

Patient Education

In addition to providing emergency care for respiratory emergencies in older adults, the EMS provider should encourage prevention for this population. Specifically, older adults need to have their immunizations, including flu and pneumococcal vaccines, up to date. The moment just following an emergency is a good opportunity to remind patients and families of the importance of these measures. Immunizations prevent disease, reduce hospitalizations, save lives, and are extremely cost effective. Some EMS systems provide these vaccinations to the community (**Figure 8-6**).

Healthcare providers who have contact with the older population can also prevent flu infection in their patients by getting themselves vaccinated regularly. Studies have shown that vaccination of nursing home staff is even more effective in preventing flu infections in patients than vaccination of the patients themselves. This is likely true for EMS providers as well.

Cigarette use is the major cause of lung disease (and many other causes of death) in the country today. It is never too late to quit. Patients who stop smoking often note immediate benefits, such as decreased cough, sputum, and dyspnea. The risk of heart attack and lung infection also drops after cessation of smoking. Once the immediate stress of an acute event is solved, take time to provide counseling regarding prevention. A few moments dedicated to such a discussion may save a life.

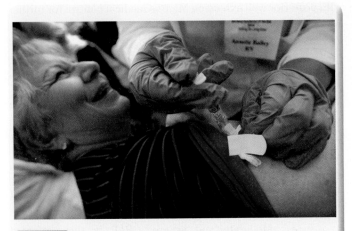

Figure 8-6 Many EMS systems provide vaccinations to the community. Immunizations prevent disease, reduce hospitalizations, save lives, and are extremely cost effective.

© Mario Tama/Getty Images News/Thinkstock

Summary

The differential for respiratory distress is complex. EMS calls for the older population may be due to acute issues or exacerbation of chronic issues. Due to the various co-morbidities, medications, and risk factors associated with this population, the patient's baseline may be altered. Providers must be able to sift through this information and attempt to identify the root cause of the patient's current dyspnea.

The goal of managing respiratory emergencies for older patients is to maintain the airway and ensure adequate ventilations and perfusion. With a thorough understanding of pulmonary physiology, respiratory pathophysiology, and treatment goals, EMS providers should be able to help manage the various types of patients suffering from breathing difficulty, one of the most common complaints resulting in EMS calls.

References

1. American Lung Association. March 2013. *Trends in COPD Chronic Bronchitis and Emphysema: Morbidity and Mortality.*
2. Health People 2020. December 5, 2013. *Sleeping, Breathing, and Quality of Life: A Healthy People 2020 Progress Review.* Retrieved from http://www.healthypeople.gov/2020/learn/Progress_Review_120513_Slides.pdf
3. Ibid.
4. Centers for Disease Control and Prevention. January 23, 2013. *Influenza Update for Geriatricians and Other Clinicians Caring for People 65 and Older.* Retrieved from http://www.cdc.gov/flu/professionals/2012-2013-guidance-geriatricians.htm
5. Ibid.
6. Jackson LA, Neuzil KM, et al. Effectiveness of pneumococcal polysaccharide vaccine in older adults. *N Engl J Med* 2003; 348: 1747-55.
7. Centers for Disease Control and Prevention. June 8, 2012. *Deep Vein Thrombosis (DVT)/Pulmonary Embolism (PE)—Blood Clot Forming in a Vein.* Retrieved from http://www.cdc.gov/ncbddd/dvt/data.html
8. Office of the Surgeon General (US). *The Surgeon General's Call to Action to Prevent Deep Vein Thrombosis and Pulmonary Embolism.* (2008). Rockville, MD: National Heart, Lung, and Blood Institute (US).
9. American Cancer Society. April 30, 2014. *Lung Cancer (Non-Small Cell).* Retrieved from http://www.cancer.org/acs/groups/cid/documents/webcontent/003115-pdf.pdf
10. Gambert SR. Prevention of tuberculosis reactivation in an elderly patient: a complex case. *Clin Geriatr* 2011:19(9).
11. American Lung Association. 2014. Lung Disease. *Understanding Acute Respiratory Distress Syndrome (ARDS).* Retrieved from http://www.lung.org/lung-disease/acute-respiratory-distress-syndrome/understanding-ards.html
12. Elsevier. 2012. *Acute Respiratory Distress Syndrome.* Retrieved from https://www.clinicalkey.com/topics/pulmonology/acute-respiratory-distress-syndrome.html

CASE STUDY SUMMARIES

Case Study 1 Summary

This case presentation is typical of a patient with emphysema. Those with emphysema will often report having some degree of breathing difficulty for many years. Many of these patients are, or were, long-term smokers and are on home oxygen. In this presentation, the patient has experienced increased difficulty over the past 3 days. Many people with emphysema have a barrel-chested appearance. This implies that the patient needs to take big, deep breaths to get in enough oxygen because the lungs are so diseased. Patients with COPD may also breathe with pursed lips. This action creates expiratory pressure within the lungs to keep the alveoli open, which increases gas exchange. The patient's wife reports morning sputum production. This is typical of a smoker. Villi within the airways that normally help to clear sputum become paralyzed by substances inhaled through cigarettes, so the smoker must produce a forceful cough to clear the sputum from the airways. Pulmonary assessment of this patient reveals diminished lung sounds throughout with some expiratory wheezing heard. Though wheezing is a classic finding in patients with emphysema, no wheezing at all can be an ominous sign: the worse the patient gets, the less they may wheeze. This is because there is not enough air moving to cause the wheezing sound.

Initial treatment for this patient should include high-flow oxygen by mask until a nebulizer treatment (albuterol/Atrovent) can be prepared and administered. The use of CPAP should also be considered if there is no improvement (and the patient meets the criteria). If the patient does not improve, the administration of epinephrine 1:1000 IM should be considered. Additional interventions include initiation of an intravenous line, steroid administration, and ECG monitoring. The patient's work of breathing must be monitored closely. A patient who continues to deteriorate may need to be intubated.

Case Study 2 Summary

This patient is presenting with symptoms of pneumonia. In this case, the initial presenting symptom, as reported by the nurse, was a change in mental status. Recall that delirium may be the only manifestation of pneumonia in this patient's age group. Additional symptoms of pneumonia in older people include new or worsening cough, newly purulent sputum, a respiratory rate greater than 25 breaths per minute, tachycardia, pleuritic chest pain, changes in respiratory exam, and fever or temperature instability. This patient is presenting with a majority of these symptoms.

Treatment should include oxygen therapy to support adequate oxygen saturation, initiation of an intravenous line, and ECG monitoring. This patient will also require a chest X-ray and antibiotic therapy.

CHAPTER 9

Cardiovascular Emergencies

LEARNING OBJECTIVES

1. Discuss the epidemiology of cardiovascular diseases in the older population.

2. Discuss the assessment of the older patient with complaints related to the cardiovascular system, including coronary artery disease, acute myocardial infarction, valvular heart disease, congestive heart failure, arrhythmias, hypertension, and syncope.

3. Given a list of signs and symptoms, identify the need for intervention and transport, and formulate a treatment plan for the older patient with cardiovascular complaints, including coronary artery disease, acute myocardial infarction, valvular heart disease, congestive heart failure, arrhythmias, hypertension, and syncope.

4. Discuss the signs and symptoms, precipitating factors, and management of cardiac arrest in the older patient.

Introduction

Cardiovascular disease is the most common cause of morbidity and mortality among people age 65 years and older.[1] With older adults representing one of the fastest-growing populations in the United States, it is not surprising that the number of people afflicted with cardiovascular disease seems to be growing as well. Coronary artery disease and congestive heart failure are the most common cardiovascular diseases found in older adults. Coronary artery disease accounts for approximately 70% to 80% of deaths among men and women in this age group, and congestive heart failure is the most common cause of hospitalizations among older patients, with the incidence continuing to increase as people live longer and the population of older adults grows.[2,3,4] This means that EMS providers need to be prepared to manage older adults with cardiovascular diseases. While the *Changes with Age* chapter reviewed the normal changes that occur with aging in the cardiovascular system, this chapter will discuss the specific cardiovascular disorders that commonly occur in the older population.

Coronary Artery Disease

Coronary artery disease (CAD), the leading cause of death in older people in the United States, is responsible for more than two-thirds of all cardiac deaths.[5] The principal feature of CAD is diminished blood flow to the myocardium caused by atherosclerosis. Atherosclerosis is a disorder in which cholesterol and other fatty substances build up and form a plaque inside the walls of blood vessels, obstructing flow and interfering with the vessels' ability to dilate or contract (**Figure 9-1**). Eventually, atherosclerosis can cause complete occlusion, or blockage, of a coronary artery. Other arteries of the body may also be involved.

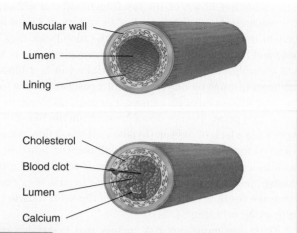

Figure 9-1 Atherosclerosis, the buildup of fatty plaque on arterial walls, may progress to the point that the plaque—or a migrating clot or a piece of plaque that broke off elsewhere—occludes the artery.

The problem begins when the first deposit of cholesterol is laid down on the inside of a coronary artery. This may happen during the teenage years; as a person ages, more of this fatty material is deposited, and the lumen, or the inside diameter of the artery, narrows. As the cholesterol deposits grow, calcium deposits may form as well. The inner wall of the artery, which is normally smooth and elastic, becomes rough and brittle with these atherosclerotic plaques. Damage to the coronary arteries may become so extensive that they cannot accommodate increased blood flow at times of increased need, resulting in an inappropriate circulating volume.

For reasons that are still not completely understood, a brittle plaque will sometimes develop a crack, exposing the inside of the atherosclerotic wall. Acting like a torn blood vessel, the jagged edge of the crack activates the blood-clotting system, just as it does when an injury has caused bleeding.

CASE STUDY 1

Mrs. Johnson is an 82-year-old female that was persuaded by her neighbor and close friend to call 911. Over the past two days, the chronic abdominal pain she has suffered for two years (with no clear diagnosis) has worsened. Mrs. Johnson also has complaints of nausea with two episodes of vomiting.

The patient's past medical history includes hypertension, type 2 diabetes, and coronary artery disease status post myocardial infarction 4 years ago. There is no complaint of chest pain or shortness of breath, and vital signs are as follows:

- Blood pressure: 210/100
- Pulse: 78
- Respirations: 12
- Glucose: 180

Other than the increase in abdominal pain, the patient's examination is not remarkable.

- What is the most likely diagnosis for this patient?
- What is your treatment plan?

In this situation, however, the resulting blood clot will partially or completely block the lumen of the artery. If this does not occlude the artery at that location, the blood clot may break loose and begin floating in the blood, becoming what is known as a **thromboembolism**. A thromboembolism is a blood clot that floats through blood vessels until it reaches an area too narrow for it to pass through, causing it to stop and block the blood flow at that point. Tissues downstream from the blood clot will experience a lack of oxygen (hypoxia). If blood flow is resumed in a short time, the hypoxic tissues will recover; however, if too much times goes by before blood flow is restored, the tissues become necrotic (dead). If a blockage occurs in a coronary artery, the result is damage or death of the heart muscle (**acute myocardial infarction [AMI]**).

There are numerous risk factors that make this process more likely to occur (**Table 9-1**). Some of these factors, such as hypertension, diabetes, cigarette smoking, and high cholesterol, present an even greater risk to the older patient because their effects grow worse with time. Hypertension is an important risk factor for the development of CAD in the older adult; however, the morbidity and mortality associated with cardiovascular disease can be reduced with aggressive treatment of hypertension. In patients whose blood pressure remains poorly controlled over a longer period of time, the heart muscle can **hypertrophy**, or become enlarged. Hypertrophy of the heart muscle, also known as hypertensive heart disease, can be a risk factor for the development of other forms of cardiac disease, such as congestive heart failure.

Older people with a history of diabetes may have disease involvement with the cardiovascular system, as well as the peripheral nervous system, eyes, and kidneys. Because diabetes can affect the peripheral nerves, a diabetic patient may not experience chest pain when having an AMI. Additionally, diabetics, as well as older patients in general, may have a different perception of pain, so a heart attack may present with vague symptoms or may be totally symptom free.

Smoking is a common risk factor in older people. While there is a current trend aimed at decreasing cigarette smoking in the United States, the long-term effects of smoking are likely to have caused irreversible cardiovascular damage to the older patient, even if the patient quit smoking several years ago. Data from a major study found that smoking alone is associated with a 64% increase in the risk of developing cardiovascular disease.[6]

Acute Coronary Syndrome

Acute coronary syndrome (ACS) affects more than one million people in the United States annually; many older patients who call for EMS assistance because of chest pain will have this condition.[7] Acute coronary syndrome is the term used to describe any group of symptoms consistent with acute myocardial ischemia. Myocardial ischemia is a decrease in blood flow to the heart, which leads to chest pain through reduction of oxygen and nutrients to the tissues of the heart. This can be a temporary situation known as **angina pectoris**, or a more serious condition such as an AMI. Because the signs and symptoms of these two conditions are very similar, they are basically treated the same under the designation of acute coronary syndrome. To understand them better, we will look at each condition separately.

Angina Pectoris

When, for a brief period, heart tissues are not getting enough oxygen (**ischemia**), chest pain known as angina pectoris, or angina, may be felt. Angina pectoris is defined as a brief discomfort that has predictable characteristics and is relieved promptly. The pain is typically described by the patient as crushing, squeezing, or "like somebody standing on my chest." It is usually felt in the midchest, under the sternum (substernal); however, it can radiate to the jaw, arms, midback, or epigastrium. The pain usually

Table 9-1	Risk Factors for Atherosclerosis	
Irreversible Factors	**Reversible Factors**
■ Aging	■ Cigarette smoking*
■ Male gender	■ Hypertension*
■ Genetic traits: family history of atherosclerosis before 50 years of age in a male relative or before 60 years of age in a female relative*	■ Obesity
	■ High cholesterol level*
	■ High levels of triglycerides
	■ Diabetes*
	■ Low levels of high-density lipoproteins (HDLs)
*Indicates a major risk factor	

lasts from 3 to 8 minutes, rarely longer than 15 minutes, and it may be associated with shortness of breath, nausea, or sweating. It disappears promptly with rest, supplemental oxygen, or nitroglycerin, all of which increase the supply of oxygen to the heart.

It is often thought that the presentation of CAD varies in older patients; however, findings have shown that angina pectoris is the presenting symptom in over 80% of older patients with a known medical history of CAD. Still, when evaluating persons age 65 years and older who have risk factors for CAD, it is important to keep in mind that atypical presentations do occur. When an older person complains of chest pain, the pain may be less localized, vague, and not the classic "crushing or squeezing" feeling. Some patients will deny experiencing any pain at all. Be sure to ask the patient about any chest discomfort, tightness, dizziness, **palpitations**, or other symptoms. Silent ischemia is also known to exist at a much higher rate in the older population.[8]

Communication Tip

Because some older patients may not experience pain during an episode of cardiac ischemia or infarction, it is especially important to identify other signs. Ask about symptoms such as fatigue, syncope, nausea, and anorexia. In patients with a prior myocardial infarction, ask specifically whether their current symptoms are similar to those they experienced with their prior infarction.

Angina is generally classified as stable or unstable. Stable angina occurs at a relatively fixed frequency and is usually relieved by rest and/or medication, while unstable angina occurs without a fixed frequency and may or may not be relieved by rest and/or medication. The first episode of angina is called initial angina. Progressive angina is stable or unstable angina that is accelerating in frequency and duration.

 ### Assessment

Angina may be difficult to distinguish from other causes of chest discomfort. Thoracic aorta dissection, pneumonia, pleurisy, gastroesophageal reflux, and pulmonary embolism are all conditions that may cause chest discomfort and are more common in the older population. Maintaining a high index of suspicion and carefully reviewing medications and risk factors may help with assessment (**Table 9-2**). Medications are especially critical to document, as failing to take a medication or taking it incorrectly can contribute to the problem. Because the older patient may be on multiple medications, bringing all of the patient's medications to the hospital is also very helpful. This allows the medical staff to identify the dosage, frequency, strength, and adherence to the medication.

Past medical history provides clues to the cause of the problem when the results of the physical examination are inconclusive. Some older people may find it difficult to communicate

information about their past medical history, perhaps as a result of hearing difficulties or acute delirium. Consider asking family or neighbors who may know about the patient's medical history. Additionally, the phone number of the patient's doctor may be posted on cabinets or refrigerators, along with a list of medical problems or medications.

A 12-lead electrocardiogram (ECG) should be performed on all patients with chest discomfort or suspected cardiac symptoms. Combine the ECG findings with your clinical exam to form a better picture of the disease process. If the patient's signs and symptoms are nonspecific, an ECG may help determine the issue.

Management

Approach all patients by addressing circulation, airway, and breathing and managing immediate life threats. Begin by making sure that the patient is as comfortable as possible, which may require moving him or her to a sitting position. Provide reassurance without offering false hope; patient anxiety can increase cardiac stress, and thus exacerbate pain and heart damage. Obtain a set of vital signs to help guide therapy, and provide supplemental oxygen for any patient who is experiencing trouble breathing or who has oxygen saturation less than 94%.

Obtain a 12-lead ECG and, if there are no contraindications, consider administering nitroglycerin to help relieve chest pain (**Figure 9-2**). Standard therapy is 0.4 mg sublingual nitroglycerin every 3 to 5 minutes as needed. Unless contraindicated, you should also consider orally administering 162 mg to 324 mg aspirin to older patients with chest pain. A caveat for the older population is that patients tend to be on multiple medications that may interact with nitrates and aspirin. For example, many antihypertensive agents will act in concert with nitrates and precipitously lower blood pressure. If this should occur, administer a fluid bolus of 250 ml crystalloid solution intravenously if there is no chest congestion, and reassess the patient. Aspirin may also interact with other antiplatelet drugs or with warfarin (Coumadin), causing excessive bleeding. As always, be sure to follow local protocols for medication administration, and consult with medical direction regarding angina pectoris to inform the emergency department that a potentially critical patient is arriving soon.

Communication Tip

Patients with angina may not be able to communicate clearly about their medical history. Ask family or caregivers who may be able to give you more information.

Acute Myocardial Infarction

Approximately 500,000 episodes of AMI occur annually in the United States. Each year, about 6 out of every 1000 men and 2 out of every 1000 women in the country have an acute myocardial infarction. Increasing age is considered to be the most

Table 9-2 Medications Commonly Prescribed for Heart Disease

Drug Type	Usage	Examples
Angiotensin-converting enzyme (ACE) inhibitors	Lower blood pressure	Captopril (Capoten); enalapril (Vasotec); lisinopril (Prinivil, Zestril); ramipril (Altace)
Angiotensin-receptor blockers (ARBs)	Lower blood pressure	Irbesartan (Avapro); losartan (Cozaar); valsartan (Diovan)
Antiadrenergic agents	Inhibit the signals of epinephrine and norepinephrine	Clonidine (Catapres); doxazosin (Cardura); prazosin (Minipress)
Antiarrhythmics	Control chronic disturbances in cardiac rhythm	Amiodarone (Cordarone); digoxin (Lanoxin); quinidine sulfate (Quinaglute)
Anticoagulants	Diminish the ability of the blood to clot	Heparin; warfarin (Coumadin)
Antihyperlipidemic agents	Promote reduction of lipid levels in the blood	Atorvastatin (Lipitor); lovastatin (Mevacor); pravastatin (Pravachol)
Antiplatelet drugs	Keep the platelets in blood from sticking together	Aspirin; clopidogrel (Plavix); dipyridamole (Persantine); ticlopidine (Ticlid)
Beta-blockers	Decrease the rate and strength of cardiac contractions	Atenolol (Tenormin); labetalol (Normodyne); metoprolol (Lopressor); propranolol (Inderal)
Calcium channel blockers	Prevent spasm of the coronary arteries and weaken cardiac contraction	Amlodipine (Norvasc); diltiazem (Cardizem); nifedipine (Procardia); verapamil (Calan)
Diuretics	Cause kidneys to excrete more sodium and water than usual	Furosemide (Lasix); hydrochlorothiazide (Hydrodiuril); spironolactone (Aldactone)
Nitrates	Decrease work of heart	Nitroglycerin (Nitrostat, Nitrolingual, Nitro-Bid, Nitro-Dur, Nitrol, Nitroglyn); isosorbide dinitrate (Isordil, Sorbitrate)
Potassium supplements	Treat or prevent low potassium levels in the blood	KCl (K-Dur, KLyte)

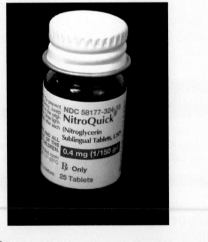

Figure 9-2 Nitroglycerin can help relieve the pain of an angina attack.
© Scott Camazine/Science Source

significant risk factor for AMI, with individuals aged older than 45 years having an eight times greater risk for an AMI than younger patients. Older individuals also have a higher risk for mortality after suffering an AMI.

Assessment

When a coronary artery becomes occluded due to rupture and thrombosis of an atherosclerotic plaque, the decreased blood flow to the heart muscle causes a decrease in oxygen perfusion to the tissue. The decreased perfusion can produce ischemia, pain, or, if it is substantial and sustained, death of the heart muscle (myocardial infarction). Older patients tend to be able to tolerate ischemia better than younger patients due to collateral circulation, which is the development of new blood vessels around tissue that is subjected to low flow rates of blood. The purpose of collateral circulation is to increase perfusion: The new vessels allow blood to shunt around occluded areas and supply oxygen to ischemic tissue.

The pain of AMI signals actual death of cells in the area of the heart where blood flow is obstructed. Once dead, the cells cannot be revived. Instead, they will eventually turn into scar tissue and become a burden to the beating heart. About 30 minutes after blood flow is cut off, some heart muscle cells begin to die. After about 2 hours, as many as one-half of the cells in the area may be dead; in most cases, after 4 to 6 hours, more than 90% of them will be dead. This is why fast action is so crucial in treating a heart attack: The sooner the blockage can be cleared, the fewer cells will die. Studies show that, in many cases, opening the coronary artery with "clot-busting" medications (fibrinolytics) can prevent or minimize damage to the heart muscle if administered no later than 12 hours after the onset of symptoms. If performed promptly, angioplasty or percutaneous coronary intervention (PCI), which is the mechanical clearing of the artery, has been shown to be the most effective treatment for a patient experiencing an AMI. Therefore, immediate recognition, treatment, and transport to an emergency department with cardiac capabilities are essential.

Remember, older patients who are experiencing an AMI may have atypical presentations, such as the following:

- Dyspnea
- Worsening of heart failure (acute or chronic)
- Pulmonary edema
- Vertigo
- Syncope (fainting)
- Stroke
- Acute onset of confusion and/or altered mentation (thinking process)
- Palpitations
- Excessive weakness
- Change in eating pattern

As many as one-third of older victims suffer from silent myocardial infarctions, in which the usual chest pain is not present. The patient may complain of epigastric or abdominal pain along with persistent nausea, vomiting, and/or weakness. A review of the patient's past medical history, medications, and risk factors will help you focus on a cardiac problem when heart disease is suspected.

Management

As with all patients, management of the patient suffering from an AMI begins with addressing circulation, airway, and breathing; forming a general impression; and making a transport decision. The patient should be placed on supplemental oxygen if he or she has an oxygen saturation that is less than 94% or is exhibiting signs of respiratory distress.

After obtaining the patient's blood pressure and pulse rate, a 12-lead ECG should be obtained as early as possible for all patients complaining of chest pain or discomfort. If the ECG identifies signs of a myocardial infarction or ischemia, the receiving hospital should be immediately alerted, as the patient may be a candidate for PCI or thrombolytic therapy. A focused history should be obtained from the patient, with a special emphasis on cardiac risk factors. If the patient is actively having chest pain or discomfort, consider administering nitroglycerin and aspirin in accordance with local protocols. Before administration, have the patient rate the pain on a scale from 0 to 10, with 10 being the worst pain of his or her life and 0 being no pain at all. This rating scale will help guide the effectiveness of your therapy, and allow you to make decisions on the next treatment to be given. However, you should remember from the *Changes with Aging* chapter that older people often have a decrease in pain sensation, and so an older patient who reports a low qualifying number can still be in acute distress. In addition, an older patient in distress or with cognitive decline may not be able to qualify their pain using a pain rating scale. Consider asking the patient about his or her "discomfort" rather than "pain."

Patients suspected of experiencing a myocardial infarction or demonstrating ECG changes consistent with an acute MI should be transported to a facility capable of performing PCI. Contacting the receiving hospital early in the process will give the emergency department more time to ensure that an appropriate bed and staff are available. The facility may have a cardiac catheter team readily available to open an occluded vessel; however, this team usually requires ample time to prepare for the patient. Speed is of the essence, as is suggested by the phrase "time is muscle." By suspecting an AMI in the prehospital setting and relaying this information to the emergency department, the

CASE STUDY 2

You are dispatched to a long-term care facility for a patient with shortness of breath. Upon arrival, you encounter Mrs. Gray, an 84-year-old woman who is on Coumadin (warfarin) and has a past medical history of chronic obstructive pulmonary disease, rheumatoid arthritis, congestive heart failure, hypertension, coronary artery disease status post coronary artery bypass grafting, and atrial fibrillation. The patient was recently admitted to the long-term care facility for rehabilitation after being discharged from the hospital with exacerbation from chronic obstructive pulmonary disease.

Physical assessment reveals a thin, frail woman who is visibly short of breath and using accessory muscles to breath. The patient is tachypneic at 34 breaths per minute and tachycardic at 100 beats per minute. She has an oxygen saturation of 85% on 2 liters of oxygen and a blood pressure of 160/100. Pulmonary assessment reveals decreased air entry and crackles. There is no edema in the legs.

- What is this patient likely experiencing?
- What are your treatment priorities?

door-to-balloon time can be greatly reduced, with a consequent rise in survival probability.

In order to help speed up the process, some locales have checklists prepared so the appropriate questions for PCI or thrombolytic therapy may be asked and the information quickly assessed and relayed to the receiving emergency department. Important questions for therapy consideration include:

1. When did the pain begin?
2. Do you have any bleeding disorders?
3. Have you ever had brain cancer/masses or a stroke?
4. Are you on any blood thinners?
5. Have you had any recent surgery or trauma?

An older person has a high probability of answering "yes" to one of the above questions, as these medications and problems are more common in this age group. However, age alone is not a major contraindication for PCI or thrombolytic therapy: patients up to 75 years of age are treated in a similar fashion to the younger population, and PCI and thrombolytic therapy are still considered to be acceptable, safe, and useful interventions for patients older than 75 years of age.

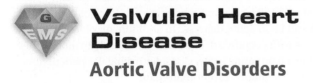

Valvular Heart Disease
Aortic Valve Disorders

Aortic Stenosis

Aortic **stenosis** is the abnormal narrowing of the aortic valve, which results from the thickening, calcification, and/or fusion of the aortic valve leaflets, and produces an obstruction to the outflow of blood from the left ventricle. An estimated 1.5 million people in the United States suffer from aortic stenosis.[9] In older patients, degenerative change in the valve leaflet is the most common factor leading to aortic stenosis. As the valve area becomes smaller, the left ventricle attempts to compensate by contracting harder to eject blood through the stenosis; however, the ability to efficiently compensate may be decreased by underlying coronary heart disease; previous heart failure; or certain medications, such as beta-blockers, which reduce the workload of the heart muscle. An inability to compensate could lead to angina or even syncope.

Assessment

Stenosis of the aortic valve leads to impairment of the valve opening, creating a pressure overload in the left ventricle. As a result, the left ventricle attempts to compensate by increasing the muscle mass (hypertrophy), allowing the left ventricle to maintain adequate cardiac output to meet the needs of the body. If the hypertrophy of the left ventricle is not sufficient to overcome the increased pressure from the stenosis, the overall cardiac output will decrease. This decrease increases stress on the heart muscle itself and can eventually lead to heart failure.

Patients may present with symptoms such as chest pain, increased shortness of breath with exertion, and syncope. Due to the increase in myocardial oxygen demand, symptoms similar to angina or ACS may be present, even in patients without CAD. Heart failure, also common in patients with aortic stenosis, can result from peripheral vasodilation or development of dysrhythmias, such as atrial fibrillation. In these cases, a reduction in the filling pressures of the ventricles makes it difficult for the heart to maintain adequate cardiac output to meet the demands of the body, and symptoms of heart failure can be noted. A hallmark exam finding in a patient with aortic stenosis is a systolic heart murmur, heard loudest along the right sterna border. Additionally, patients may have tachycardia, hyper/hypotension, peripheral edema, jugular venous distention, and pulmonary crackles. An underlying diagnosis of aortic stenosis should be considered when a field diagnosis is developed. The diagnosis of aortic stenosis can be made by either echocardiography or cardiac catheterization.

Management

EMS providers may not necessarily know the patient is suffering from aortic stenosis, as symptoms that indicate ACS or acute heart failure may be the only indication that an underlying cardiac issue is present. Providers should assess for potential life threats and address any issues that compromise circulation, airway, or breathing. Patients experiencing chest pain or signs of heart failure should be managed in the standard fashion; however, keep in mind that patients with aortic stenosis may not respond to conventional prehospital treatment. With that said, management of pain, volume resuscitation to improve cardiac output, and optimizing oxygenation should be considered in any patient suspected of having aortic stenosis. Prompt transport to a facility capable of handling cardiac emergencies should be a priority in the management of these patients.

Aortic Regurgitation

Aortic regurgitation is the leakage of blood from the aorta into the left ventricle. This condition results from abnormalities in the aortic valve leaflets or from dilation of the aorta, preventing leaflet closure. Leaflet abnormalities can result from calcific degeneration, congenital anomalies, and damage from an infection such as **endocarditis**.

Assessment

Aortic regurgitation may result from an acute or chronic event. Acute aortic regurgitation is usually caused by endocarditis or a dissection. From these processes, the aortic valve acutely becomes incompetent and causes a back-pressure of blood filling into the left ventricle. The increase in pressure inhibits the left ventricle from functioning properly, leading to acute heart failure, **cardiogenic shock**, or pulmonary edema. Chronic aortic regurgitation is slower in onset, and the left ventricle is initially able to compensate for the back-pressure of blood. This results in progressive dilation of the ventricle with increased stress on the muscle. Even with severe aortic regurgitation, most patients remain asymptomatic for years due to the heart's ability to compensate. Eventually, however, the increase in compensation and stress will lead to ventricular failure, resulting in cardiogenic shock and pulmonary edema.

Regardless of whether it is acute or chronic, the patient with aortic regurgitation may present with chest pain, dyspnea, hypotension, tachycardia, pulmonary edema, and diaphoresis. In addition, patients typically have a high-pitched murmur that is noted during filling of the heart.

Management

The treatment of aortic regurgitation in the prehospital setting is mainly supportive. While the EMS provider may not realize the patient is suffering from aortic regurgitation, other clues of a cardiac problem will most likely be apparent. The goal of therapy is to treat life threats, optimize oxygenation, and transport the patient to the closest appropriate facility. In addition, EMS providers should be prepared to aggressively resuscitate any patient in acute distress with suspected aortic regurgitation, as sudden cardiac death is not uncommon in these patients.

Mitral Valve Disorders

Mitral Stenosis

Mitral stenosis in the older population almost exclusively occurs as a result of rheumatic fever. Thickening of the valve leaflets and other structural changes gradually reduce the size of the mitral valve opening, which leads to decreased blood flow into the left ventricle. Mitral stenosis is a slow, progressive process that may not produce symptoms for several decades. Once a patient develops significant symptoms, the likelihood of survival is very poor unless surgical intervention is performed.

Assessment

As stated, most cases of mitral stenosis are related to rheumatic fever. This infection causes inflammation in the connective tissues of the skin, joints, brain, and heart. When the tissue of the mitral valve becomes affected, the inflammation disrupts the flow of blood and the overall effectiveness of the left ventricle. Eventually, the valve may scar, leading to stenosis. Similar to aortic stenosis, the reduced blood flow across the mitral valve affects the left ventricle's ability to circulate blood to the body. The restriction in flow causes back-pressure to the pulmonary circulation and can result in heart failure and shock. In addition, patients may develop atrial fibrillation as a result of the increased pressure in the left atrium.

EMS providers should suspect mitral stenosis in a patient with symptoms of right-sided heart failure (i.e., jugular venous distention, peripheral edema), shortness of breath, pulmonary

edema, and fatigue accompanied by a murmur (described as an opening "snap") noted during ventricular filling.

Management

Many patients with mitral stenosis are already aware of their condition and receiving treatment by a cardiologist. The involvement of EMS typically surrounds an event leading to acute heart failure. These patients will present with acute or worsening dyspnea, peripheral and/or pulmonary edema, hypotension, and possible atrial fibrillation. As with all patients, the primary goal of prehospital treatment is to immediately manage circulation, airway, and breathing. The EMS provider should initiate treatment of heart failure based on local protocols and rapidly transport the patient to the closest appropriate facility. In addition, the possible etiology of the acute heart failure should be considered. For example, the patient may be experiencing a dysrhythmia (such as atrial fibrillation) that is contributing to the heart failure. If this is the case, the dysrhythmia should be managed according to advanced cardiac life support (ACLS) guidelines and local protocol.

Mitral Regurgitation

Mitral valve regurgitation results when the heart's mitral valve fails to close appropriately, causing a backward flow of blood from the left ventricle into the left atrium. Moderate or severe regurgitation is frequent, and its prevalence increases with age. Causes of this condition include rheumatic heart disease, myocardial infarction, left-sided heart failure, endocarditis, and mitral valve prolapse.

Assessment

Acute mitral regurgitation is usually the result of a myocardial infarction or endocarditis. Normally, when the left ventricle squeezes, blood is pumped through the aortic valve to the rest of the body. When the mitral valve becomes incompetent, blood from the left ventricle is pumped out through the aortic valve and the mitral valve, resulting in a backward flow of blood through the heart. This backward flow causes increased filling pressures and strain on the left side of the heart. The heart attempts to compensate, eventually leading to pulmonary edema and cardiogenic shock.

Chronic mitral regurgitation develops over time, allowing the heart to compensate for the incompetent valve. Initially, compensation increases the left ventricular output to the body. Over time, however, the left side of the heart becomes stressed and unable to continue the compensatory mechanisms needed to maintain adequate output, leading to heart failure.

Patients with mitral regurgitation present with fatigue, weakness, and dyspnea with exertion. If mitral regurgitation is severe, the patient will likely present with signs of heart failure as well. If heart failure is present, the patient may also have signs of pulmonary edema and cardiogenic shock. A loud murmur is usually appreciated as a result of the turbulent blood flow crossing the incompetent valve.

Management

The definitive treatment for patients with signs of heart failure is surgical intervention, with either a valve repair or replacement. In the prehospital setting, optimizing oxygenation and managing life threats are the immediate goals of therapy. Heart failure should be treated as directed by local protocol and the EMS provider should be prepared to aggressively resuscitate should the patient develop cardiogenic shock. If the patient is in severe respiratory distress and meets all the criteria, continuous positive airway pressure (CPAP) may be beneficial.

Congestive Heart Failure

Congestive heart failure (CHF) is a common cardiovascular condition in older people, in which the heart is unable to maintain adequate output to meet the metabolic needs of the body. The prevalence of this disease increases dramatically with age. For people age 65 years and over, CHF is the most common reason for admission to an acute care hospital, and 10% of people over the age of 80 will suffer from CHF.[10]

Assessment

With CHF, the heart muscle fails to pump sufficiently. This occurs as the aging heart and vessels undergo structural and physiologic changes, particularly stiffening of the muscle. The three leading disease processes associated with CHF in older patients are hypertension, coronary artery disease, and **atrial fibrillation**. There are many ways to categorize CHF, but for prehospital purposes, the easiest is left- and right-sided heart failure.

With left-sided heart failure, the pumping function of the left ventricle is damaged by CAD, diseased heart valves, or chronic hypertension. When the myocardium can no longer effectively contract, the heart attempts to maintain adequate cardiac output in other ways. Two specific changes occur: heart rate increases, and the left ventricle enlarges in an effort to increase the amount of blood pumped each minute. When these adaptations can no longer make up for the decreased heart function, CHF eventually develops. The lungs become congested with fluid and blood tends to back up in the pulmonary veins, increasing the pressure in the capillaries until it exceeds a certain level and fluid (mostly water) passes through the walls of the vessels and into the alveoli. This condition is known as **pulmonary edema**. Pulmonary edema may occur suddenly, as in an AMI, or slowly over months, as in chronic CHF. Sometimes, in patients with an acute onset of CHF, severe pulmonary edema will develop; in this case, the patient will have pink, frothy sputum and severe dyspnea.

With right-sided heart failure, the right side of the heart has been damaged, causing fluid to collect in the body and often showing up as swelling (edema) of the feet and legs. Dependent edema is the collection of fluid in the part of the body that is closest to the ground (for patients who are bedridden, this may be in the sacral area of the back); pedal edema is swelling specifically in the feet and legs. This swelling causes relatively few symptoms other than discomfort; however, chronic pedal edema may indicate underlying heart disease (right-sided heart failure) even in the absence of pain or other symptoms.

Patients with CHF generally require multiple medications, so a review of medications may be helpful during assessment (**Table 9-3**). Those patients often develop problems associated with fluid overload, which could be secondary to worsening heart function from a myocardial infarction or an **arrhythmia**. An increase in dietary salt or failure to take medications, especially diuretics, can also lead to worsening heart failure. Salt increase, which can cause fluid overload, may occur if the patient drinks too much fluid or has a diet that is high in sodium. The risk of medication errors occurring in the older person may be increased by memory impairment, poor vision, and the need to take multiple medications. Additionally, a person taking diuretics may skip a dose due to the fear of being incontinent at a public event.

The most common complaint with acute or worsening CHF is shortness of breath. Patients may also experience pedal or peripheral edema, cough, fatigue, or weight gain in a short period of time. Orthopnea (dyspnea when lying down) and dyspnea on exertion are also classic findings with CHF (**Figure 9-3**). Try to

Table 9-3 Medications Commonly Prescribed for CHF	
Drug Type	**Examples**
Angiotensin-converting enzyme (ACE) inhibitors	Captopril (Capoten); ramipril (Altace)
Angiotensin-receptor blockers (ARBs)	Losartan (Cozaar, Hyaar)
Digoxin	Lanoxin
Diuretics	Furosemide (Lasix); hydrochlorothyazide (Hydrodiuril)
Nitrates	Isosorbide mononitrate (Imdur); isosorbide dinitrate (Isordil)
Potassium supplements	KCl

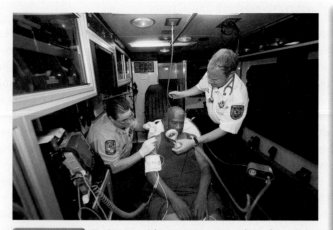

Figure 9-3 Patients with CHF may need to be transported in an upright position because shortness of breath and cough often worsen when they lie flat.
© Jones & Bartlett Learning. Courtesy of MIEMSS.

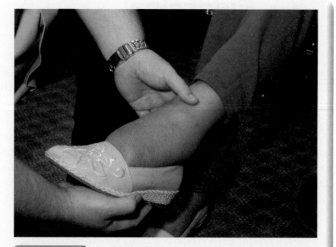

Figure 9-4 Swelling in the lower extremities, or peripheral edema, is a sign of CHF. To distinguish fluid from fat, gently press a finger along the shin bone. If this leaves an indentation, it is more likely fluid in the tissues; if not, it is more likely fatty tissue.
© Jones & Bartlett Learning. Courtesy of MIEMSS.

find out if these are new or chronic problems. Ask questions that compare the most recent episode to how the patient functioned one month ago (e.g., "How far can you walk before you get out of breath? How far were you able to walk a month ago?"). The patient may report a productive cough with pink, frothy sputum. This typically suggests pulmonary edema.

Patients in acute heart failure may present in acute respiratory distress. The respiratory exam is crucial in the evaluation of the CHF patient. Auscultation will reveal bilateral crackles in the patient with pulmonary edema. In isolated or severe cases, breath sounds may be diminished or wheezes may be present (cardiac asthma). When describing the lung sounds, note how high the crackles are auscultated (e.g., 1/3 up, 1/2 up, etc). Be careful not to confuse crackles with signs of consolidation, like rhonchi. Isolated rhonchi accompanied with wheezing and a fever may indicate an infectious process like pneumonia, which is a common diagnosis in the older population. Care must be taken not to misdiagnose CHF for pneumonia.

Auscultation of the heart or palpation of the pulses may reveal tachycardia. Additional abnormalities commonly found when checking vital signs include hypertension, low pulse oximetry, and increased respiratory rate. A good axiom to remember is that hypertension in combination with shortness of breath is CHF until proven otherwise. When heart failure is severe, however, blood pressure will be low, because the heart is not strong enough to generate a pressure. Round out your focused exam by checking for jugular venous distention, enlargement of the liver, and peripheral and dependent edema (the sacral area and abdominal area are common sites) (**Figure 9-4**).

Once CHF develops, it can be treated but not cured. Regular use of medications may alleviate the symptoms; however, patients often will become ill again and are frequently hospitalized. Approximately one-half of these patients will die within 5 years of the onset of symptoms.

Medication Tip

Patients with CHF usually take multiple medications. Watch for diuretics, potassium supplements, and other medication categories.

Management

Dyspnea is usually the presenting complaint of patients with an acute exacerbation of CHF. This is due to pulmonary edema and problems with oxygenation. Vital signs should be obtained and circulation, airway, and breathing should be addressed. If the situation permits, the patient should be positioned upright to allow gravity to shunt some of the fluid away from the lungs. Oxygen therapy should be provided, as well as an intravenous line and ECG monitor. Obtaining a 12-lead ECG should be considered in patients exhibiting signs of CHF, especially if the patient is complaining of chest pain. Acute coronary syndrome may be the underlying cause of heart failure; if AMI is suspected from the 12-lead ECG, the patient should be transported to a facility with a cardiac catheterization lab capable of PCI.

The medical management for CHF is covered in the *Respiratory Emergencies* chapter. Patients experiencing symptoms of CHF are typically very ill. Be sure to follow local protocol to inform the emergency department that you are en route with a CHF patient. This will allow the emergency department ample time to mobilize any necessary resources for the patient.

Electrical Disturbances

With aging, changes in the cardiovascular system can lead to conduction system abnormalities. These abnormalities result in a disturbance of the normal heart rhythm (arrhythmia) or heart rate. An arrhythmia may be asymptomatic or may present with chest pain, dyspnea, palpitations, dizziness, change in mental status, syncope, or even sudden death. There are many types of arrhythmias, and entire textbooks have been dedicated to their recognition and management. A discussion of all the different types of arrhythmias is beyond the scope of this text; instead, the focus will be on atrial fibrillation.

Assessment

Atrial fibrillation is the most commonly sustained arrhythmia found in the older population (**Figure 9-5**). About 5% of people age 65 years and older are afflicted with this condition, and incidence and prevalence increase with age.[11] Atrial fibrillation is usually classified as acute (paroxysmal) or chronic. It may be precipitated by acute systemic illnesses such as pneumonia or electrolyte abnormalities, or it may be caused by chronic, previously undiagnosed systemic problems such as thyroid disease, poorly controlled chronic obstructive pulmonary disease, or kidney failure (**Table 9-4**). Additionally, atrial fibrillation is a major contributor to stroke in the older population. Whereas a 50-year-old with atrial fibrillation has a 1% to 2% risk of stroke per year, the risk jumps to 8% to 12% per year for a person over 80 years.

Management

Prehospital management focuses on recognition of atrial fibrillation and control of rapid ventricular response. A calcium channel blocker, such as diltiazem (Cardizem), is effective for rate control. A standard loading dose of diltiazem is 0.25 mg/kg (20 mg maximum) by IV bolus administered slowly over 2 minutes. If response is inadequate, diltiazem can be repeated with a dosage of 0.35 mg/kg (25 mg maximum) over 2 minutes. For patients older than 50 years of age or with borderline blood pressure (90 mm Hg systolic), an initial bolus of 5 mg to 10 mg administered IV over 2 minutes should be considered. Cardioversion may be required if the patient presents with serious signs and symptoms, such as chest pain, shortness of breath, decreased level of consciousness, hypotension, hypoperfusion, pulmonary congestion, CHF, and/or AMI. Although a rhythm strip is helpful, a 12-lead ECG will also be helpful in determining the cause of the arrhythmia.

Medications for rate control of atrial fibrillation may also include calcium channel blockers and digoxin. For patients who are considered to be at minimal risk for medication interaction, adherence issues, or falls, treatment with an anticoagulant such as warfarin (Coumadin), dabigatran (Pradaxa), or rivaroxaban (Xarelto) should also be considered. In certain situations, aspirin is a good alternative to these medications to prevent stroke.

Many older people with heart disease have cardiac pacemakers to maintain a regular cardiac rhythm and rate. Pacemakers are inserted when the electrical conduction system of the heart is so damaged that it cannot function properly. These battery-powered devices deliver an electrical impulse through

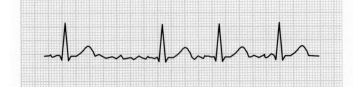

Rate:	Variable, ventricular response can be fast or slow
Regularity:	Irregularly irregular
P wave:	None; chaotic atrial activity
P:QRS ratio:	None
PR interval:	None
QRS width:	Normal
Grouping:	None
Dropped beats:	None

Putting it all together:
Atrial fibrillation is the chaotic firing of numerous pacemaker cells in the atria in a totally haphazard fashion. The result is that there are no discernible P waves, and the QRS complexes are innervated haphazardly in an irregular pattern. The ventricular rate is completely guided by occasional activation from one of the pacemaking sources. Because the ventricles are not paced by any one site, the intervals are completely random.

(A)

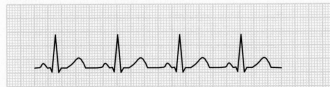

Rate:	60–100 BPM
Regularity:	Regular
P wave:	Present
P:QRS ratio:	1:1
PR interval:	Normal
QRS width:	Normal
Grouping:	None
Dropped beats:	None

Putting it all together:
This rhythm represents the normal state with the SA node as the lead pacer. The intervals should all be consistent and within the normal range. Note that this refers to the atrial rate; normal sinus rhythm (NSR) can occur with a ventricular escape rhythm or other ventricular abnormality if AV dissociation exists.

(B)

Figure 9-5 (A) Atrial fibrillation. (B) Normal sinus rhythm.

Table 9-4	Possible Causes of Atrial Fibrillation
Underlying structural heart defect	■ Conduction abnormalities ■ Valvular heart defects ■ Myocardial infarction
Acute systemic illness	■ Pneumonia ■ Electrolyte abnormalities ■ Pulmonary edema (cardiogenic or noncardiogenic) ■ Pulmonary embolism
Chronic systemic illness	■ Thyroid disease ■ Asthma ■ Chronic obstructive pulmonary disease ■ Chronic renal disease

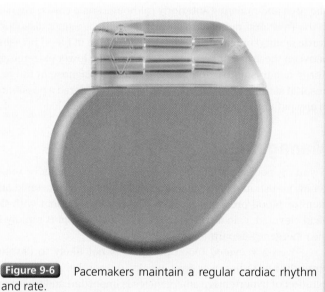

Figure 9-6 Pacemakers maintain a regular cardiac rhythm and rate.
© Carolina K. Smith, MD/ShutterStock, Inc.

wires that are in direct contact with the myocardium. The generating unit typically resembles a small silver dollar and is generally placed under a heavy muscle or a fold of skin in the left upper part of the chest (**Figure 9-6**).

Normally, the EMS provider does not need to be concerned about problems with pacemakers. Thanks to modern technology, an implanted unit will not require battery replacement for years, and wires are well protected and rarely broken. In the past, pacemakers were sometimes known to malfunction when a patient got too close to an electrical radiation source such as a microwave oven; however, this is no longer the case. Patients should still be aware of precautions, if any, which must be taken to maintain proper functioning.

If a pacemaker does not function properly—as when the battery wears out—the patient may experience syncope, dizziness, or weakness because of an excessively slow heart rate. Without the stimulus of the pacemaker, the pulse will likely be less than 60 beats/min because the heart is beating without the regulation of its own electrical conduction system, which may be damaged. In this circumstance, the heart tends to assume a fixed slow rate that is not fast enough to allow the patient to function normally. A patient with a malfunctioning pacemaker should be promptly transported to the emergency department for evaluation and possible repair of the pacemaker. If an automated external defibrillator (AED) or manual defibrillator is used on a patient with a pacemaker, the pads should not be placed directly over the device. This will ensure a better flow of electricity through the patient's body.

Many older patients who survive ventricular fibrillation cardiac arrest have a small automatic implantable cardiac defibrillator (AICD). Patients who are at particularly high risk for a cardiac arrest may also have an AICD implanted. This device attaches directly to the heart to continuously monitor the heart's rhythm, delivering shocks as needed (**Figure 9-7**). Regardless of whether a patient having an AMI has an AICD or not, he or she should be treated like all other AMI patients. Treatment should include performing CPR, beginning with chest compressions, and using an AED or manual defibrillator if the patient goes into cardiac arrest. Generally, the electricity from an AICD is so low that it will have no effect on rescuers and, therefore, should not be of concern to you.

Hypertensive Emergencies

According to the Centers for Disease Control and Prevention (CDC), 67 million adults in the United States have high blood pressure.[12] Hypertensive emergencies are generally regarded as elevated blood pressure occurring with evidence of organ damage, with commonly afflicted organs including the heart, eyes, brain, and kidneys; damage manifests as chest pain,

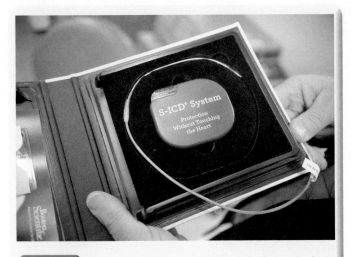

Figure 9-7 An AICD continuously monitors the heart rhythm, delivering shocks as needed for patients who develop a lethal arrhythmia.
© STEPHEN FLOOD/Express-Times/Landov

visual changes, mental status changes, or urinary abnormalities, respectively. Blood pressure cutoffs vary from textbook to textbook, and, as such, there are no set-in-stone criteria for the level of blood pressure that needs to be reached in order for a hypertensive emergency to exist. However, the American Heart Association defines a hypertensive emergency as a systolic reading of 180 mm Hg or higher, or as a diastolic reading of 110 mm Hg.[13]

Previous teachings stressed that, in order to protect the patient having a hypertensive emergency, blood pressure should be lowered as quickly as possible to low or "normal" levels. Subsequent studies have shown this to be potentially harmful to the patient, as rapid lowering of blood pressure can result in stroke, MI, or death. Newer thinking dictates lowering blood pressure about 30% from the initial mean arterial pressure.

 Assessment

Because blood pressure cannot be directly felt by the patient, the signs and symptoms of a hypertensive emergency are related to the effects of the hypertension. Some patients with chronic hypertension may not experience signs or symptoms until their systolic pressure is significantly high. One of the most common signs is a sudden severe headache, often described as "the worst headache" the patient has ever felt. This may also be a sign of cerebral hemorrhage. Other signs and symptoms include a strong bounding pulse, ringing in the ears, nausea and vomiting, dizziness, warm skin (dry or moist), nosebleed, altered mental status, and even the sudden development of pulmonary edema. Untreated hypertensive emergencies can lead to a stroke or a dissecting aortic aneurysm.

An aortic aneurysm is a weakness in the wall of the aorta. The aorta dilates at the weakened area, making it susceptible to rupture. A dissecting aortic aneurysm occurs when the inner layers of the aorta become separated, allowing blood to flow (at high pressures) between the layers. The separation of layers weakens the wall of the aorta significantly, making it more likely to rupture under conditions of continued high blood pressure. If the aorta ruptures, the amount of internal blood loss will be so large that the patient will die almost immediately.

The primary cause of a dissecting aneurysm is uncontrolled hypertension. Signs and symptoms include very sudden chest pain located in the anterior part of the chest or between the shoulder blades in the back. It may be difficult to differentiate the chest pain of a dissecting aortic aneurysm from that of an AMI, but a number of distinctive features can help. For example, the pain from an AMI is often accompanied by other symptoms—nausea, indigestion, weakness, and sweating—and tends to come on gradually, getting more severe with time and often described as "pressure" rather than "stabbing." By contrast, the pain of a dissecting aortic aneurysm usually comes on full force from one minute to the next, and is more consistently described as a "tearing, burning sensation" originating in the back or scapular area and radiating anteriorly (although some cases originate in the front and radiate posteriorly). A patient with a dissecting aortic aneurysm may also exhibit a difference in blood pressure between the arms, or diminished pulses in the lower extremities. Aortic aneurysms are almost impossible to diagnose in the prehospital setting; however, they should be considered a possibility in any patient with significant hypertension.

Management

If you suspect a patient is experiencing a hypertensive emergency, you should attempt to make him or her comfortable and monitor blood pressure regularly. Position the patient with the head elevated, gain intravenous access, and transport rapidly to the emergency department.

Severely elevated blood pressure is not likely to develop abruptly, but rather over days, weeks, or months. Although recognition of hypertensive emergencies is important and treatment in the field is sometimes necessary, in many cases more harm than good is done by aggressively attempting to lower the blood pressure. Aggressive dosing with intravenous medications or fast-acting oral agents can lead to hypotension, and reducing severely elevated blood pressure below the autoregulatory zone too quickly can result in markedly decreased perfusion to the brain and eventually ischemia or infarction. In addition, the rapid lowering of blood pressure is usually unnecessary in asymptomatic patients.

 Syncope

Syncope becomes increasingly common with aging and can be attributed to many causes. While **vasovagal syncope** is the most common culprit in the younger population, the older population tends to have a wider variety of causes. Those of most concern involve neurologic and cardiac causes. Keep in mind that older patients may be much more sensitive to dehydration and antihypertensive medications than their younger counterparts.

Assessment

You should assume that syncope in an older person is life threatening until proven otherwise, with the most important cardiac problems to investigate being myocardial infarction, arrhythmias, and valvular disease. A myocardial infarction may cause enough damage to pump action to decrease blood flow to the brain and precipitate syncope. An AMI may also precipitate an arrhythmia that produces syncope; heart rates that are too slow or too fast can decrease blood flow to the brain to the point that the flow is no longer adequate to sustain consciousness. Aortic stenosis (stiffening of the aortic valve) can impair the left ventricle's ability to pump blood, and is a common and serious cause of cardiac syncope in the older patient. A history of cardiac disease is a very important clue to a cardiac cause; without it, a cardiac cause is extremely unlikely.

Management

An older patient with syncope is much more likely to be injured than a younger patient. Older patients who experience a syncopal episode require a thorough focused history and physical examination. Patients should receive cardiac monitoring (including a 12-lead ECG), intravenous access, and glucose testing. Treatment is based upon findings.

Cardiac Arrest

Cardiac arrest has been described as the number one killer in the United States, and is estimated to account for 350,000 to 500,000 deaths per year.[14] Many EMS providers encounter a moral dilemma when faced with resuscitating older cardiac arrest patients. Our duty as prehospital professionals is to provide each patient with appropriate care. Resuscitative efforts should not be withheld from the older patient due to concerns of ineffectiveness. Age is not a determinant for CPR effectiveness and, therefore, it should not be considered as an independent predictor of survival.

Attitude Tip

When comparing the value and benefit of resuscitation efforts for a younger patient versus an older patient, remember that older patients *do* benefit from aggressive resuscitation efforts, heart attack and stroke risk-reduction efforts, and other treatment modalities, such as thrombolytics, coronary artery bypass surgery, and angioplasty.

Summary

Cardiac emergencies tend to happen with greater frequency in the older population than in any other age group. The signs and symptoms do not always conform to the classic presentation we read about in textbooks, so remember to take a detailed medical history, including a list of medications the patient is taking, and pay close attention to what the patient tells you. In addition, a 12-lead ECG should be performed in all cardiac emergencies involving older patients. The patient may have very vague complaints that do not necessarily point to a cardiac cause. By keeping an open mind and looking a little deeper, you may find a cardiac problem when you initially did not suspect it.

References

1. Centers for Disease Control and Prevention, National Center for Injury Prevention and Control. (October 15, 2012.) *10 Leading Causes of Death by Age Group, United States–2011.* Retrieved from http://www.cdc.gov/injury/wisqars/leadingcauses.html
2. Cannon LA, Marshall JM. Cardiac disease in the elderly population. *Clin Geriatr Med.* 1993; 9:499–525.
3. Ghali JK, Cooper R, Ford E. Trends in hospitalization rates for heart failure in the United States, 1973–1986: Evidence for increasing population prevalence. *Arch Intern Med.* 1990;150: 767–773.
4. O'Connell JB, Bristow MR. Economic impact of heart failure in the United States: Time for a different approach. *J Heart Lung Transplant.* 1993;13: S107–S112.
5. Gillespie CD, Wigington C, Hong Y. Coronary heart disease and stroke deaths–United States, 2009. *MMWR.* 2013;62(03): 157–160.
6. Umachandran V, Ranjadayalan K, Ambepityia G, et al. Aging, autonomic function, and the precipitation of angina. *Br Heart.* 1991;66: 15–18.
7. Kolansky DM. Acute coronary syndromes: morbidity, mortality, and pharmacoeconomic burden. *Am J Manag Care.* 2009;15: S36–41.
8. O'Connell JB, Bristow MR. Economic impact of heart failure in the United States: Time for a different approach. *J Heart Lung Transplant.* 1993;13: S107–S112.
9. "U.S. Aortic Stenosis Disease Prevalence & Treatment Statistics." (July 8, 2013). University of Maryland Medical Center. Retrieved from http://umm.edu/programs/heart/services/programs/surgery/valve-surgery/facts

10. Wolf PA, Abbott RD, Kannel WB. Atrial fibrillation: A major contributor to stroke in the elderly. *Arch Intern Med.* 1987;147: 1561–1564.

11. Follman DF. Aortic regurgitation: Identifying and treating acute and chronic disease. *Postgrad Med.* 1993;93: 83–90.

12. Centers for Disease Control and Prevention. Vital signs: awareness and treatment of uncontrolled hypertension among adults—United States, 2003–2010. *MMWR.* 2012;61(35): 703–709.

13. "High Blood Pressure." (April 4, 2012). American Heart Association. Retrieved from http://www.heart.org/HEARTORG/Conditions/HighBloodPressure/AboutHighBloodPressure/About-High-Blood-Pressure_UCM_002050_Article.jsp

14. Huerta-Alardín AL, Guerra-Cantú M, Varon J. Cardiopulmonary resuscitation in the elderly: a clinical and ethical perspective. *J Geriatric Cardiology.* 2007;4(2): 117–119.

CASE STUDY SUMMARIES

Case Study 1 Summary

It may be easy to associate Mrs. Johnson's symptoms with a gastrointestinal problem such as diverticulitis or gastroenteritis; however, the EMS provider must consider the atypical presentation of myocardial infarctions in older people. An acute myocardial infarction can be completely painless in diabetics and women (especially older women). Do not rule out the possibility of myocardial infarction simply because the patient does not have symptoms of chest pain.

Early treatment should include a 12-lead ECG. Mrs. Johnson's diagnosis is non-ST elevation myocardial infarction (non-STEMI). Cardiac enzymes were positive, showing troponin elevation. Catheterization showed a 99% occlusion of one of the branches of the circumflex artery; and two stents were placed. The right coronary artery (RCA) had a 90% proximal stenosis, but stent placement and percutaneous transluminal coronary angioplasty (PTCA) were unsuccessful. Mrs. Johnson was scheduled for a repeated catheterization for RCA stent placement in 2 to 3 weeks.

Case Study 2 Summary

The EMS provider should always take a shortness of breath complaint seriously and initiate treatment immediately. Consider the common causes of shortness of breath, including exacerbation of chronic obstructive pulmonary disease, congestive heart failure, pulmonary embolism, and myocardial infarction. Treatment consists of a 12-lead ECG, breathing treatments, and aspirin. (Aspirin provides the largest decrease in the risk of mortality for a patient with an acute myocardial infarction).

The diagnosis for Mrs. Gray is exacerbation of congestive heart failure. Some of the most common causes of congestive heart failure admission include pneumonia or respiratory processes, ischemia or acute coronary syndromes, arrhythmias, uncontrolled hypertension, nonadherence to medications, worsening renal function, and nonadherence to diet.

CHAPTER 10

Neurological Emergencies

LEARNING OBJECTIVES

1. Discuss age-related changes of the nervous system.

2. Discuss the epidemiology of nervous system diseases in the older population.

3. Discuss assessment of the older patient with complaints related to the nervous system, including stroke, generalized weakness, altered mental status, delirium, dementia, Alzheimer's disease, Parkinson's disease, seizures, and aggressive or assaultive behavior.

4. Identify the need for intervention and transport, and develop a treatment and management plan for the older patient with complaints related to the nervous system.

Introduction

Aging produces changes in the nervous system that are reflected in the neurological examination. Changes in cognitive (thinking) speed, memory, and postural stability are the most common normal findings in an older person. Often, these changes are not evident to the patient or family members, and a precise date or time of onset cannot be recalled. In contrast, diseases of the neurological system tend to produce acute changes in neurological function and frequently have a sudden onset, causing a more rapid and noticeable decrease in neurological function. Additionally, certain disease states that are common in the older population increase the chance for secondary problems that can further damage the nervous system; for example, a patient with Parkinson's disease may fall and sustain an injury.

The brain decreases in terms of weight (5% to 10%) and volume (**atrophy**) as a person ages. However, the functional significance of these changes is not clear. The human brain has an enormous reserve capacity, and having a smaller and lighter brain does not interfere with the mental capabilities of productive older people. Still, because the brain is responsible for coordinating the other systems of the body, the specific functions of other body systems may decline with mental function decline. For example, regulation of respiratory rate and depth, pulse rate, blood pressure, hunger, and thirst may all be affected by changes to the central nervous system. Reflexes often slow, resulting in the person not being able to protect themselves in normal ways. For example, an older patient with slowed responses to pain may sustain a serious burn if it takes the patient longer to remove his or her hand from a hot surface. Changes in body temperature regulation and temperature perception also occur with mental function decline, meaning that the affected person is less capable of recovering from exposure to extreme temperatures and less likely to recognize these exposures.

Attitude Tip

Avoid the ageist mistake of assuming that older people are confused and disoriented as a natural result of aging. Confusion, delirium, and dementia are not normal changes of the aging process, but rather the results of acute or chronic disease processes.

Normal Age-Related Changes in the Nervous System

Normal age-related changes in the nervous system are defined as progressive and irreversible neurological changes that develop with advancing age in most individuals without obvious disease.[1] The following sections discuss these changes in regard to their effects on various functions and body systems.

Mental Function and Status

Studies have documented age-associated decline in mental function, especially slower central processing of sensory stimuli and language and longer retrieval times for short- and long-term memory. Together, a decline in these functions typically affects performance on the mental status portion of the neurological examination. Common findings may include slow responses to questioning or requests to repeat a question. These normal changes can be confused with the symptoms associated with diseases such as Alzheimer's disease or other forms of dementia, depression, **encephalopathy** (any acute disease of the brain), or Parkinson's disease and related disorders.

The main features of normal age-related cognitive disorders are that they are relatively isolated (not associated with multiple abnormal neurological findings that suggest specific disease states) and that the onset and any progression of these findings are "in time" with the individual's aging process—that is, the findings are not sudden or extreme, and do not extend to other abnormalities.

Cranial Nerve Function

The cranial nerves provide both motor and sensory function to various parts of the head and neck, including the ears, eyes, tongue, face, and muscles used for facial expression and movement of the head. The most common changes associated with deteriorating cranial nerve function include a decline in vision, hearing, range of eye movements (especially vertical

CASE STUDY 1

You are dispatched to the home of a 74-year-old woman, Mrs. Hewett. Mrs. Hewett's husband reports that his wife had not been feeling well all day and that she went to take a nap about an hour ago. When Mr. Hewett went to wake his wife for dinner, he noted that her speech was slurred.

Your assessment reveals that the patient seems to be oriented but is now having trouble communicating. In addition to her speech being slurred, her answers to your questions are inappropriate. There is marked facial droop and weakness in the patient's right arm.

- What information should you obtain?
- What are your treatment priorities?

movements), and range of both facial expression and cervical motion. Age-related changes are mild, slow in onset, and progress gradually. It is important to distinguish these from other more exaggerated changes associated with disease states. Three features in particular—diminished eye movements, facial expression, and cervical movement (along with other neurological exam changes such as tremor and limb rigidity)—might suggest Parkinson's disease or another Parkinsonian-like disorder.

Undeniably, the performance of most of the sensory organs declines with increasing age, with decreases in the ability to see and hear being the most common sensory impairments among older people. Although these senses may not be as sharp as they once were, this does not mean you should assume that all older people are blind and deaf. If you note an inability to communicate effectively, gradually modify your technique until communication is effective.

Visual changes affect 50% of patients older than 65 years. Tear production decreases with age, which can lead to the sensation of dry or itchy eyes and increase the chance of mild eye injury (such as corneal abrasion) and infection. Visual impairment may be caused by conditions such as diabetes, age-related macular degeneration, and retinal detachment. The two most common causes of visual disturbances in older people are cataracts and glaucoma. Cataracts are a result of the lenses hardening over time. Eventually, the lenses become opaque, preventing light and images from being transmitted to the rear of the eye. Patients with cataracts may report blurred vision, double vision, spots, and/or ghost images, and surgical treatment is typically needed for improvement. Glaucoma is caused by an increase in intraocular pressure that is severe enough to damage the optic nerve, potentially resulting in permanent loss of peripheral and central vision. Treatment of glaucoma consists of oral medications and eye drops.

Gradual hearing loss is also common as people age, though not all older people experience hearing loss. A common cause of hearing impairment in the older population is presbycusis, a progressive hearing loss particularly pertaining to high frequencies, along with a lessened ability to discriminate between a particular sound and background noise. Patients with hearing loss may lose the ability to interpret speech, resulting in a decreased ability to communicate, which may lead to isolation and/or depression. Even when hearing loss is not severe enough to consistently interfere with conversation, certain activities, like going to the movies or listening to music, may be less enjoyable. In addition, hearing loss has the potential to threaten a person's safety, as many warning signals, such as smoke detectors and car horns, are auditory.

Motor Function

Changes in motor function take place in both the central and peripheral nervous systems. As these changes occur, the individual cannot initiate movement as quickly or sustain it as well, causing a decline in coordination. Mild coordination problems also result from reduced nervous system functions such as vision and balance. Motor function can also be affected by nervous system deterioration that causes a decrease in muscle bulk and possibly strength. Another common finding in the older population is benign "senile" tremor, which may be **idiopathic** (of unknown cause) or inherited. This tremor is symmetrical and mainly affects the upper limbs, hands, head, and voice.

Age-associated changes of motor function are generally symmetrical, mild, and—as in other systems—gradual in their development. One-sided, severe, or sudden symptoms more likely indicate a specific disease state such as stroke, Parkinson states, or acute inner ear disorders. When symptoms indicative of the latter occur, they must receive prompt evaluation in the emergency department.

Sensation and Reflexes

The sense of touch decreases with aging from the loss of end nerve fibers. This loss, in conjunction with the slowing of the peripheral nervous system, can result in a delayed reflex reaction. Changes in sensation and reflexes involve decreased sensitivity to vibration and reduction or loss of ankle jerk reflex. Along with declining vision, changes in sensation and reflexes make the older patient susceptible to falls from misplacement of the feet, as vibration and position sense are the main contributors to balance.

Communication Tip

Difficulty in communicating with older patients is often the result of normal effects of the aging process on sensory function. Remember, there is little the patient can do about these changes.

Posture and Gait

With aging, changes to the spinal canal typically produce forward thrusting of the head and a flexion of the thorax that result in a slightly stooped stance. An older person's **gait** (manner of walking) may change, resulting in a shortened step, wider base, and decreased arm swing; in general, walking is slower and looks "stiff." A decrease in vibration and position sense in the lower legs also causes older people to take smaller, more cautious steps, and produces more postural sway.

The sense of body position (proprioception) also becomes impaired with age. Proprioception, which enables a person to maintain postural stability, is accomplished through the use of a variety of receptors in the joints and information provided by the eyes. As these mechanisms fail with age, older people become less steady on their feet, and the tendency to fall markedly increases. This tendency may be exacerbated by any of the previously mentioned changes in sensory perception.

When evaluating and documenting an older person's gait, remember that walking requires the ability to stand, maintain position (keeping the center of gravity over the feet), and advance from the starting position. While the brain is the overall controlling mechanism of these movements, it must also coordinate with the feet, ankles, knees, and hips to bear weight. In addition, the inner ear must be able to determine the direction of gravitational pull, the eyes must be able to judge distance and compensate for other impaired sensory systems, and the peripheral nerves must be able to send information from the environment to the spinal cord.

To evaluate posture and gait, observe the older person stand up from a chair without using his or her arms. You and your partner must remain on either side of the person in case he or she falls. If the person is unable to stand without using his or her arms, allow him or her to do so. Observe how easily balance is maintained. Ask the person to walk 10 to 15 feet and observe how easily forward motion is initiated. Assess for the presence of fear when ambulating (for example, the person may take small cautious steps as if walking on ice), especially if there is a history of falling. If you note any difficulty with ambulation, report this finding to the emergency department staff.

Neurological Examination of the Older Patient

Neurologic examination for older patients is similar to that of any adult. However, non-neurologic disorders that are common among older people may complicate the exam. For example, visual and hearing deficits may impede evaluation of cranial nerves, and periarthritis (inflammation of tissues around a joint)

in certain joints, especially shoulders and hips, may interfere with evaluation of motor function. Symmetric findings unaccompanied by functional loss and other neurological symptoms and signs may be noted. Signs detected during the examination must be considered in light of the patient's age, history, and other findings.

The neurological examination begins as soon as contact is made with the patient. First, determine the patient's level of consciousness using the AVPU (alert, verbal or painful stimuli, unresponsive) scale. Once circulation, airway, and breathing have been assessed and deemed adequate, a more focused neurological examination may begin. While assessing the patient, it is essential to obtain as much information as possible about the history of the incident, as well as the patient's medical history, medications, and allergies.

During this time, a general impression of the patient's behaviors and actions should also be formed, and the patient's mental status should be evaluated in more detail. This includes asking the patient simple questions, such as the date or location, and determining if the patient's comments are logical. It may not always be appropriate, however, to ask the older person, "What day of the week is it?' or "Who is the President of the United States?" For some older people in long-term care settings, time takes on a different meaning, and it would not be unusual for the patient to not know the answers to these questions. Ask instead, "What season are we in?" or "What holiday did we recently celebrate?" **Table 10-1** summarizes additional important questions to ask the older patient during the neurological examination.

The neurological examination continues with examination of the structures of the face for symmetry, including the eyelids,

Table 10-1 Questions to Ask During the Neurological Examination
■ Does the patient have any past history of head injury?
■ Has the patient had frequent or severe headaches (if so: when, where, and how often)?
■ Has the patient had any dizziness or vertigo?
■ Has the patient had any difficulty swallowing solids or liquids? (If the patient answers yes, this is a possible clue to CN IX-X abnormality.)
■ Has the patient had any episodes of difficulty speaking (if so: when and for how long)?
■ Has the patient had any coordination problems?
■ Does the patient have any numbness or tingling?
■ Has the patient had any prior neurological issues?
■ Has the patient had any decrease in memory or change in mental function?
■ Has the patient had any tremors in the hands or face?
■ Has the patient had any sudden changes in vision or sudden blindness?
■ Has the patient had any sudden weakness on one side of the body but not the other?
■ Has the patient ever experienced loss of consciousness (if so, what were the circumstances)?
Note: Positive findings to any of these questions should be reported to the emergency department physician.

mouth, and pupils. Both pupils should be evaluated with a penlight to determine if they have an equal and symmetrical reaction to light. Next, assess the function of the nerves and muscles that control eye movements by having the patient follow the penlight with their eyes, in both horizontal and vertical directions. Sensation of the face may be quickly examined by touching both sides of the face above the eyes, below the eyes, and along the mandible, and asking the patient if the sensation is equal and normal on both sides. The nerves that control motor function in the face may be assessed by having the patient close his or her eyes, smile, and protrude the tongue. All of these actions should produce symmetrical movements, and the tongue should not deviate to either side.

Once the face has been examined, an examination of the extremities may be conducted. Begin by inspecting the extremities for muscle bulk, tremors, and abnormal movements such as rapid, uncontrolled arm movement. In addition, the upper extremities should be examined by having the patient flex and extend at the elbow, with a provider's hand supplying light resistance against this movement. Next, grip strength should be evaluated bilaterally and simultaneously so that differences in strength may be detected. Sensation may then be evaluated by touching the patient's arms at various points to determine if the stimulus is felt and if it feels normal. The lower extremity examination is similar to that of the upper extremities. The patient should flex and extend the knee, and **dorsiflex** ("toes toward the head") and **plantarflex** ("stepping on the gas") the feet against mild resistance provided by the provider's hands. Sensation may then be examined in a manner similar to that of the upper extremities.

There are many issues that have the potential to affect the neurological examination in the older adult. For example, due to decreased hearing and vision, a patient's neurological examination may be negatively affected by the environment. A complete exam may be best performed once the patient is transferred to the ambulance, where lighting and other environmental conditions can be controlled. Opioid use may also affect the examination: Pharmacokinetics is altered in older adults due to decreased liver and renal function, so opioids may stay in the body longer, increasing the risk of nervous system depression. Older adults with an infection or fluid and electrolyte imbalances (such as dehydration or hypernatremia) are also at risk for developing changes in their neurologic examination. A sudden onset of confusion or change in the level of consciousness may be the first sign of an infection in older adults, particularly a urinary tract infection. Additionally, fatigue may affect an older person's communication and motor function, and pain may limit range of motion and mobility, thus giving the impression of an altered examination.

Though the underlying disease processes involved in neurological conditions can seem complex, there are ways to simplify the hunt for a cause. The mnemonic VITAMINS C & D is a helpful reminder of the possible origins and mechanisms of nervous system pathophysiology (**Table 10-2**). The approach begins by noting the type of signs present, and then lists what might be causing these signs. This is particularly useful when the patient has neurological symptoms that might have multiple causes.

Attitude Tip

Do not merely project a caring, interested, supportive, and compassionate attitude to your older patient—embrace it and live by it. Remember that older people do not like to be patronized or treated like children. Treat them with dignity like responsible adults.

Table 10-2 VITAMINS C & D: Origins or Mechanisms of Nervous System Pathophysiology

V	*Vascular*: stroke or brain embolism
I	*Inflammation*: inflammation of the blood vessels in the brain (**vasculitis**)
T	*Toxins*: carbon monoxide poisoning *Trauma*: concussion or intracerebral hemorrhage *Tumors*: primary brain tumor or **metastasis** (developed elsewhere and spread to the brain)
A	*Autoimmune*: production of immune system components against a normal structure in the central nervous system
M	*Metabolic*: liver or renal failure, hypoglycemia, hyperglycemia, hypothyroidism, or **nonketotic diabetic acidosis**
I	*Infection*: meningitis or encephalitis
N	*Narcotics and other drugs*: many possibilities, with a higher chance of mental status changes if there is preexisting brain disease
S	*Systemic*: sepsis or hypoxia
C	*Congenital*: seizures
D	*Degenerative*: Alzheimer's disease and other dementias, or Parkinson's disease
Note: Some categories overlap.	

Complaints Related to the Nervous System

Stroke and Cerebral Vascular Disease

Of the primary neurological problems found in the older population, stroke is the most common. Each year, approximately 800,000 people suffer a stroke; nearly three quarters of these incidents occur in people over the age of 65 years, with risk more than doubling each decade after the age of 55.[2] In addition, stroke kills almost 130,000 people in the United States each year, and more than 80% of these deaths occur in persons older than 65 years.[3] The main risk factors for stroke are preventable and treatable and include hypertension; cardiac disease (especially atrial fibrillation); smoking; diabetes; and high levels of fats in the blood, including cholesterol. Other important risk factors, such as obesity and a sedentary (inactive) lifestyle, are also controllable. In addition to these factors, normal changes of aging, such as loss of vascular elasticity, place the older person at risk of hemorrhagic stroke.

There are two main types of stroke: hemorrhagic and ischemic. About 20% to 30% of all strokes are hemorrhagic. Hemorrhagic stroke occurs when a blood vessel within the brain tears and produces bleeding in or around the brain. Although hemorrhagic stroke is less common than ischemia, it is often more lethal. Ischemic stroke typically occurs when a clot obstructs blood flow in an artery that supplies a portion of the brain (**Figure 10-1**). The clot may have formed within the artery at a specific site, or developed elsewhere—in the heart, for instance—and broken off, traveled, and finally lodged in an artery serving part of the brain. Brain tissue supplied by this artery is thus deprived of oxygen and glucose, resulting in immediate brain tissue death.

A vitally important concept in the pathophysiology of ischemic stroke is that of the **penumbra**, the tissue surrounding the central area of stroke. Because this tissue is still viable if treated within a few minutes or hours, it is critical to quickly

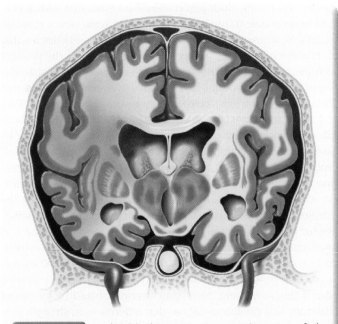

Figure 10-1 A clot blocking an artery serving part of the brain causes immediate brain tissue death. Saving tissue around the central area of stroke is the goal of immediate stroke care.

transport all patients with suspected stroke to the closest center that specializes in the care of stroke patients. The main thrust of ischemic stroke research is devoted to salvaging the penumbral tissue and thus minimizing the damage done by the stroke.

Ischemic stroke may develop slowly; often, the patient will awake in the morning presenting with signs. Hemorrhagic stroke, on the other hand, may have a rapid onset. Both forms of stroke can be life threatening; however, ischemic stroke rarely leads to death within the first hour, whereas hemorrhagic stroke can be rapidly fatal. It is vital that the EMS provider attempt to determine from the patient (if possible) or from the family or

CASE STUDY 2

You are called to the home of Mrs. Walker, an 81 year-old female with a fall injury. The patient's son is present and explains that after being unable to reach his mother, he drove to her residence to find her lying on the floor in the garage. The son reports Mrs. Walker lives alone and is very independent, but slipped and fell while taking the trash out that evening. The patient is conscious, alert, and oriented, and complaining of right shoulder pain. Your assessment reveals a possible fractured right shoulder; other assessment findings are unremarkable. You splint the patient's arm and prepare to transport her to the emergency department. The son advises you that he will not be coming to the hospital, as he must get to work.

A week later, you are called back to Mrs. Walker's residence by her son. He reports that his mother is not acting right: she seems vague, distracted, and confused; her house is a mess; and he thinks she has not changed her clothes in several days. The son states that he had no concerns about his mother up until she fell and broke her shoulder, but that this is a vast departure from his mother's usual behavior. Having treated and transported Mrs. Walker previously, you also notice that her mental status is markedly altered and that she is suffering from delirium.

- What are your concerns about Mrs. Walker?
- What information would you like to gather?

caregiver when the patient was last known to be well (baseline mental status) to establish the exact time of the onset of symptoms (**Table 10-3**). The importance of obtaining a history of the stroke patient cannot be overemphasized. Inquire of the patient (if possible), family, or caregiver about any history of cardiovascular disease, hypertension, diabetes, previous stroke, sickle cell disease, or cigarette smoking.

Assessment

Assessment of the older patient with suspected stroke is the same as for all other patients experiencing an acute emergency—adequate maintenance of circulation, airway, and breathing. With severe symptoms of hemorrhagic stroke, patency of the airway and adequate circulation are vital. Be prepared to provide ventilatory support. Time of symptom onset is crucial, especially when considering interventions.

In addition to noting abnormal findings during the neurological examination, the EMS provider can use a stroke scale to assess a possible stroke patient. The simplest and easiest stroke scale to use is the Cincinnati Prehospital Stroke Scale (**Table 10-4**). This scale tests speech, facial droop, and arm drift:

- Speech: Ask the patient to repeat a simple phrase such as, "The sky is blue in Cincinnati." If the patient is able to do this correctly, the patient can understand and repeat speech.
- Facial droop: Ask the patient to smile. Observe whether both sides of the face around the mouth move equally. If only one side moves well, there may be weakness in the muscles that control the other side.
- Arm movement: Ask the patient to hold both arms out in front of his or her body, with palms facing up, eyes closed, and without moving. Over the next 10 seconds,

Table 10-3 Symptoms of Ischemic Stroke Versus Hemorrhagic Stroke

Ischemic Stroke	Hemorrhagic Stroke
Weakness (hemiparesis) or paralysis (hemiplegia) on one side of the body	Headache (often described as the worst headache of the patient's life)
Numbness on one side of the body	Nausea and vomiting
Dysarthria (slurred speech)	Change in mental status; patient may become restless, agitated, or confused. Mental status changes may progress from alert to lethargic.
Aphasia	
Confusion	
Convulsions	
Visual disturbances	
Incontinence	
Numbness of the face	
Headache	
Dizziness	

Table 10-4 Cincinnati Prehospital Stroke Scale

Test	Normal	Abnormal
Speech (Ask patient to say, "The sky is blue in Cincinnati.")	Patient uses correct words with no slurring.	Patient slurs words, uses inappropriate words, or is unable to speak.
Facial droop (Ask patient to smile.)	Both sides of face move equally well.	One side of the patient's face does not move as well as the other.
Arm drift (Ask patient to close eyes and hold both arms out with palms up.)	Both arms move the same, or both arms do not move.	One arm does not move, or one arm drifts down compared with the other side.

watch the patient's hands. If one side drifts toward the ground, there is weakness on one side of the body. If both arms drift toward the ground, the patient may be experiencing a problem other than stroke.

The use of prehospital stroke scales has been well-validated by multiple studies. In fact, stroke scales are recommended by the American Stroke Association and are the standard of care in EMS systems.

Management

One of the most important management considerations for the stroke patient is rapid recognition of symptoms, early hospital notification, and rapid transport to a stroke center. Prehospital providers should identify hospitals in their region that are designated as stroke centers. Remember: *time is brain*. Circulation, airway, and breathing must be managed, as paralysis of the throat, tongue, and mouth muscles can lead to airway obstruction. Be prepared to suction the patient's airway, and provide supplemental oxygen at 2 to 6 liters via nasal cannula (unless hypoxic or in respiratory distress). Provide ventilatory support as necessary.

Position the patient with the head elevated at 30 degrees, and complete the Fibrinolytic Therapy Checklist for ischemic stroke (**Table 10-5**). If the patient is a candidate for fibrinolytic therapy and a stroke center can be reached within 3.5 hours of sign/symptom onset, the patient should be transported to that stroke center. If there is not a stroke center that can be reached within 30 minutes, the patient should be transported to the nearest

hospital. In rural areas, air medical evacuation to a stroke center should be considered. During transport, the patient should have IV access established, ECG monitored, and glucose level obtained. Basic life support (BLS) providers should not delay transport of stroke patients while awaiting advanced life support (ALS). The patient's vital signs should be frequently monitored and recorded, and a repeat neurological examination should be conducted in order to gauge the progression of symptoms.

Management of hypertension in the prehospital setting for stroke patients continues to be a controversial topic. Please refer to local protocols regarding management of these patients.

Controversy

Management of hypertension in the prehospital setting is not recommended for stroke patients.

Attitude Tip

A stroke is a traumatic and emotional event for the patient. A sensitive and compassionate approach is essential. Even though these patients may not be able to communicate with you, they may be able to understand. Communicate with them as you would any other patient—in a calm and reassuring manner.

Table 10-5 Fibrinolytic Therapy Checklist for Ischemic Stroke
All of the **"YES"** boxes and all of the **"NO"** boxes must be checked before a patient is transported to a "Designated Stroke Center."

INCLUSION CRITERIA

(**All** of the **"YES"** boxes must be checked)

YES
- 18 years of age or older
- Signs and symptoms of stroke with neurologic deficit (abnormal Cincinnati Stroke Scale)
- Patient can be delivered to a stroke center within 3.5 hours of sign/symptom onset

EXCLUSION CRITERIA

(**All** of the **"NO"** boxes must be checked)

NO
- Active internal bleeding (e.g., GI or urinary bleeding within the last 21 days)
- Known bleeding disorder
- Within 3 months of intracranial surgery, serious head trauma, or previous stroke
- Within 14 days of major surgery or serious trauma
- History of intracranial hemorrhage
- Witnessed seizure at stroke onset
- History of cancer of the brain

Transient Ischemic Attack

Transient ischemic attacks (also known as TIAs or ministrokes) are temporary disturbances of blood supply to the brain that result in sudden, temporary decrease in brain function. The symptoms of a TIA are the same as those for a stroke, but generally last less than 1 hour. Although lasting brain damage does not occur, the gravity of this condition should not be minimized in the field, as it is a warning sign of a future stroke.

Because of the short amount of time that you often have with your patient, you most likely will not be able to determine whether the patient is experiencing a stroke or a TIA. For this reason, any patient experiencing stroke-like symptoms should be treated as though he or she is having a stroke. Furthermore, patients who report a history of previous TIAs should be considered at much higher risk of having a stroke rather than another TIA, as the risk of experiencing a stroke within the 48 hours following a TIA is about 1% to 8%.

EMS providers play a pivotal role in the outcome of a stroke patient. Effective prehospital acute stroke care includes early recognition, discovery of conditions that mimic stroke (such as hypoglycemia or hypoxia), and timely transport to the most appropriate facility. Use a stroke assessment tool as appropriate, taking the patient's history into account when you are assessing the components of the scale. An older person with severe arthritis may not move as well on one side, or damage from a previous stroke may make his or her speech difficult to assess. Always ask family or caregivers for information that may help you identify deviations from the patient's normal pattern of behavior or activity.

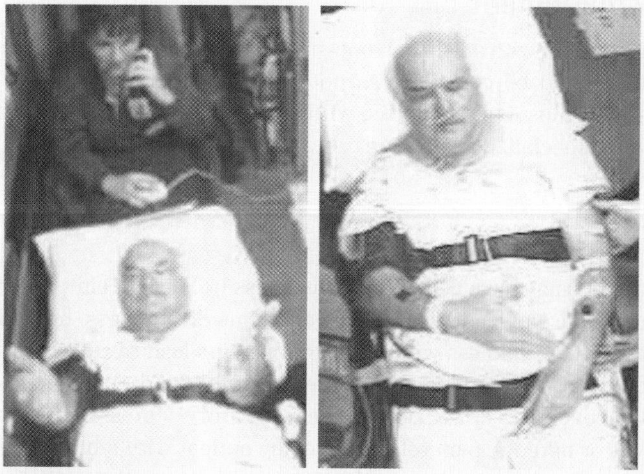

Sudden Loss of Focal Neurological Function

Loss of focal neurological function may include loss of vision, language expression, or comprehension; dysarthria (slurred speech); facial or unilateral weakness; or loss of balance in conjunction with one of these (**Figure 10-2**).

Assessment

When assessing the patient with loss of focal neurological function, consider the following key questions:

- When was the patient last known to be well (not the time the patient was *discovered* to be abnormal)?
- Are risk factors for stroke present, such as hypertension, coronary artery disease, high cholesterol, diabetes, smoking, or prior stroke or TIA? Did the patient have a previous "mini stroke" or brief loss of vision suggestive of a TIA? (Think stroke as a cause of the deficit.)
- Is there history of preceding trauma? (Think brain contusion or intracerebral hemorrhage.)
- Is there a known or previously treated cancer, or an immunocompromised state caused by cancer,

Figure 10-2 Over an 8-minute period, this patient's left arm dropped, indicating weakness from an evolving stroke. The patient survived thanks to rapid recognition and transport by EMS providers, and appropriate treatment at the hospital.

Dr. LaMonte and research team members of Telemedicine for the Brain Attack Team, University of Maryland School of Medicine

chemotherapeutic drugs, or HIV disease? (Think brain metastasis, primary tumor, or abscess.)
- Is there a preceding or current infection? (Think meningitis or encephalitis.)

In addition to taking the patient's history, assess the patient's circulation, airway, and breathing. Most patients with one-sided neurological deficits will be able to manage their airway and respiratory effort, but they may not be able to protect their airways from secretions. Mental status should also be assessed. For example, if the patient is alert, can he or she speak and understand commands? The patient who is alert but not responsive may have **aphasia**, which can be caused by stroke. See the *Communication* chapter for information on communicating with patients that have aphasia.

The following tests help to get an even better idea of what may be causing the patient's problem:

- *Speech and language.* Have the patient repeat the phrase "Take me out to the ballgame," and check for slurred speech. This test evaluates the patient's ability to understand commands, as well as formulate speech.
- *Facial strength.* Have the patient smile widely, or ask them to "show me all of your teeth." If the patient's face appears asymmetrical while performing this task, it suggests a stroke on the opposite side of the brain.
- *Body strength.* Have the patient squeeze both hands, and raise both arms and legs, equally. This test evaluates the patient's ability to perform and coordinate gross motor functions.

Management

Any patient with an abrupt, one-sided loss of a neurological function should be considered a potential stroke patient. All such patients must be transported with priority to the nearest medical center specializing in stroke care.

Generalized Weakness

Patients may have generalized weakness because of either a primary neurological disease or a general medical illness. In many cases, the weakness will be progressive and lead to a decreased ability to breathe and possible exhaustion from expending so much energy to do so. Do not give respiratory depressants (sedatives or narcotic pain relievers) to any patient with motor weakness unless you are prepared to intubate and provide ventilatory assistance. These patients are extraordinarily sensitive to any medication that interferes with the metabolism or function of nervous system tissue.

> **Medication Tip**
>
> Remember, generalized weakness can be caused or worsened by certain medications.

Assessment

For the patient who has a new complaint of general motor weakness, ask the following questions:

- Was the patient exposed to alcohol, drugs, or toxins?
- Did the patient experience preceding trauma (such as spinal cord damage)?

After establishing adequate circulation, airway, and breathing, assess the patient further for respiratory weakness, as this is the area of motor function that can most quickly create an emergency. Check for evidence of severe respiratory compromise such as paradoxical breathing, which occurs during inhalation when the patient's chest moves out while the abdomen moves in (**Figure 10-3**). Common causes of respiratory muscle weakness include acute toxin exposure and unusual diseases, such as **Guillain-Barré syndrome** and **myasthenia gravis**. Guillain-Barré syndrome typically occurs after a patient has had a viral respiratory illness. It begins with weakness in the lower extremities that progresses toward the patient's head, and may lead to respiratory insufficiency or aspiration of stomach contents from the inability to cough. For patients with myasthenia gravis, complaints will focus on rapid muscle fatigue and loss of strength following the use of a muscle or group of muscles. This condition occurs when immune system antibodies form against the patient's neurotransmitter (acetylcholine) receptors—the

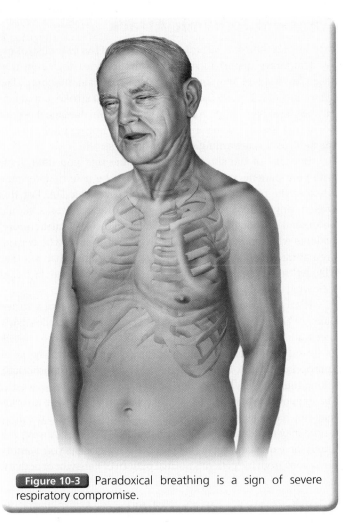

Figure 10-3 Paradoxical breathing is a sign of severe respiratory compromise.

receptors that normally allow muscles to receive the signal to contract.

Management

Even without initial signs of respiratory trouble, patients with a new complaint of weakness may deteriorate quickly. Be ready to provide oxygen as needed. If ventilatory status is inadequate and worsening, patients may benefit from intubation to protect the airway from aspiration and ventilatory support to assist with breathing.

Altered Mental Status

Altered mental status is a symptom, not a disease. As a consequence, the assessment and subsequent management of its numerous causes is complicated. Confused or disoriented patients make poor historians. They may also be unable to speak and follow commands, making assessment even more difficult.

Remember: An altered mental status is not normal. When attempting to determine a cause, the prehospital provider must consider all neurologic causes (such as Alzheimer's disease, Huntington disease, and Parkinson's disease) and endocrine changes (such as diabetes or blood glucose level fluctuations). Consideration should also be given to the possibility of a head injury (medical or traumatic), tumor, emotional disorder, eye or ear problem, heart rhythm disturbance, dementia, medication, fluid balance change (such as blood loss), respiratory disorder (such as hypoxia), hyperthermia or hypothermia, and infection.

Assessment

During assessment, rapidly determine if the patient requires immediate transport. If the patient is exhibiting signs of altered mental status, determine the onset of symptoms. Ascertain what is normal for this patient and whether the patient has a pertinent history that may be attributed to the complaint. For example, if the patient is a diabetic, has he or she taken the appropriate medications? Is it possible the patient may have taken the wrong medication or taken alcohol with medication? Could the patient possibly have taken a medication that was not prescribed to them? Because of cost concerns, many older patients try medications that are prescribed to a spouse or loved one who has a similar problem—or worse, a completely different problem.

Table 10-6 lists additional questions to ask about altered mental status.

Assess circulation, airway, and breathing. Many patients with drug intoxication, overdose, or mental status changes related to drug combinations and side effects will also have compromised vital functions and vital signs. For example, an overdose of some types of seizure medication will produce a decreased level of consciousness as well as changes in heart rate, ECG, blood pressure, and respiratory rate. Therefore, in order to identify potentially fatal changes, vital signs should be monitored closely in any patient who has overdosed on a medication.

As with loss of consciousness, examination of the patient with altered mental status centers on the AVPU scale. Always

Table 10-6	**Altered Mental Status: Key Questions**
■ Was the patient exposed to alcohol, drugs, or toxins?	
■ What is the patient normally like? When was the last time the patient was noted as having his or her baseline mental status?	
■ Did the patient complain of headache, or does the patient have a headache now?	
■ Did the patient have a preceding infection?	
■ Did the patient, or does the patient, have a fever?	
■ Has the patient had any falls?	
■ Is the patient feeling ill in any way?	
■ Is the patient adequately nourished?	

assume that an older individual who is behaving erratically, unreasonably, irrationally, or aggressively is suffering from an organic (physical) disorder until proven otherwise, as it is uncommon for mental disorders of strictly psychiatric origins to begin late in life. Most commonly, even in older individuals with a known or long-standing psychiatric disorder, a change in the usual pattern of behavior or thinking that brings the patient to the attention of EMS is a "red flag" for a medical problem. Special consideration should be given to the patient with an abnormal level of consciousness and any one of the following signs and symptoms:

- Fever
- Headache
- Neck stiffness
- Body rash

Patients with these signs and symptoms most likely have meningitis, encephalitis, or another central nervous system (CNS) infection that may be transmitted to EMS providers or future patients via respiratory droplets or contact with contaminated equipment. If a patient is suspected of having a CNS infection, appropriate protective equipment, such as masks, should be used and the ambulance should be thoroughly cleaned after the patient is transferred to the hospital staff. It may also be prudent to leave a contact number with the hospital staff, so that EMS providers can be alerted to take measures to reduce the likelihood of developing an infectious disease if the patient is diagnosed with one.

Management

For the older patient with an altered mental status, prehospital treatment should focus on ensuring adequacy of circulation, airway, and breathing. Provide supplemental oxygen. Assess for the presence of a stroke or recent trauma as the possible cause of the altered mental status. Hypotension should be managed with IV fluids, but be alert for signs of fluid overload. Lung sounds should be monitored prior to fluid therapy and frequently thereafter. Consider the possibility of hypoglycemia or a narcotic overdose. Monitor the patient's blood glucose level and provide dextrose as necessary. If a narcotic overdose is suspected, administer naloxone (Narcan) per local protocol.

Delirium

Delirium (also known as acute brain syndrome or acute confusional state) is a symptom, not a disease. This temporary state is generally a reflection of an underlying disturbance to a person's well-being (usually a physical or mental illness) and, although usually treatable and reversible, it is a true medical emergency in the older adult.

Delirium is characterized by disorganized thoughts, inattention, memory loss, disorientation, striking changes in personality and affect, hallucinations, delusions, or a decreased level of consciousness. The confusion and disorientation fluctuate with time, and hallucinations may lead to bizarre, uncharacteristic, or confusing behavior. The patient experiences a rapid alteration between mental states (such as lethargy and agitation), serious attention disruption, disorganized thinking, and changes in perception and sensation. Symptoms of delirium may mimic intoxication, drug abuse, or severe psychological disorders such as schizophrenia.

The assessment and subsequent management of delirium's numerous causes is complicated. In older people, delirium often replaces or confounds the typical presentation caused by a medical problem, an adverse medication effect, or drug or alcohol withdrawal. The EMS provider should assess for recent changes in the patient's level of consciousness or orientation, specifically looking for an acute onset of anxiety, an inability to think logically or maintain attention, and an inability to focus. Also assess for changes to vital signs, temperature (indicating infection), glucose level, and medication—all of which are frequent causes of delirium.

With delirium, the onset of confusion or disorientation is abrupt (occurring within hours to days) and generally resolves with treatment of the underlying problem. Therefore, treatment is focused on resolution of the causative disease or disorder, which may be complicated by the patient's uncooperative behavior and inability to provide an accurate medical history.

Possible causes of delirium can be determined by using the DELIRIUMS mnemonic (**Table 10-7**).

Dementia

Dementia is a condition that produces irreversible brain failure, and is diagnosed when two or more brain functions are impaired. These functions include language, memory, visual perception, emotional behavior and/or personality, and cognitive skills. Dementia affects 5% to 7% of persons aged 65 years and older, and 40% to 50% of those 90 years and older, with two thirds of assisted-living and the majority of nursing home residents having a dementia syndrome. Patients with dementia have progressive loss of cognitive function, impairments in long-term and/or short-term memory, loss of communication skills, inability to perform activities of daily living (ADLs), an increased ability to become lost (even in familiar places), and changes in temperament and affect, specifically increased anger. While dementia is not synonymous with delirium, a patient with dementia may also suffer from an acute delirium.

Signs and symptoms of dementia may take months to years to become apparent and include short-term memory loss or shortened attention span, jargon aphasia (talking nonsense), hallucinations, confusion, disorientation, difficulty in learning

Table 10-7 DELIRIUMS Mnemonic

Potential Causes	Management
D Drugs and toxins	Manage symptoms based upon the specific drug, and administer naloxone (Narcan) for respiratory depression.
E Emotional (psychiatric)	Provide emotional support.
L Low PO2 (carbon dioxide poisoning, chronic obstructive pulmonary disease [COPD], congestive heart failure [CHF], acute myocardial infarction [AMI], pneumonia, pulmonary edema)	Provide oxygen and bronchodilators as necessary and according to local protocol.
I Infection (pneumonia, UTI, sepsis)	Provide IV fluids as necessary for hypotension.
R Retention of stool or urine	Provide supportive care.
I Ictal (seizures)	Provide seizure control (per local protocol), monitor airway and respiratory effort, and provide glucose as necessary.
U Undernutrition/dehydration	Provide IV fluids and glucose as necessary.
M Metabolism (thyroid/endocrine, electrolytes, kidneys)	This cause will often be unknown in the prehospital setting, as determination requires lab values. If cause of delirium cannot be determined, vital signs should be supported, glucose and ECG should be monitored, and IV access should be established.
S Subdural hematoma (an estimated 50% of people with dementia do not remember falling)	Treat all injuries and immobilize accordingly. Consider referral to a trauma center.

and retaining new information, and personality changes such as social withdrawal or inappropriate behavior. Occasional forgetfulness such as forgetting where the car keys were put is not a sign of dementia, but locating the car keys and not knowing what they are used for is a sign of dementia.

Risk factors that may predispose a patient to dementia include a low level of education, female gender, and African American ethnicity, although these are more accurately described as correlating factors rather than causes of dementia. Disorders that cause dementia include conditions that impair vascular and neurologic structures within the brain, such as infections, strokes, head injuries, poor nutrition, and medications. The two most common degenerative types of dementia in older people are Alzheimer's disease (one of the fastest-growing health problems in the United States) and multi-infarct or vascular dementia, both of which cause structural damage to the brain. Dementia may also be the result of tumors within the brain, emotional disorders, Parkinson's disease, or **Huntington chorea**. While most causes of dementia cannot be prevented, some experts suggest that low-fat diets and exercise may help ward off vascular dementia.

Because dementia is a chronic condition, most requests for emergency care will be related to new presentation of dementia-related symptoms or inability to manage behavioral disruptions, such as angry outbursts. There is no definitive treatment for dementia, but an acute change in mental status may be related to underlying medical problems that can be treated. It is important to ascertain from caregivers the patient's baseline behaviors and abilities and to ask specifically about the changes that led them to request emergency services. Patients may provide inaccurate or conflicting information about their own conditions; information provided by the patient with advancing dementia should be checked against information provided by caregivers.

Despite the weakened physical condition of patients with dementia, you should be cautious when caring for patients with dementia-related complaints because these patients may not be able to rationally evaluate the impact of their behaviors and may attempt to harm you because of confusion or anxiety. Patients with dementia are also at an increased risk of victimization at the hand of caregivers because they are unable to accurately report injury or neglect. Caregiver stress is an additional concern when caring for patients with dementia. Over 50% of caregivers suffer from depression. Referrals to home health agencies, respite care programs, and other community services may be helpful.

Delirium Versus Dementia

Distinguishing delirium from dementia in the prehospital setting may be difficult (**Table 10-8**). The key difference is that delirium presents with a new onset and dementia is progressive. Delirium is an abrupt disorientation to time and place, usually with illusions. The mind wanders, speech may be incoherent, and the patient is in a state of mental confusion. Dementia, on the other hand, is a slow, progressive loss of awareness of time and place, usually with the inability to learn new things or remember recent events, although remote memories may be intact. Total loss of function and a regression to an infantile state may result.

To differentiate between delirium and dementia, ask the patient's family member or caregiver, "How was the patient yesterday? One hour ago?" Remember, an acute, rapid deterioration signals delirium; and a slow progression signals dementia. Furthermore, while delirium is a reversible and potentially life-threatening problem that requires extreme emergency care, dementia is a slow, progressive problem that requires support. If you suspect that the patient is experiencing delirium, the DELIRIUMS mnemonic will help in determining the cause.

Alzheimer's Disease

The most common type of dementia in the United States is Alzheimer's disease. In 2014, an estimated 5 million people in the United States had the disease and more than 500,000 older people died because of it.[4] Experts have not identified a single cause for Alzheimer's disease, but most believe it is not a normal part of the aging process. Although age is a significant risk factor (with the disease typically affecting patients older than 60

Table 10-8 Delirium Versus Dementia

Delirium	Dementia
Abrupt onset	Gradual onset
Reduced attention	Impaired recent memory
Disorganized thinking	Regression
At least two of the following:	
Reduced level of consciousness	Disjoined thinking
Perceptual disturbances (hallucinations, illusions)	Poor judgment
Increased or decreased psychomotor activity	Loss of mental function

years), it is not the cause. Additional risk factors include genetics (there is a 40% likelihood that a twin will develop the disease if his or her twin sibling has it) and decreased education (<12 years). African Americans are also more likely to develop Alzheimer's disease earlier on in life.

Alzheimer's disease begins with subtle symptoms, such as frequently losing items or difficulty recalling the names of people. With time, patients lose their ability to think, reason clearly, solve problems, and concentrate. They may forget the identities of close family members, including their spouses and children, and they may also forget their own past experiences. Alzheimer's disease symptoms may present as confusion (lack of familiarity with surroundings); changes in personality or judgment; and extreme difficulty with daily activities, such as feeding, bathing, and bowel and bladder control.

The disease cannot be cured or reversed by any known treatment or intervention, and disease progression is classified into stages. The earliest stage, mild cognitive impairment (MCI), is more accurately described as a pre-Alzheimer's stage because not all patients who develop MCI will progress to Alzheimer's disease. MCI is characterized by forgetfulness (especially forgetting earlier conversations or recent events), difficulty performing more than one task at a time, diminished problem-solving skills, and slowness performing more difficult tasks.

Early-stage Alzheimer's disease, which involves more cognitive impairment than MCI, includes having problems with language; misplacing items; getting lost on familiar routes; having personality changes; losing social skills; losing interest in previously enjoyed activities; and having difficulty performing moderately complex tasks that were once easy, such as balancing a checkbook or preparing food using a recipe.

As Alzheimer's disease progresses, symptoms become more profound and include forgetting details about current events and components of a person's life history; difficulty reading and writing; impairment in assessing danger and risk; disorganized language use and construction of nonsensical sentences; hallucinations and delusions; dangerous or violent behaviors and agitation; and difficulty performing basic tasks, like preparing simple foods, choosing proper clothing, and driving.

Another profound symptom of Alzheimer's disease is changes in sleep patterns, sometimes called "**sundowners**" (also referred to as Sundowner's Syndrome or sundowning). EMS providers may be called to a home or other residential setting for a patient who is experiencing sundowners. This symptom is defined as changes in mood and behavior that occur a few hours before or during twilight. Sundowners may be temporary or prolonged, and mild or severe. Behaviors associated with sundowners include the following:

- Pacing and/or rocking
- Restlessness and/or agitation
- Fear
- Anger
- Crying
- Depression

- Stubbornness
- Shadowing (following around a family member or caregiver)

Other, more extreme symptoms associated with sundowning include:

- Paranoia
- Wandering
- Violence
- Hallucinations
- Hiding objects

Severe or end-stage Alzheimer's disease involves forgetting things learned in the first 2 or 3 years of life. Patients in this stage can no longer understand language; recognize even close family members; or perform basic self-care tasks such as eating, dressing, and bathing. These patients may no longer interact verbally with family members or caregivers. In addition, they may require the use of medical devices, such as gastric tubes and urinary catheters, to facilitate the tasks that they can no longer perform on their own, such as eating and voiding.

Alzheimer's disease is not diagnosed by a specific test, but rather by the exclusion of other causes of dementia. The only way to truly diagnose Alzheimer's disease is by evaluating the brain tissue after death.

Treatment of Alzheimer's disease in the prehospital setting will generally revolve around supportive care and treatment of symptoms. Communicate slowly with these patients and consider other illnesses. Antipsychotics or benzodiazepines may be used for combative patients who are a danger to themselves or others; however, the use of chemical restraints should only be considered after other means of verbal containment have proven ineffective.

There are several medications used to treat Alzheimer's disease; however, none of these medications can stop the disease from ultimately progressing (**Table 10-9**). Cholinesterase inhibitors are prescribed for mild to moderate Alzheimer's disease and may help to delay or prevent symptoms from becoming worse for a limited time. They may also help control some behavioral symptoms. Cholinesterase inhibitors include Razadyne (galantamine), Exelon (rivastigmine), and Aricept (donepezil). Namenda (memantine), an N-methyl D-aspartate (NMDA) antagonist, is prescribed to treat moderate to severe Alzheimer's disease. Namenda's main effect is to delay the progression of some of the symptoms of moderate to severe Alzheimer's. It is believed to work by regulating the brain chemical glutamate. Aricept is also approved for the treatment of moderate to severe Alzheimer's disease.

Parkinson's Disease

Parkinsonism is a general term used to describe brain dysfunction that causes loss of flexibility and fluidity of posture and movement, and development of a tremor in the hands. Patients with signs of Parkinsonism, regardless of the cause, typically have decreased function of the neurons that produce the neurotransmitter dopamine in the brain. The most common primary source of this dysfunction is **Parkinson's disease**, a chronic and progressive movement disorder, caused by the loss of dopamine-producing nerve cells in the brain. The four cardinal signs of Parkinson's disease are resting tremors (the most common sign, affecting almost 70% of patients), rigidity, slowness of movement (**bradykinesia**), and postural instability.[5] Possible secondary causes of the disease include exposure to carbon monoxide, multiple strokes, brain injury such as that which occurs with boxing, and the use of antipsychotic medications to treat schizophrenia (such as haloperidol and other dopamine antagonists). The difference between Parkinsonism and Parkinson's disease is that Parkinsonism is a group of signs and symptoms associated with a decreased level of dopamine in the brain, while Parkinson's disease is a primary cause for the decreased levels of dopamine in the brain.

There is approximately 7 to 10 million people worldwide living with Parkinson's disease. An estimated one million of these people live in the United States, with 60,000 people diagnosed each year. The occurrence rate increases dramatically in patients older than 55 years, and men are 1.5 times more likely to be diagnosed with the disease.[6]

There are several medications used to treat Parkinson's disease. Sinemet (levodopa/carbidopa) is the most commonly prescribed and most effective drug for controlling the associated symptoms, particularly bradykinesia and rigidity. Dopamine agonists (Requip, Mirapex, Neupro) may be taken alone or in combination with Sinemet. Generally, dopamine agonists are prescribed first and levodopa is added if the patient's symptoms cannot be controlled sufficiently.

Symmetrel may be a helpful treatment for people with mild Parkinson's disease, as it increases the amount of available dopamine in the brain, therefore reducing the symptoms of the disease. However, Symmetrel often causes significant side effects, including confusion and memory problems. Eldepryl and Azilect help to conserve the amount of available dopamine by preventing it from being destroyed. Catechol-O-methyltransferase (COMT) inhibitors (such as Tasmar and Comtan) work by blocking COMT, another enzyme that helps break down dopamine. When COMT is blocked, dopamine can be retained and used more effectively, reducing the symptoms of Parkinson's. COMT inhibitors can also increase the effectiveness of levodopa.

Seizure Disorders

Seizures are defined as an intermittent derangement of the central nervous system due to a sudden, excessive, disorderly discharge of cerebral neurons. The discharge of neurons results in an almost instantaneous disturbance of sensation, convulsive movements, altered or impaired cognition, or a combination

Table 10-9 Medications Used to Treat Alzheimer's Disease

Drug Name	Drug Type and Use	How It Works	Common Side Effects
Namenda (memantine)	N-methyl D-aspartate (NMDA) antagonist prescribed to treat symptoms of moderate to severe Alzheimer's	Blocks the toxic effects associated with excess glutamate and regulates glutamate activation	Dizziness, headache, constipation, confusion
Razadyne (galantamine)	Cholinesterase inhibitor prescribed to treat symptoms of mild to moderate Alzheimer's	Prevents the breakdown of acetylcholine and stimulates nicotinic receptors to release more acetylcholine in the brain	Nausea, vomiting, diarrhea, weight loss, loss of appetite
Exelon (rivastigmine)	Cholinesterase inhibitor prescribed to treat symptoms of mild to moderate Alzheimer's (patch is also for severe Alzheimer's)	Prevents the breakdown of acetylcholine and butyrylcholine (a brain chemical similar to acetylcholine) in the brain	Nausea, vomiting, diarrhea, weight loss, loss of appetite, muscle weakness
Aricept (donepezil)	Cholinesterase inhibitor prescribed to treat symptoms of all ranges of Alzheimer's	Prevents the breakdown of acetylcholine in the brain	Nausea, vomiting, diarrhea

Source: Reproduced from Alzheimer's disease Medication Fact Sheet, National Institute on Aging, January 2014.

of these symptoms. Although once considered rare, seizures in patients aged 65 years and older are now remarkably common. In fact, with the exception of neonates, the highest incidence of new-onset seizures occurs in the older population. In addition, seizures are the third most common cause of neurological disorder in older people, with cerebrovascular accidents being the most common precipitant.[7]

Clinically, seizures in older people are not different from those in children, adolescents, and younger adults, except for petit mal seizures (also referred to as absence seizures), which almost never occur in older persons. However, the onset of seizures after age 65 years is more often symptomatic and associated with injury, and incidence progressively increases with each decade.

The cause of a seizure depends to a large extent on the patient's age and cognitive integrity. The most common causes in older people include cerebrovascular disease, brain cancer, head trauma, Alzheimer's disease, metabolic disorders, central nervous system infection, or multiple causes. Patients with advanced Alzheimer's disease are six times more likely to experience an unprovoked seizure.

Assessment

Obtain patient history, including answers to the following key questions:

- Was there preceding trauma?
- Has the patient had a prior stroke?
- Does the patient have a known immune-compromised state (such as from cancer, chemotherapy, organ transplant, or HIV)?
- Is the patient diabetic? (Think hypoglycemia.)
- Does the patient have other organ failure such as renal or liver failure, or myocardial infarction? (Think hypoxia or electrolyte abnormality.)
- Does the patient use alcohol? If so, when was the last drink? (If the patient is an alcoholic, consider the possibility of withdrawal as a cause of the seizure.)

Assess the patient's level of alertness. A period of confusion (postictal period) lasting minutes to hours accompanies all generalized seizures, but may not be present for partial seizures. Examine the patient for head and body trauma. Assess for fever and skin rash, as these may be clues to meningitis. Assess the pupils: They should be equal in both size and reactivity. Unequal pupils may be a sign of a serious underlying brain condition.

When the patient is alert, examine for speech, language, or motor deficit, as you would for a possible stroke patient. A focal deficit is a sign of a serious underlying brain disorder; however, patients who have had a partial seizure may show a deficit in the part of the body supplied by the area of the brain where the seizure occurred, such as in the eyes or an extremity. Immobilize the neck and spine if head or neck trauma may have occurred during a fall produced by the seizure.

Management

Patients who have an abnormal neurological examination following a seizure—especially those with fever, stiff neck, unequal pupil size, or focal motor weakness—should be urgently transported. An abnormal neurological examination may indicate the presence of an underlying medical condition such as meningitis. Remember that there will be a postictal period following the seizure; the patient will gradually become more alert and oriented, but will continue to be confused and act in an awkward manner.

All patients who are actively seizing should be protected from further injury. Remove objects around the patient and prevent the patient from falling. Patients who are seizing should never be forcefully restrained, as this may lead to injury. Once the seizure has stopped, the patient should receive oxygen. If the patient is uncooperative (which is likely because of postictal confusion), a provider can deliver the oxygen to the patient by holding a nonrebreathing mask near the patient's face.

Blood sugar should be determined if a glucometer is available, as hypoglycemia is a potential cause of seizures. If blood glucose levels are found to be low, dextrose or glucose should be administered in accordance with local protocols. An IV should also be established on the patient, in case the patient develops multiple seizures without a return to full level of consciousness between each seizure; this is a potentially fatal condition known as **status epilepticus**. If it is determined that a patient is in status epilepticus, the administration of benzodiazepines should be considered based upon local protocols, and the patient should be emergently transported to the closest appropriate hospital. In this case, pad all hard objects near the patient with pillows and blankets.

Controversy

The use of restraints is not recommended in older patients. Restraints can injure an older person's fragile skin and threaten their sense of control and independence, which is often already a major concern. However, if you are alone with a violent patient who is a threat to himself or herself, or to you, and you have tried to calm the patient without success, restraints may be considered as a last resort. If restraints are necessary, place them on the patient with extreme gentleness and care. Continue to try to calm the patient by looking him or her in the eye and using a low-pitched soothing voice. Again, this should only be done as a last resort measure, as the use of restraints is not condoned.

Lowered Level of Consciousness

The major concerns for patients with a lowered level of consciousness are airway protection and ventilator support as needed. A lowered level of consciousness may result from several causes, including trauma to the head; hypoglycemia; drug overdose; or expanding lesions within the cranium, such as an epidural hematoma. Brain herniation is a particularly dire condition that may progress from mild lethargy to coma and respiratory insufficiency in minutes. For patients who are suspected of having brain herniation, it is essential to protect the airway and provide aggressive ventilation with supplemental oxygen by nonrebreathing mask or bag-valve-mask device. These patients should also be provided IV fluids to maintain a systolic blood pressure of 100 mm Hg. Hyperventilating the patient can help reverse—or at least slow—the increase in intracranial pressure.

After attending to circulation, airway, and breathing and providing supplemental oxygen, consider determining the patient's blood glucose if a glucometer is available. If the blood glucose is low, glucose or dextrose should be administered to the patient. When a glucometer is not available and the cause of the lowered level of consciousness is unknown, consider administering glucose or dextrose and naloxone (Narcan) to the patient. After appropriate therapy has been provided in the prehospital setting, patients with a continued lowered level of consciousness should be transported emergently to the closest appropriate medical facility.

Many conditions that lead to a lowered level of consciousness are amenable to successful treatment if recognized early. Conditions that may be rapidly reversed if recognized and treated early include meningitis, encephalitis, subarachnoid hemorrhage, drug overdose, hypoxia, carbon monoxide poisoning, hypoglycemia, hypothermia, and alcoholic encephalopathy. EMS providers must recognize the need to provide immediate treatment in the prehospital setting and/or rapid transport to the hospital.

Loss of Consciousness
Assessment

History is especially important in older patients who have lost consciousness (**Figure 10-4**). Specifically, conditions for which the individual is being treated and the drugs prescribed can give significant clues to the cause. Be sure to ask about any conditions the patient might have, and document all medications the patient is taking. **Table 10-10** lists key questions to ask.

Assess the patient's circulation, airway, and breathing. Check for airway patency, chest wall motion, and adequacy of breathing and pulse. If any of these are insufficient, follow standard BLS and ALS procedures. Assess the patient's mental status using the AVPU scale. Inspect the patient's head and neck for evidence of

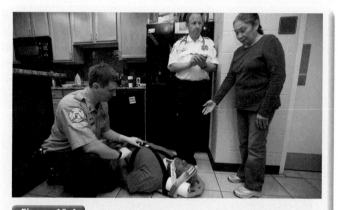

Figure 10-4 History is especially important in older patients who have lost consciousness.
© Jones & Bartlett Learning. Courtesy of MIEMSS.

Table 10-10 Loss of Consciousness: Key Questions

- Is there any possibility that the patient has experienced trauma?
- Has the patient had, or does the patient have, an infection?
- Does the patient have risk factors for cerebrovascular disease (such as hypertension, atrial fibrillation, diabetes, smoking, heart disease, or high cholesterol)?
- Did the patient complain of sudden, severe headache?
- Does the patient have a known immunocompromised state, such as from HIV, cancer, an organ transplant, or another serious chronic disease?
- Does the patient have a seizure disorder?
- Could the patient have had a drug overdose or toxin exposure? Could the patient have a problem with alcohol abuse?
- Does the patient have a history of an unstable medical condition, such as:
  - Myocardial infarction or insufficiency
  - Diabetes
  - Liver or renal failure
  - Chronic obstructive pulmonary disease (COPD) with increased carbon dioxide levels
  - Electrolyte and acid–base disorders

Source: Alzheimer's Disease Medication Fact Sheet, National Institute on Aging, January 2014.

trauma such as lacerations, **Battle's sign** (bruising behind an ear), or other hematomas or contusions, and palpate the skull for fracture (**Figure 10-5**). In addition, check the nose and ears for leaking cerebrospinal fluid or blood. Check for fever or rash suggestive of meningitis or encephalitis and, if no trauma can be assured, check for a stiff neck by having the patient touch chin to chest.

Assess further for the origin of unresponsiveness. Examine the pupils for size and reactivity: Small, reactive pupils and respiratory depression suggest narcotic overdose. If a narcotic overdose is suspected, administer naloxone (Narcan) according to local protocol. Unequal pupils may indicate **brain herniation** (protrusion of the brain through the opening at the base of the skull) caused by a space-occupying lesion, such as an intracerebral hemorrhage, in which swelling causes a rapid rise in intracranial pressure (**Figure 10-6**). A brain herniation may also appear as two fixed (unreactive) and dilated pupils if intracranial pressure is increasing on both sides. Additional conditions that can cause brain herniation include trauma, brain tumor, or brain abscess. Ultimately, a patient with brain herniation will have depressed or absent respirations and fluctuations in blood pressure and heart rate. (An increase in systolic pressure, widened pulse pressure, decrease in pulse, and irregular respiratory pattern is known as Cushing's triad.)

Never underestimate a patient with a lowered level of consciousness, as changes can rapidly occur. With proper management, however, they may be reversible.

Paraplegia and Quadriplegia

Paraplegia and **quadriplegia** are major, severe neurological deficits that require immediate and full attention. Paraplegia is paralysis of the lower half of the body, while quadriplegia is paralysis of all four limbs. Although these conditions are most often injury-related, an acute onset of paraplegia or quadriplegia may occasionally occur when an infection or disease process affects the spinal cord.

Assessment

If the patient is alert, ask if there is pain in a specific area of the spine. If the onset of the neurological deficit is not related to trauma, other causes should be explored, such as an infection along the spinal column, cancer, or a progressive disease process such as Guillain-Barré syndrome. A history of fever, weight loss, pain along the spinal column, or decreasing strength over the past several days may suggest a medical cause for the patient's neurological deficit. Regardless of the suspected cause of the deficit, all patients who present with paraplegia or quadriplegia should be moved using the logroll technique.

Circulation, airway, and breathing assessment may show signs of either respiratory compromise (high spinal cord injury) or neurogenic shock (mid- to low-cord injury). Carefully look for protrusions or areas of trauma in or around the spine. Ask if the patient has sensation in the arms and legs, and test with your fingertips (**Figure 10-7**). In addition, ask if the patient can wiggle the toes and fingers.

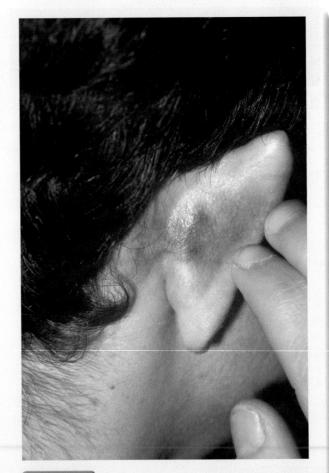

Figure 10-5 Inspect the head and neck for evidence of trauma such as lacerations, Battle's sign (shown here), or other hematomas or contusions.
© Mediscan/Visuals Unlimited

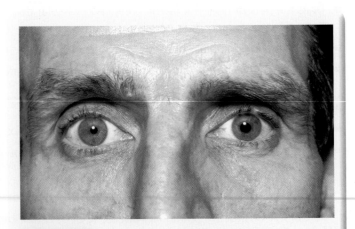

Figure 10-6 Unequal pupils may indicate rising intracranial pressure caused by brain herniation.
© Mediscan/Corbis

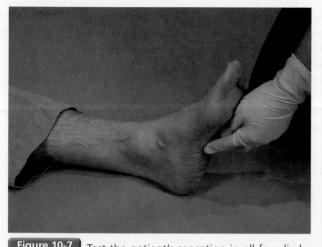

Figure 10-7 Test the patient's sensation in all four limbs by using your fingertips.
© Jones & Bartlett Learning. Courtesy of MIEMSS.

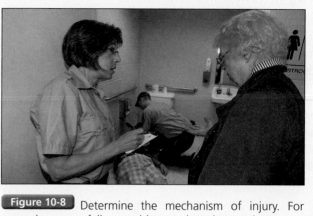

Figure 10-8 Determine the mechanism of injury. For example, was a fall caused by an altered mental status, a seizure, or poor vision or balance?
© Jones & Bartlett Learning. Courtesy of MIEMSS.

Management

If spinal cord injury is suspected, begin full-spine immobilization as soon as it is practical, using a cervical collar and backboard or other full-spine device. Because curvature of the spine is common in the older patient, forcing the patient to lie flat may lead to further injury. Instead, immobilize the patient with pillows, rolled blankets, and tape.

Head and Spine Trauma

Assessment

Determine the nature and mechanism of the injury. For instance, if caused by a motor vehicle crash, was the patient the driver or a passenger? Did the airbag deploy? If the patient was a passenger, was he or she in the front seat or the back seat? Was the patient belted or unbelted? If the cause of trauma was a fall, was the fall caused by altered mental status, a seizure, or poor vision or balance (**Figure 10-8**)? Was the individual behaving normally before the trauma? If not, what were the preceding events and behavior? If the patient is conscious, ask if there is a specific area of pain.

Assess the patient's circulation, airway, breathing, and mental status (AVPU). Check for **raccoon eyes** (bruising around the eyes), Battle's sign, blood draining from the ears, or clear spinal fluid leaking from the nose—all of which may indicate a basilar skull fracture. Check for the size and symmetry of pupils and their reaction to light. Ask the patient to repeat a sentence to assess language and speech, and then ask the patient to smile or show all of his or her teeth to evaluate facial movement. Assess sensation by testing the hands and legs with light touch. Ask about specific areas of numbness. Check whether the patient can wiggle the toes and fingers. While examining the patient, maintain spinal alignment by using the logroll technique to move the patient, and apply a cervical collar and full spinal immobilization according to standard protocol.

Management

Emergency care of head and spine trauma is covered in the *Trauma* chapter. Remember to always assume that both the brain and the spinal cord have been injured when an older person falls or is found on the ground; and transport to the nearest neurosurgical trauma center, if one is available.

Secondary Neurological Disorders

Secondary neurological disorders are disorders of the central nervous system that are caused by the influence of factors originating from outside the CNS. These disorders may be caused by toxins; hypoxia; diseases, such as cancer, that have spread to the CNS; and trauma to the brain.

Metabolic Encephalopathies from Systemic Illness

Nervous system response to systemic (bodywide) disorders is by far the most common secondary cause of neurological problems in older persons. Disorders in other organs of the body can produce secondary effects on any part of the nervous system. For example, patients with liver or kidney failure may accumulate toxins in the blood, leading to profound effects on the brain, such as confusion and stupor. Cardiovascular disorders may also present with nervous system dysfunction as the principal symptom. Patients with hypertension may complain of headache, dizziness, or confusion, and those who have cardiac disease may present with syncope. Patients with diabetes also may have signs and symptoms of central and/or peripheral nervous system dysfunction. Blood glucose levels outside the normal range may cause a change in the patient's behavior or level of consciousness.

Drug Interactions and Toxins

Drug interactions and toxin exposure are significant problems for the older population. Treatment of medical problems often involves medications that are metabolized in the liver. Thus, prior liver disease, or liver damage from chronic use of alcohol, can lead to elevated blood levels of these medications and a higher risk of adverse reactions and dangerous interactions (**Figure 10-9**). In addition, because of normal declines in liver and kidney function with aging, doses of medications that are safe in younger adults can build up to toxic levels in older adults. Many cancer therapies (chemotherapies) are also toxic to the nervous system, and effects may not be reversible.

> **Medication Tip**
>
> Liver disease or damage puts patients at higher risk for a variety of problems involving medications metabolized in the liver.

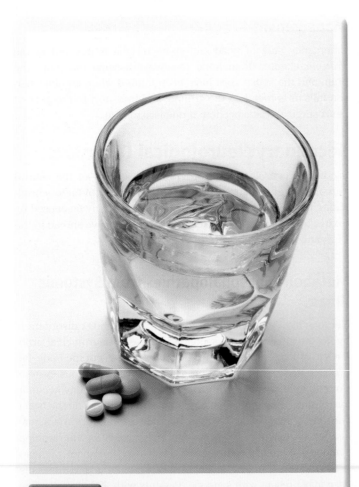

Figure 10-9 Chronic alcohol use is one cause of liver damage that can lead to elevated blood levels of liver-metabolized medications.
© DNY59/iStockphoto.com

Chronic alcohol use or abuse results in many possible secondary neurological disorders. Both acute intoxication and delirium tremens can be deadly due to their effects on the nervous system itself or from resulting trauma. Alcohol withdrawal, for instance, can produce life-threatening seizures. Chronic alcohol use contributes to a higher risk of stroke and leads to dementia, acute encephalopathy, memory loss, balance disorder due to specific effects on the cerebellum, and neuropathy and myopathy (damage to cardiac and skeletal muscle) that result in pain and weakness.

Disorders Related to Trauma

Trauma to the head and spine consumes a large portion of medical costs in the older population. Many factors contribute to injury in the older population, including diminished sensations, mental response, and physical agility. Medical disorders, depression, and drug side effects add to the older person's risk of trauma. Like stroke and dementia, brain and spinal cord injury often result in disability for the older person and the need for long-term care due to the loss of ability to perform ADLs.

Infections

Systemic disorders that occur frequently in the older population and affect nervous system function include pneumonia, urinary tract infection, cellulitis, sepsis, **meningitis**, and **encephalitis**. Each of these infections can lead to a change in mental status, presenting with signs that range from confusion to coma. Patients who have a localized infection in the brain, such as an abscess, may present with general or focal neurological dysfunction.

Cancer in the Nervous System

Most malignant tumors within the brain of adults and older patients result from metastases from other parts of the body to the brain. Tumors of the brain, whether malignant or benign, may result in general or focal neurological dysfunction due to the effect that the mass has on the surrounding structures. Brain cancer might first manifest as headache or symptoms suggestive of stroke.

Behavioral Emergencies: Intervention, Management, and Transport
Behavior That Is Potentially Threatening to the Patient

The first step in intervening and managing self-directed aggressive behavior is recognition. Be vigilant for signs of depression, such as depressed mood and somber affect. All patients suspected of depression should be assessed for suicidal thoughts. In a tactful but direct manner, ask the patient whether they have thoughts of doing self-harm; if they have a plan to enact such thoughts; and, if so, whether they have a means by which to enact the plan. (For example, "Do you think you might harm yourself?" "Have you thought about how you might harm yourself?" "Do you have a type of weapon?") Provide reassurance and stay within arm's length of a patient who has suicidal thinking (or closer if the patient is actively attempting self-harm). The *Psychosocial Aspects of Aging* chapter addresses depression and suicide in more depth.

Behavior That is Potentially Threatening to the Caregiver

Older individuals with severe depression or dementia may react with aggressive behavior toward caregivers. Patients with advanced brain disease may also become aggressive or severely agitated because they do not perceive the world normally. Aggressive behavior is often the result of internal fears that are outwardly directed. Assess the situation and the patient's response to a calm, nonthreatening manner and verbal reassurance. If the patient does not respond to these primary strategies, consider administering medication prior to transport. Haloperidol (Haldol) and midazolam (versed) are carried by some EMS systems as anxiolytic agents, as they are very effective in the management of aggressive and violent patients; however, haloperidol should be avoided in older patients (and is contraindicated in patients with Parkinson's disease). If either medication must be utilized, the initial loading dose should be reduced for the older patients.

If the situation is potentially explosive, call for police assistance. A "show of force" by a backup team provides realistic and visual assurance to the patient that aggression will be controlled, and may be all that is needed to encourage the patient to abandon the aggressive attitude.

Controversy

The sedation of violent patients (chemical restraint) is a procedure that must be undertaken carefully and only in a limited number of circumstances, especially for those older patients who may be at higher risk for adverse reactions to sedatives. Some EMS systems do not allow sedation at all. If yours does, follow local protocol and monitor the patient closely.

Uncooperative Patients and Refusal of Transport

When faced with an obviously ill patient who is uncooperative with the history and examination part of the assessment, the EMS provider will need to attempt to ascertain important information from environmental clues and witnesses. Be sure to examine the area for any medications. If head or spinal trauma is suspected in the uncooperative patient, use a cervical collar and backboard.

When a patient appears ill and refuses transport, the EMS provider must quickly assess the patient's ability to make appropriate decisions **(Figure 10-10)**. For instance, a patient with dementia may not be able to accurately judge his or her own safety. Relay this information to the appropriate supervisor or individual responsible for assisting with these decisions. In extreme cases, assistance from police officers may be appropriate.

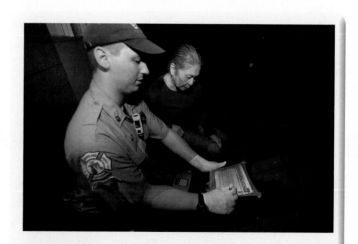

Figure 10-10 When an older patient appears ill and refuses transport, the EMS provider must assess the patient's ability to make appropriate judgments.
© Jones & Bartlett Learning. Courtesy of MIEMSS.

Summary

Neurological emergencies are the most complex aspects of geriatric emergency care. Older adults may present with abnormal neurological findings that are "baseline" for them, so it is up to the prehospital provider to determine what has changed for the patient and in what way. Do not assume the patient's problem is isolated; acute abnormal neurological signs can be the result of more than one problem.

Abnormalities that can be quickly fixed (i.e., hypoglycemia) must be treated immediately upon discovery. However, because there are so many causes of altered mental status, it is not beneficial to the patient to spend time in the field attempting to determine the underlying etiology. Remember, when treating stroke emergencies, *time is brain*. Utilizing the assessment techniques and tools identified in this chapter will greatly enhance the care of an older patient suffering a neurological emergency.

References

1. Olney RK. The Neurology of Aging, in Aminoff MJ (ed): *Neurology and General Medicine*, ed 3. Philadelphia, PA, Churchill Livingstone, 2001.
2. Centers for Disease Control and Prevention. Stroke Facts. 2014. Available from: http://www.cdc.gov/stroke/facts.htm
3. Ibid.
4. Alzheimer's Association. Alzheimer's Facts and Figures. 2014. Available from: http://www.alz.org.
5. Hauser R, Zesiewicz T. *Parkinson's Disease: Questions and Answers*, ed 3. Merit Publishing International, 2000.
6. Parkinson's Disease Foundation. Statistics on Parkinson's. 2014. http://www.pdf.org.
7. Smith M, Burns D, Robinson D. Geriatric seizures [letter to the editor]. *J Am Geriatr Soc* 2002:50(5):974–975.

Resources

Alzheimer's Association (www.alz.org)

Parkinson's Disease Foundation (www.pdf.org)

CASE STUDY SUMMARIES

Case Study 1 Summary

Your first priority, of course, is circulation, airway, and breathing. You should also be sure to obtain a thorough medication history, specifically in regards to any previous history of neurological disorders. Note any abnormal findings during the neurological examination, and utilize the Cincinnati Prehospital Stroke Scale. Based upon Mrs. Hewett's presentation, your assessment should lead you to a possible ischemic stroke. Determining when the patient was last determined to be well, or at her baseline, is critical.

If the patient can be delivered to a designated stroke center within 3.5 hours, she may benefit from fibrinolytic therapy. Determine if the patient meets all of the inclusion criteria consistent with the Fibrinolytic Therapy Checklist for Ischemic Stroke (and is ruled out for all exclusion criteria). The two most important things that prehospital providers can do for stroke patients is (1) determine that a stroke has occurred and (2) transport the patient to a designated stroke center. Other interventions for Mrs. Hewett included providing low flow oxygen via nasal cannula (maintaining oxygen saturation between 94% to 99%), obtaining a blood glucose level, and establishing intravenous access. These interventions should be completed during transport. Remember, *time is brain*.

Case Study 2 Summary

Delirium is a syndrome with multiple causes. Since you have treated Mrs. Walker previously, it is important to find out what is different since your last encounter with the patient. You know from the previous transport, the patient only takes a baby aspirin every day. She has no significant medical history and does not seem to have any significant risk factors. However, when the son provides you with his mother's hospital discharge papers from the prior week, you notice that Mrs. Walker was prescribed a narcotic analgesic for the pain caused by the shoulder fracture. You recall from the DELIRIUMS mnemonic that drugs and toxins are often the cause of a delirium state in older people, as co-morbidities and polypharmacy can make it challenging to limit side effects while controlling the older patient's pain.

You also recall that delirium is a medical emergency, and early diagnosis and treatment offers the best chance of recovery. Gathering a thorough patient history, including the patient's medication use, will aid the emergency department physician in determining the cause of the patient's delirium. In this case, you also have detailed knowledge of the patient's recent injury and change in behavior; be sure to share this information, as it will also be valuable to other healthcare providers.

CHAPTER 11

Other Medical Emergencies

LEARNING OBJECTIVES

1. Discuss the epidemiology and pathophysiology of infectious diseases in older people, including HIV and hepatitis.

2. Discuss the epidemiology, pathophysiology, assessment, intervention, and transport of older patients with sepsis and urinary tract infections.

3. Discuss age-related changes of the endocrine system, as well as the epidemiology, pathophysiology, assessment, intervention, and transport of older patients with endocrine emergencies, including diabetes and thyroid disorders.

4. Discuss age-related changes of the integumentary system, as well as the epidemiology, pathophysiology, assessment, intervention, and transport of older patients with integumentary emergencies, including pressure ulcers.

5. Discuss age-related changes of the gastrointestinal system, as well as the epidemiology, pathophysiology, assessment, intervention, and

transport of older patients with gastrointestinal emergencies, including gastroesophageal reflux disease (GERD), gastrointestinal bleeding, gallbladder disease, and problems with elimination.

6. Discuss the epidemiology, pathophysiology, assessment, intervention, and transport of older patients with nutritional emergencies, including malnutrition and dehydration.

7. Discuss age-related changes in temperature regulation, as well as the epidemiology, pathophysiology, assessment, intervention, and transport of older patients with environmental emergencies, including hypothermia and hyperthermia.

8. Discuss the epidemiology, pathophysiology, assessment, intervention, and transport of older patients with burns.

9. Discuss the epidemiology and pathophysiology of cancer in older adults.

Introduction

There are a number of medical conditions that deserve consideration in the study of geriatric prehospital care, in addition to those discussed in the *Respiratory Emergencies*, *Cardiovascular Emergencies*, and *Neurological Emergencies* chapters. This chapter discusses medical conditions that EMS providers commonly encounter when responding to the needs of older people, including conditions involving the endocrine and integumentary systems, malnutrition and dehydration, environmental emergencies, and burns.

Infectious Diseases

Older people are at increased risk of acquiring and/or dying from nearly every serious infectious disease. Many of these diseases are preventable and, if diagnosed and treated promptly, are not necessarily associated with greater mortality than those in younger adults.[1] However, in order to ensure prompt treatment is provided, EMS providers must be aware of the unusual presentation infections can have in older people.

Age-Related Changes of Immune Function

Almost every aspect of immune function is affected by age. The immune system does not wear out with age; instead, it becomes dysfunctional. Although the process is insidious and often goes unnoticed until times of physiological stress (i.e. acute illness), it causes older people to be more prone to infection and secondary complications than younger adults.[2] Chronic conditions such as diabetes, dementia, malnutrition, cardiovascular disease, chronic pulmonary disease, and cancer place older individuals at even greater risk of serious infection (**Table 11-1**).

Older people manifest infections differently than younger people. Although fever is often present in younger adults with minor illness, fever in older persons usually indicates serious infection. In many cases, the older person with infection will not have a fever; some older adults will even have hypothermia (some older adults have an oral baseline temperature of 97.4°F).[3] Therefore, when the older person's temperature is either too high or too low, the EMS provider should think infection. In many cases,

Table 11-1	Age-Related Risk Factors for Infection

- Decreased pulmonary function and cough reflex
- Decreased gastric acidity and GI motility (activity)
- Heart disease
- Thin, easily traumatized skin; skin ulcers
- Impaired immune mechanisms
- Inadequate nutrition and hydration
- Chronic use of medications
- Chronic diseases
- Urinary retention or incontinence
- Institutional living
- Need for invasive medical devices (e.g., catheters)
- Impaired access to healthcare

the only sign of underlying infection may be an acute decline in baseline functional status, with symptoms such as anorexia, fatigue, weight loss, falls, or mental status change.

Infection in Community-Dwelling Versus Nursing Home Residents

Infections in independent, community-dwelling older people often differ from those of institutionalized residents. Nursing home residents tend to acquire more serious infections because they are exposed to antibiotic-resistant bacteria that infect or colonize fellow nursing home patients. It is also easy to pass infection from person to person in the close confines of a nursing home, and health care providers with poor handwashing techniques and lack of universal precautions may carry bacteria from one patient to the next. Additionally, patients who reside in a nursing home are often sicker than those living in the community and, therefore, cannot fight off infection as well. Adding to the atypical presentation, about 50% of nursing home residents have dementia and are unable to describe symptoms.[4]

CASE STUDY 1

© 123dartist/Thinkstock

You are called to the home of a "sick person." On arrival you find a semiconscious 80-year-old female. The patient's skin is cool, moist, and pale; and she has delayed capillary refill. Her vital signs are: BP: 120/60; P: 160 and thready; R: 28 and nonlabored with an oxygen saturation of 94% on room air. You hear no audible wheezes or rales. Family members are present and concerned.

- What do you think is the problem?
- What do you need to assess?
- What would you like to ask the family?

HIV

Approximately 1.1 million people in the United States are living with HIV. In 2011, 37% of these people were older than age 50; this percentage is expected to jump to 50% by 2015.[5] Older adults are more likely than younger adults to be diagnosed with HIV infection late in the disease process. The later diagnosis may be the result of health care providers not always testing older people for HIV infection; additionally, older people may mistake HIV symptoms for those of normal aging and not consider HIV as a cause. Regardless, the occurrence leads to a late start in treatment, which can result in a poorer prognosis and a quicker progression to AIDS. An estimated 24% of people in the United States aged 25 to 29 years who were diagnosed with HIV infection in 2010 progressed to AIDS in 12 months, compared with an estimated 53% of people aged 65 and older.[6]

Many older adults are sexually active and have the same risk factors for HIV infection as younger adults, including a lack of knowledge about HIV, inconsistent condom use, and multiple sexual partners. Women and men who no longer worry about pregnancy may also be less likely to use a condom, and age-related thinning and dryness of vaginal tissue can increase the risk for HIV infection. Additionally, older adults are less likely than younger adults to discuss their sexual habits with their doctors, and doctors are often less likely to ask their older patients about these issues. The stigma associated with HIV may prevent older patients from seeking HIV care or disclosing their HIV status.[7]

Hepatitis

There are some unique differences in the epidemiology and presentation of viral hepatitis in older adults versus in younger individuals. Older adults with viral hepatitis have higher mortality rates, partly due to a higher prevalence of comorbid conditions. Additionally, physiological changes associated with aging, such as diminished immune response, metabolic derangements, nutritional deficiencies, and greater cumulative exposure to environmental toxins may also contribute to worse outcomes of viral hepatitis in older people.[8]

Data from the third National Health and Nutrition Examination Survey indicated that 31% of the United States population had previously been infected by the hepatitis A virus, with 75% of those individuals being older than 70 years of age.[9] Recovery from acute hepatitis A virus infection is usually uneventful, especially in children and younger adults, in whom the infection is often nearly or completely asymptomatic. Older adults, on the other hand, are likely to have more profound dysfunction of the liver cells, frequent jaundice and coagulopathy, and a higher incidence of complications such as prolonged **cholestasis** (slowed or blocked flow of bile from the liver), pancreatitis, and ascites.[10]

Older persons with acute hepatitis B virus infection are also likely to present differently than younger adults with the infection. For example, during an outbreak of the virus in a nursing home, most infected residents were asymptomatic; only a few presented with jaundice and non-specific symptoms such as anorexia, nausea, and vomiting.[11] Vaccination against hepatitis B virus is recommended in older persons at risk for infection, including all nursing home residents, as the risk of transmission is higher in these facilities.

Despite a decrease in the incidence of acute hepatitis C, the prevalence of chronic hepatitis C infection is increasing among older adults.[12] Most older adults with chronic hepatitis C virus infection acquired the disease earlier in life, such as from receiving blood transfusions, using injection drugs, and receiving tattoos. These patients often present with liver disease complications, mainly cirrhosis and hepatocellular carcinoma.

Sepsis

Sepsis, also referred to as septicemia or bacteremia, is the disease state that results from the presence of microorganisms or their toxic byproducts in the bloodstream. Every year, severe sepsis strikes about 750,000 people in the United States, killing an estimated 28% to 50% of these individuals.[13] Sepsis is more frequent and more often fatal in older persons. The most common infection sites in these patients are the urinary tract, abdominal cavity, skin, and respiratory tract. Risk factors include exposure to instrumentation and procedures, institutionalization, comorbid illnesses, **immunosenescence** (gradual deterioration of the immune system), malnutrition, and poor performance status.[14]

The diagnosis of infection in older people is challenging. While the presentation may be more severe in older patients than younger patients, it more commonly consists of nonspecific signs such as altered mental status, delirium, weakness, anorexia, malaise, falls, and urinary incontinence. Fever may be blunted in up to 50% of older patients with sepsis.[15] Additionally, while tachypnea and altered mental status are common among older patients with sepsis, one study reported that the incidences of tachycardia and hypoxemia were significantly lower among septic patients who were older than 75 years of age.[16]

Management

Know the subtle findings compatible with sepsis and treat abnormal vital signs. Administer high-flow oxygen for respiratory complaints, especially those accompanied by tachypnea. When patients are hypotensive, administer a fluid bolus and consider septic shock. If the patient is hot, flushed, and hypotensive, circulation is being shunted peripherally and not reaching the vital organs. In this case, fluid administration is essential. Consider sepsis whenever you encounter a hot, flushed patient who is also tachycardic and tachypneic.

The most important life-saving intervention, after ensuring circulation, airway, and breathing, is to transport the patient to definitive care for intravenous antibiotics. Just as acute myocardial infarction patients are put on the fast track to a cardiac intervention center, septic patients should be put on the fast track to receive antibiotic therapy. Be sure to get a thorough history of medications, especially antibiotics, including the type and when it was last taken. Also, obtain a thorough history of immunizations. Has the patient received a flu shot or pneumonia vaccination? Ask about the patient's exposure to disease: What illnesses is he or she in contact with? It is especially important to find out about infections in a nursing home patient's roommate and others on his or her floor.

It is essential for EMS providers to maintain universal precautions for the protection of older people. Universal precautions help to prevent the horizontal spread of infection between patients (that is, infection being spread to patients by EMS providers). For example, *Clostridium difficile* (*C. diff*) is reaching epidemic proportions in the older population due to close quarters in long-term nursing facilities, overuse of broad spectrum antibiotics, and less than optimal health care provider compliance with hand washing. Alcohol-based hand sanitizers do not kill *C. diff* fomites; only hand washing with soap and water and strict adherence to contact precautions prevents the spread of this potentially lethal disease. Be sure to disinfect equipment such as the stethoscope so it does not serve to spread bacteria. Use respiratory precautions on any patient with cough or congestion to protect yourself from infection. Congested, coughing patients usually will benefit from supplemental oxygen. Be sure to provide the correct liter flow for the device being used. An oxygen mask, fitted well to the patient's face, can serve as respiratory isolation to protect against droplet spread; however, an oxygen mask should never be used solely for respiratory isolation.

As an EMS provider, you should also make sure to receive immunizations, including a flu shot every year. This measure is more to protect the frail older person than yourself, but you will also benefit. If you do have the flu, be sure to wear a mask to stop the spread of respiratory droplets. What is a minor nuisance to you may cause sepsis in an older person.

Urinary Tract Infections

A urinary tract infection (UTI) occurs when bacteria accumulates in the bladder or kidney and causes an infection. Older people are more likely to experience UTIs as a result of having a suppressed immune system due to age and certain age-related conditions. Additionally, older adults may have weakened bladder muscles, making it more difficult to completely empty their bladder upon urination. Urine retention can result in bacteria accumulation and subsequent infections, as the bladder can serve as a **nidus** for infection and bacterial

overgrowth. Certain medical conditions can also make older persons susceptible to UTIs:

- Diabetes results in a low resistance to infections, such as UTIs.
- Urinary catheter use or surgery in an area around the bladder may cause contamination to the bladder.
- Bowel incontinence may also cause contamination to the bladder.
- An enlarged prostate can obstruct urine passage, causing urine retention.
- Kidney stones may result in inflammation and obstruction of urine passage.[17]

The typical signs and symptoms of a UTI include a frequent urge to urinate; pain or burning upon urination; cloudy or bloody urine; strong or foul-smelling urine; pressure or pain in the lower pelvis; fever; and night sweats, shaking, or chills. However, due to the effects of age, the immune system may not initiate a typical response to the infection; therefore, like with sepsis, an older person with a UTI may not present with a fever. Instead, he or she is more likely to present with poor motor skills, dizziness and falling, frequent touching of themselves, a new onset of incontinence, and behavioral changes similar to those seen in the early stages of dementia or Alzheimer's disease.[18]

Management

If left untreated, UTIs can lead to acute or chronic kidney infections that can permanently damage the kidneys and eventually result in kidney failure. These infections are also a leading cause of sepsis. Prehospital management of a patient with a UTI is symptomatic. Treatment in the hospital setting includes antibiotic therapy and the removal of infected catheters.

Endocrine Emergencies
Diabetes

The percentage of diabetic adults age 65 years and older in the United States remains high at 25.9%, with Type 2 diabetes being the most prevalent type of diabetes in this age group.[19] Diabetes in older adults is linked to higher mortality, reduced functional status, increased risk of institutionalization, and increased risk of acute and chronic microvascular and cardiovascular complications. Older adults with diabetes are less likely to present with the classic triad of diabetic symptoms: polyuria, polydipsia, and polyphagia. Instead, nonspecific symptoms, such as anorexia, weight loss, altered sleep patterns, fatigue, incontinence, and cognitive impairment, are more likely to manifest.

Diabetic complications, which occur more often in older patients, may be the presenting problem. For example, diabetic older adults have higher rates of lower-extremity amputation, myocardial infarction, visual impairment, and end-stage renal disease than any other age-group. Additionally, death from hyperglycemic crisis is significantly higher in older adults, and persons aged greater than 75 years are twice as likely as other diabetics to visit the emergency department for hypoglycemia.[20] Factors that predispose older type 2 diabetic patients to hypoglycemia include:

- Poor or irregular nutritional intake
- Altered mental status that impairs the perception or response to hypoglycemia
- Increased polypharmacy and medication noncompliance
- Dependence or isolation that prevents early treatment
- Impaired renal or hepatic metabolism
- Comorbid conditions that mask or lead to misdiagnosis of hypoglycemia (e.g., dementia, delirium, depression, sleep abnormalities, seizures, myocardial infarction, and stroke)[21]

Management

A thorough assessment, including a glucometer reading, must be performed on any older patient who presents with an altered mental status. Older patients with hypoglycemia should be treated with oral glucose or intravenous dextrose. A bolus of normal saline (500 ml/hour) should be immediately administered to older patients with hyperglycemia. Older patients receiving fluid therapy should be monitored for signs of fluid overload. In the hospital setting, patients often require many liters of fluid administration to correct dehydration and metabolic abnormalities. Admission to an intensive care setting is usually necessary due to the requirement for intravenous insulin infusions and large volume fluid resuscitation, as well as the need for close monitoring during correction of severe metabolic disturbances.

Thyroid Disorders

The main function of the thyroid gland is to secrete appropriate amounts of the hormones tetraiodothyronine (T4) and triiodothyronine (T3) (**Figure 11-1**). Thyroid hormones result in the following:

- Promotion of normal fetal and childhood growth and development
- Regulation of heart rate, myocardial contractility, and cardiac output
- Maintenance of ventilator responses to hypoxia and hypercapnia in the bloodstream
- Modulation of body energy expenditure, heat generation, and weight
- Regulation of lipid and carbohydrate metabolism
- Stimulation of bone turnover and increasing of bone resorption and formation
- Affection of gastrointestinal motility and renal water clearance

Thyroid disease is often overlooked in the older population; however, prevalence is twice that of the younger population, with **hypothyroidism** (low levels of thyroid hormones) occurring at a rate of 2% to 7% and **hyperthyroidism** (high levels of

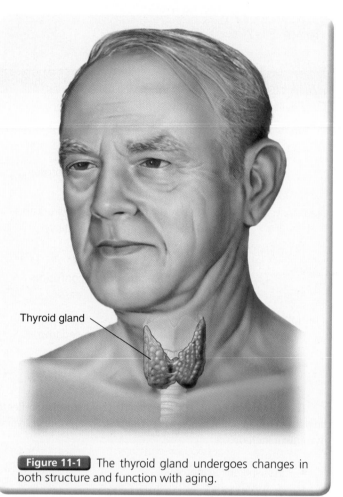

Thyroid gland

Figure 11-1 The thyroid gland undergoes changes in both structure and function with aging.

thyroid hormones) occurring at a rate of 2% in the older population. Thyroid disease manifests itself with symptoms derived from the patient's most compromised organ system; therefore, the existence of other disease(s) and the use of multiple medications often masks or mimics the presentation of thyroid disease.

Hypothyroidism in older people is most commonly the result of chronic autoimmune thyroiditis, radioactive iodine ablation, thyroid surgery, or iodine deficiency. Other possible causes include the use of amiodarone and lithium. The clinical presentation of hypothyroidism often represents the most compromised organ system in the individual affected by the disease (**Table 11-2**). Additionally, 50% of those with hypothyroidism complain of fatigue and weakness. Weight gain is usually not more than 10 to 20 pounds. Signs of hypothyroidism include:

- Puffy face
- Hoarseness of voice
- Coarse hair and hair loss
- Edema
- Dry skin
- **Macroglossia**
- Atrophic thyroid gland
- Delayed relaxation phase of deep tendon reflexes

Table 11-2	Clinical Presentation of Hypothyroidism
System	**Presentation**
Cardiovascular	■ Bradycardia ■ Diminished cardiac output ■ Low voltage QRS ■ Diastolic hypertension ■ Increased low-density lipoproteins ■ Pericardial effusion
Neuropsychiatric	■ Lethargy, fatigue, sleep disturbance ■ Poor concentration, cognitive impairment ■ Depression ■ Myxedema madness (confusion, paranoia) in severe disease
Pulmonary	■ Sleep apnea ■ Exquisite sensitivity to sedative medications

The clinical presentation of hyperthyroidism also reflects the patient's most vulnerable organ systems. Symptoms of hyperthyroidism include:

■ Nonspecific symptoms
   ■ Anorexia
   ■ Weight loss and loss of appetite
   ■ Constipation
■ Cardiovascular symptoms
   ■ Tachycardia and tremulousness
   ■ Dyspnea
   ■ Angina
   ■ Congestive heart failure and myocardial infarction
■ **Apathetic thyrotoxicosis**
■ Muscle weakness and proximal muscle wasting

Severe hyperthyroidism can lead to **thyrotoxicosis**, a condition often marked by fever, tachycardia, tremulousness, and altered mental status. Thyroid storm, the most severe form of thyrotoxicosis, is associated with organ failure and can be lethal if not promptly treated.

Treatment

When treating the older patient for hypothyroidism, full thyroid hormone replacement should not be given too rapidly, as it may put stress on the heart and central nervous system. Instead, the older patient may be given a partial daily dose of hormone at the beginning of treatment, allowing the heart and central nervous system to adjust. Side effects of treatment include increased angina, shortness of breath, confusion, and a change in sleep habits.[22]

During the treatment of hyperthyroidism, the disease's effects on other body systems should be closely monitored, as co-existing diseases are likely in older people. As with the treatment of hypothyroidism, cardiac function must be specifically observed. The patient may also receive beta-adrenergic blockers in order to control symptoms of the condition. Angina and congestive heart failure are treated at the same time in order to bring thyroid function under control.[23]

Integumentary System Emergencies

The skin, hair, and nails make up the integumentary system, the largest organ or system in the human body. Like any other body system, the integumentary system changes over time. These changes may be due to either the normal aging process or a disease state.

Age-Related Changes in the Integumentary System

The skin has two main layers: the **epidermis** (outer, protective layer) and the **dermis** (inner, living layer) (**Figure 11-2**). These layers stretch over the body, protect it from losing fluid, and provide a barrier against harmful external substances.

The epidermis is only a few cells thick (0.07 to 1.4 mm) and contains pores, pigments, and ducts. Normal changes occur to the epidermis with age. One of these changes is flattening of the dermal–epidermal junction. The dermal–epidermal junction is the connection between the two main layers that helps with communication and nutrient transfer between the layers. Flattening of the junction increases the tendency of the skin to tear or blister. In addition, the epidermis is continually shedding dead cells and gaining new cells as part of a process called epidermal turnover. By the time a person is in their 70s, epidermal turnover has declined by about 30% of what it was when the

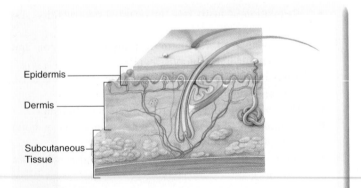

Epidermis
Dermis
Subcutaneous Tissue

Figure 11-2 The skin has two main layers, the epidermis and dermis, which are connected by the dermal–epidermal junction.

person was in their 20s. The slowing of this process affects the amount of time it takes for a wound to heal.

Attitude Tip

Proper use of a device such as a blood pressure cuff is an excellent alternative to a constricting band (tourniquet), which can damage an older person's skin during IV therapy. Another alternative to preserving the skin during IV therapy is to apply the constricting band over clothing.

The dermis has many functions, but the main ones are mechanical protection and thermoregulation, meaning this layer of skin protects the body against trauma and changes in external temperatures. Changes that occur to the dermis with age include decreases in thickness (atrophy) and blood flow. Deterioration of the ability to regulate blood flow, combined with other changes in the dermis, also impacts wound healing.

Subcutaneous fat is the layer beneath the dermis. Its major purposes are also protection and thermoregulation. The subcutaneous fat layer protects the body against trauma and pressure of the dermis, and limits conductive heat loss in order to help the body control temperature. The thickness of the subcutaneous fat layer decreases with age, affecting these functions. (Subcutaneous fat is different from total body fat, which often increases with age.) **Table 11-3** presents a summary of the changes that occur to the skin with age.

Attitude Tip

Older people are more sensitive to the cold. It is important to protect the aging patient, particularly the older trauma patient, against heat loss. Hypothermia is one of the three components of the lethal triad in trauma patients, with coagulopathy and acidosis completing the triad.

Table 11-3 Age-Related Skin Changes

Age-Related Change	Clinical Implications
Epidermis thins, with flattening of dermal–epidermal junction, limiting transfer of nutrients and making separation of layers easier.	▪ Increased tendency to blister ▪ Increased skin tearing
Slower cell turnover	▪ Slower healing of wounds
Less **melanocyte** activity, with slower DNA repair	▪ Increased photosensitivity, with increased tendency toward skin malignancy
Altered epidermal protein profile	▪ Dry, rough, and flaky skin more common ▪ Abnormal skin barrier, so more prone to irritant contact dermatitis
Altered connective tissue structure and function	▪ Reduced elasticity and strength of skin
Decreased blood flow through dermal vascular beds	▪ Skin appears cooler and paler ▪ Thermoregulation is less efficient ▪ Hair and gland growth and function slow
Subcutaneous fat decreases in volume and is distributed differently (i.e. more abdominal fat)	▪ Thermoregulation is less efficient ▪ Protection against pressure injury decreases ▪ Facial features appear more aged due to loss of facial fullness
Number of cutaneous nerve endings decreases	▪ Cutaneous sensation blunts (i.e. fine touch, temperature, proprioception) ▪ Pain threshold increases
Fewer cutaneous glands	▪ Thermoregulation is less efficient
Nail bed function decreases	▪ Nails become thick, dry, brittle, and yellow, with longitudinal ridges
The immune functioning of the skin decreases	▪ Increased risk of skin infections and malignancies

Data from Durso, Samuel C.; Bowker, Leslie K.; Price, James D.; Smith, Sarah C. *Oxford American Handbook of Geriatric Medicine*. New York: Oxford University Press, 2010, p. 610.

Pressure Ulcers

A **pressure ulcer**, also known as a decubitus ulcer, pressure sore, or bedsore, is caused by pressure that compromises the blood supply to an area of tissue, resulting in the death (infarction) of that area of tissue. This condition mainly occurs to immobile or debilitated patients, with prevalence in the United States ranging from 3.5% to 29% among hospitalized patients, 2.4% to 26% among long-term care patients, and 10% to 12.9% among home health care patients. Health care costs associated with pressure ulcers are estimated at 5 billion dollars per year for 1.5 million patients in the United States.[24]

Pressure ulcers are usually localized in areas close to a **hard site** (bony prominence), such as around the sacrum, greater trochanter, ischial tuberosity, heel, scapula, and fibular head (**Figure 11-3**). Approximately 95% of pressure ulcers occur in the lower part of the body. In addition to pressure, three key factors contribute to the development of pressure ulcers: friction, moisture, and shearing forces (forces sliding past each other in opposite directions). Shearing forces and friction may occur when an older person slides down in bed, causing the subcutaneous tissues to stretch and the blood supply to be compromised. Moisture may result from incontinence or perspiration and can lead to tissue maceration, making the skin more susceptible to pressure, friction, and shearing forces.

Pressure affects blood flow and oxygenation to the tissues between the bony prominence and the skin, first causing a failure in oxygenation and nutrient delivery to the area, followed by an accumulation of waste products, and ultimately tissue damage or death (necrosis). Time and the amount of pressure exerted are important factors in this process. For example, tissue damage can occur after enough pressure to affect the blood flow is applied for approximately 2 hours, but with higher pressure, the amount of time required to cause damage decreases. The damage also depends on the person's general health and the type of tissue affected. Muscle and subcutaneous tissues are more susceptible to pressure and hypoxia than epidermal tissues. Therefore, damage usually first occurs in the underlying tissues and is not clearly visible in the epidermis.

Any factor that increases exposure to pressure in the hard sites of the body increases the risk for pressure ulcers. Conditions that affect mobility, such as spinal cord injury, brain injury, neuromuscular disorders, or any acute or chronic illness that makes the person less active, increase the risk for a pressure ulcer. Problems with nutrition, fecal or urinary incontinence, and neuropathies also can significantly increase the risk for pressure ulcers.

Clinical Stages

Pressure ulcers can be classified in four different stages (**Table 11-4**). These stages represent the severity of the sore (**Figure 11-4**). A Stage I pressure ulcer is a **nonblanching erythema**. At this stage, the skin will be intact, as the damage is occurring underneath the skin. Additionally, applying gentle pressure with a finger to the area of tissue redness will not produce blanching (whiteness) during Stage I. In Stage II, the sore may appear as a superficial ulcer or blister, as the damage

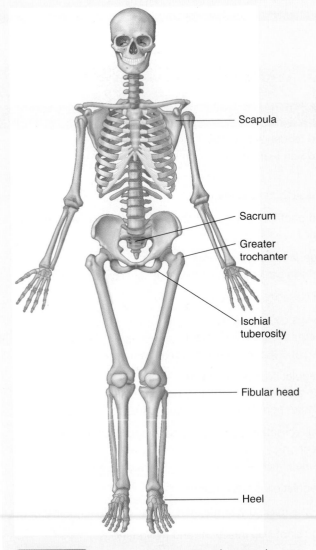

Figure 11-3 Pressure ulcers commonly occur in areas around the scapula, sacrum, greater trochanter, ischial tuberosity, fibular head, and heel.

Table 11-4	Pressure Ulcer Stages
Stage	**Description**
I	Nonblanching erythema, with damage beneath the skin
II	Blister or ulcer affecting the epidermis and dermis
III	Ulcer exposing the fat down to the fascia
IV	Ulcer exposing muscle or bone

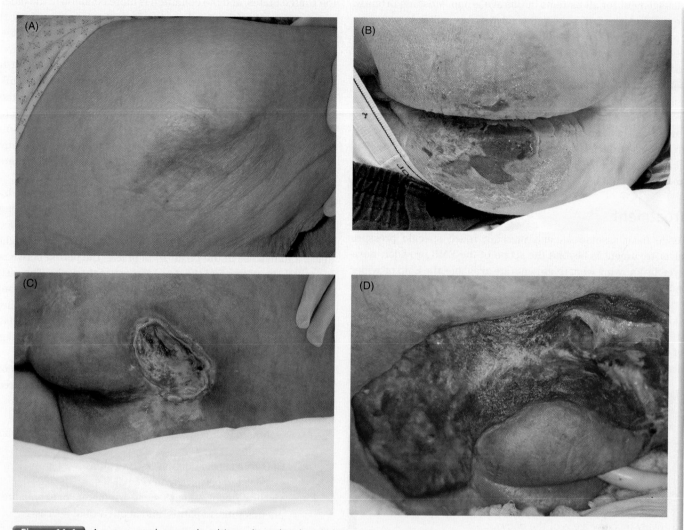

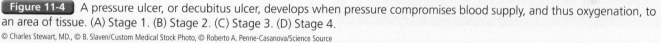

Figure 11-4 A pressure ulcer, or decubitus ulcer, develops when pressure compromises blood supply, and thus oxygenation, to an area of tissue. (A) Stage 1. (B) Stage 2. (C) Stage 3. (D) Stage 4.

© Charles Stewart, MD., © B. Slaven/Custom Medical Stock Photo, © Roberto A. Penne-Casanova/Science Source

extends through the epidermis and dermis. In Stage III, the epidermis, dermis, and subcutaneous tissues are affected, and fat is visible at the base of the ulcer. In Stage IV, the ulcer extends into muscle, tendons, or bone.

On occasion, an ulcer cannot be classified due to scar tissue formation or a covering of black, dead tissue (**eschar**), which makes it difficult to know how deep the ulcer is. Therefore, in addition to noting the stage of the ulcer, it is important to describe the surrounding structure, location, appearance, and size. This will help in treating the sore, following its progress, and communicating with other health care professionals.

Complications

Development of pressure ulcers has been associated with an increased risk of death, due to either an underlying clinical problem that led to the ulcer, or as a complication of the ulcer itself. Approximately 60,000 people die each year from pressure ulcer complications. In addition to pain and discomfort in the affected area, complications include bleeding, cellulitis, sepsis, and **osteomyelitis** (inflammation of the bone caused by infection)—all of which occur more commonly in Stage III and Stage IV. Any nonhealing ulcer should be evaluated for signs of infection, especially osteomyelitis, as this condition can affect healing of the infection if not appropriately treated. The diagnosis of osteomyelitis is made with x-rays or a nuclear medicine bone scan. A secondary complication, wound-related **bacteremia**, can increase the risk of mortality to 55%.[25]

Prevention and Care

Prevention should be targeted at persons with risk factors for pressure ulcers, but because nearly all older people will have thinning skin, it is prudent to practice good preventive skin care management for all patients in this age group. Most importantly, decreasing pressure, especially on hard sites, will help prevent a pressure ulcer from developing. One way EMS providers can help decrease pressure is by placing a blanket on the backboard prior to immobilizing older patients. Prevention can also be achieved with careful positioning prior to long transports. The goal is to spread the maximal areas of pressure over a large region, with frequent changes of position to promote mobility and use of pillows to cushion areas of high risk, such as the sacrum and heels, from hard surfaces. It is also important to inspect the skin regularly and avoid friction or tearing forces, excessive moisture, and skin irritants.

Treatment

Aside from assessment and pressure relief, specific pressure ulcer treatment is beyond the scope of the EMS provider; however, by knowing what treatments are available, the EMS provider is better able to educate patients, family members, and caregivers. The primary treatment is relieving pressure from the area of skin damage to allow the growth of new skin. Infections must be treated, and dressing will depend on the stage and characteristics of the ulcer. In addition, all of the preventive measures previously discussed must be followed during treatment (**Table 11-5**).

> ### Attitude Tip
>
> A patient can develop pressure ulcers after lying on a hard surface, such as a backboard, for 2 hours. Anytime you are caring for an immobile patient for 2 hours or more, relieve discomfort and reduce risk by finding safe ways to reposition the patient. When possible, avoid hard surfaces and package the patient with pillows to relieve pressure, particularly on bony areas of the body.

Infection in the Aging Skin

Herpes Zoster

Herpes zoster (shingles) is caused by the reactivation of the varicella zoster virus, the virus that causes chickenpox, on nerve roots. Infection rates have gradually increased among adults in the United States, and the condition is more common in the older population, with risk sharply increasing after 50 years of age.[26] Most people with herpes zoster are in good health, but those with cancer or immunosupression are at higher risk.

People with herpes zoster most commonly have a rash on one or two adjacent areas of skin, particularly in the trunk area. This is known as localized zoster. Less commonly, the rash is more widespread, affecting three or more areas of skin; this is known as disseminated zoster, a condition that is difficult to distinguish from varicella. Disseminated zoster generally occurs only in people with compromised or suppressed immune systems.

The rash caused by herpes zoster is usually accompanied by pain, itchiness, or tingling, with symptoms sometimes preceding the rash by days to weeks. Some people may also experience headaches, photophobia (an intolerance or sensitivity to bright light), and malaise in the **prodromal** phase (the period between the initial symptoms and the development of the rash). The rash develops into clusters of clear **vesicles**, with new vesicles forming over three to five days and progressively drying and crusting over. Although there may be permanent pigmentation changes and scarring on the skin, the rash usually heals in two to four weeks.

Postherpetic neuralgia is the most common complication of herpes zoster and is characterized by a persistent pain in the area where the rash once was. Additional complications include:

- Ophthalmic involvement with acute or chronic ocular **sequelae**
- Bacterial superinfection of the lesions
- Cranial and peripheral nerve palsies
- Visceral involvement, such as meningoencephalitis, pneumonitis, hepatitis, and acute retinal necrosis[27]

In addition to these complications, people with compromised or suppressed immune systems are more likely to have severe, longer lasting rashes.

People with active lesions caused by herpes zoster can spread the varicella zoster virus to susceptible people, such as those who have not had chickenpox and never received vaccination. The virus spreads through direct contact with active herpes zoster lesions. If this occurs, the person is at risk of developing varicella rather than herpes zoster.

Table 11-5	Pressure Ulcer Treatment
1.	Assess the stage of the ulcer.
2.	Relieve pressure.
3.	Assess and manage nutritional status.
4.	Cleanse ulcer at each dressing change.
5.	Provide pain relief.

Gastrointestinal Emergencies

Age-Related Changes in the Gastrointestinal System

Although aging does not have as much of an effect on the gastrointestinal system as it does on other organ systems, there are certain changes worth noting. For example, older adults are prone to having poor dentition, a factor that closely relates to the gastrointestinal system. Poor dentition results in an increased risk of aspiration (due to an inability to chew food properly) and all forms of pneumonia (aspiration and non-aspiration type pneumonias). A decrease in the strength of the esophageal sphincter also weakens the ability to hold back stomach contents. The stomach lining is no longer able to resist damage as it once was, increasing the older person's risk of developing peptic ulcer disease. Additionally, the stomach cannot accommodate as much food due to a decrease in elasticity, and gastric emptying occurs at a slower rate.

Function of the small and large intestine changes little as a consequence of age, although the incidence of certain bowel disease increases. The movement of contents through the large intestine slows and the strength of the rectal sphincter muscles decrease; for this reason, along with the result of dehydration, medication side effects, and low fiber intake, constipation is a common condition in the older population.

The liver undergoes a number of changes with age, many of which play a role in medication absorption. For example, there is a decrease in the liver's blood flow and ability to metabolize many substances, causing some drugs to stay active longer and have more side effects than they would in younger people. Additionally, the liver becomes less able to withstand stress and repair damage; therefore, toxic substances are likely to cause more damage than in younger people. The gallbladder also changes with age, with the production and flow of bile decreasing, making older adults more likely to develop gallstones.

Gastroesophageal Reflux Disease (GERD)

Gastroesophageal reflux disease (GERD) is a chronic digestive disease that occurs when stomach acid or, occasionally, stomach content, flows back into the esophagus. The backwash (reflux) irritates the lining of the esophagus. Reflux may increase with use of medications that alter esophageal sphincter tone and gastric emptying (such as alpha-adrenergic antagonists, calcium channel blockers, nitrate vasodilators, and anticholinergic agents).[28]

GERD is common in older people, with typical symptoms including dysphagia (difficulty swallowing), vomiting, and breathing difficulties. Less frequent symptoms include acid regurgitation and heartburn.

Treatment

The condition is treated with proton pump inhibitors, prokinetic drugs, and bicarbonated mineral water hydration (**Table 11-6**).[29] Additionally, symptoms may be relieved or avoided if the patient takes the following measures:

- Eating smaller low-fat meals
- Not eating late at night
- Maintaining an upright position after eating
- Sleeping propped up in bed

Table 11-6 Proton Pump Inhibitors

Generic Name	Brand Name
Dexlansoprazole	Dexilant
Esomeprazole	Nexium
Lansoprazole	Prevacid
Omeprazole	Prilosec, Zegerid
Pantoprazole	Protonix
Rabeprazole	Aciphex

- Smoking cessation
- Avoiding alcoholic and/or carbonated beverages

Gastrointestinal Bleeding

Gastrointestinal bleeding becomes more common with age for a number of reasons. Physiologic changes may lead to an increased likelihood of bleeding systemically. Additionally, pathologic processes may impact the digestive system, and co-morbid illnesses are more likely. Older adults are also more likely to take ulcerogenic medications such as NSAIDs. Minor gastrointestinal bleeding in the older population is often caused by hemorrhoids and colorectal cancer, whereas major bleeding may be the result of peptic ulcer disease, diverticular disease, or angiodysplasia.[30]

Upper Gastrointestinal Bleeding

Upper gastrointestinal bleeding occurs when there is bleeding from the esophagus, stomach, or duodenum (**Figure 11-5**). Most older patients with acute upper gastrointestinal bleeding present with either hematemesis (vomit with blood), melena (blood in the stool), or both; however, the initial presentation may be light-headedness, postural hypotension, or syncope.

Peptic ulcer disease is the most common cause of upper gastrointestinal bleeding in older adults, accounting for more than 90% of hospitalizations for upper gastrointestinal bleeding.[31] The risk of bleeding from this disease increases with the use of anticoagulation therapy. There has also been a significant increase in patients presenting with upper gastrointestinal bleeding while on NSAIDs or aspirin, with an estimated 50% or more of older adults using one of these drugs at the time of an episode.[32] Additionally, chronic alcohol use can lead to cirrhosis of the liver, which may cause large veins (varices) to form in the esophagus. These veins can rupture and result in massive bleeding. Stomach cancer or esophageal cancer can also produce upper gastrointestinal bleeding. Recent weight loss or difficulty swallowing should raise suspicion of an underlying cancer as the source of bleeding.

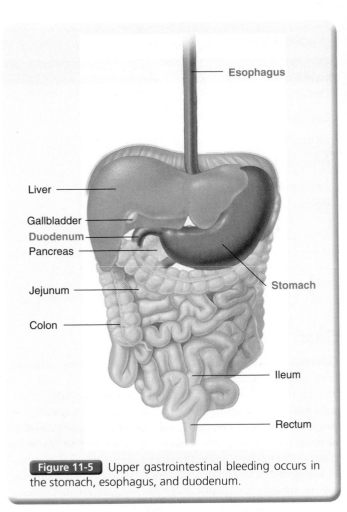

Figure 11-5 Upper gastrointestinal bleeding occurs in the stomach, esophagus, and duodenum.

Patients may report **dyspepsia** as a presenting symptom of peptic ulcer disease; however, a gnawing, burning pain in the upper abdomen can also signal a myocardial infarction. A 12-lead ECG should be obtained in older patients presenting with these symptoms. The use of NSAIDs may decrease the pain from peptic ulcer disease and, as a result, the patient may not report abdominal pain. The absence of abdominal pain often delays diagnosis of the disease until complications, such as hemorrhage, perforation, or pyloric stenosis, have developed. These complications, along with the presence of a serious comorbid illness (such as cardiovascular disease, chronic obstructive pulmonary disease, and renal failure), are associated with higher mortality rates in the older patient.

In assessing older patients with upper gastrointestinal bleeding, note any underlying risk factors such as NSAID or alcohol use. Determine the severity of the bleeding based on the history, physical presentation, and vital signs. Tachycardia and hypotension in an older patient with hematemesis or melena represents severe upper gastrointestinal bleeding, and is a true medical emergency. Additionally, remember that many older people are more likely to take blood-thinning medications such as warfarin (Coumadin), which can make the bleeding even more severe.

Medication Tip

Medications can be major contributors to gastrointestinal bleeding problems. Nonsteroidal anti-inflammatory drugs and alcohol often cause gastrointestinal bleeding, and blood thinners such as warfarin make it more severe.

Lower Gastrointestinal Bleeding

Lower gastrointestinal bleeding primarily describes bleeding from the colon and rectum (**Figure 11-6**). The incidence of lower gastrointestinal bleeding increases with age due to an increased incidence of diverticular disease, colonic neoplasms, angiodysplasia, and ischemic colitis.

Diverticulosis, a condition characterized by the presence of diverticula (pouchlike protrusions from the bowel), is primarily found in older people (**Figure 11-7**). The prevalence of diverticula increases from less than 5% at age 40 to 65% by age 85. Most patients with the condition are asymptomatic; however, an estimated 3% to 5% will present with **hematochezia** (bright red blood in the stool). Risk factors include the use of NSAIDs, a

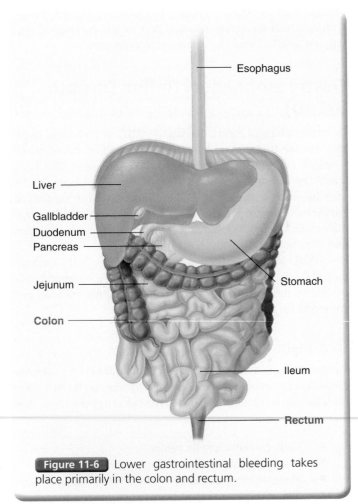

Figure 11-6 Lower gastrointestinal bleeding takes place primarily in the colon and rectum.

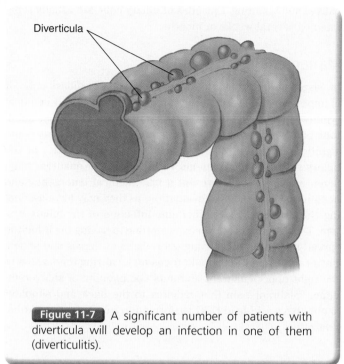

Diverticula

Figure 11-7 A significant number of patients with diverticula will develop an infection in one of them (diverticulitis).

lack of fiber in the diet, constipation, and age. Diverticular hemorrhage carries a morbidity and mortality of 10% to 20% in older people.[33]

Some people with diverticulosis will develop an infection within a diverticulum, a condition known as diverticulitis. The typical symptoms of diverticulitis are left lower quadrant abdominal pain and fever. Rarely, the pain will be in the right lower quadrant. Diarrhea may also be reported. Chronic inflammation around the walls of the colon may result in fistula (an abnormal connection) formation between the colon and surrounding organs. For example, people who describe the release of fecal material when they urinate have developed a fistula between the colon and bladder. Diverticulitis can also result in perforation of the colon and spillage of fecal material into the abdominal cavity. These patients will often present with peritonitis and septic shock.

When assessing patients with left lower quadrant pain, ask if there is a known history of diverticulosis. Many older people have undergone colon cancer screening with flexible sigmoidoscopy or colonoscopy, and may recall being told they have diverticulosis. It is also important to assess for the presence of fever. Those without fever can usually be treated as outpatients and given oral antibiotics if they are able to consume liquids without vomiting; however, those with fever will likely require a computer tomography (CT) scan and hospitalization for IV antibiotics. On abdominal exam, a palpable mass in the lower abdomen may represent a large abscess that has formed from a perforated diverticulum. The development of peritoneal signs represents a surgical emergency that requires immediate attention.

Inflammatory bowel disease (IBD) is another common cause of lower gastrointestinal bleeding. Approximately 10% to 30%

of people with IBD are older than 60 years of age, and incidence decreases with age.[34] The two main types of inflammatory bowel disease are Crohn's disease and ulcerative colitis. Studies indicate that about 33% of all new cases of **Crohn's disease** occur in the older population.[35] The inflammation caused by Crohn's disease can occur anywhere in the gastrointestinal tract but most commonly presents in the small and large intestines. Symptoms typically include abdominal pain, rectal bleeding, and weight loss.

Ulcerative colitis is characterized by inflammation and ulcer formation within the colon. The rectum is generally involved; however, inflammation may extend into the upper parts of the colon. When inflammation is restricted to the rectum, the disease is known as ulcerative proctitis; when the entire colon is involved, it is referred to as pancolitis or universal colitis. Symptoms of ulcerative colitis include bloody diarrhea and abdominal pain, which are intermittently recurring and range from mild to severe. Although the cause of the condition is unknown, treatment involves medications and, depending on the severity of the condition, surgery.

Ischemic colitis is another type of colitis. This condition is characterized by reduced blood flow to the colon due to narrowed or blocked blood vessels. Most people with ischemic colitis will present with an acute onset of mild abdominal pain and tenderness over the affected bowel. Post-prandial pain is a very common symptom of chronic mesenteric ischemia. The urge to move the bowels is also common, and passage of bright red or maroon blood, often mixed with stool, usually occurs within 24 hours.

Assessment of the patient with lower gastrointestinal bleeding should begin by identifying risk factors such as a history of previous bleeding, symptoms or signs suggestive of colon cancer, recent constipation or diarrhea, and use of medications such as blood thinners. Determine the severity of the bleeding based on the history, physical presentation, and vital signs. Minor lower gastrointestinal bleeding is characterized by small amounts of red blood covering formed brown stools, or scant amounts of red blood noticed on the toilet paper. Patients with minor lower gastrointestinal bleeding will have normal vital signs and usually do not require admission to the hospital, though they should be evaluated in the emergency department. Severe lower gastrointestinal bleeding is characterized by passing significant amounts of red blood or maroon-colored stools. Patients may describe the whole toilet bowl as appearing full of red blood. In the most severe cases, tachycardia and hypotension will be present; these findings indicate a severe medical emergency.

Treatment

Both hematemesis and hematochezia should be considered an emergency. Prehospital treatment is directed at airway maintenance, adequate oxygenation, and restoration of circulating volume. A major cause of morbidity and mortality in patients with upper gastrointestinal bleeding is breathing problems resulting from aspiration of blood; therefore, if the patient with upper gastrointestinal bleeding is unconscious or has an inadequate gag reflex, endotracheal intubation should be considered. Additionally, IV fluids should be initiated for any patient with hypovolemia or hemorrhagic shock due to upper or lower gastrointestinal bleeding. Definitive care hinges upon identifying the source of bleeding and achieving hemostasis. Most patients will have the source of bleeding identified and controlled with either an 'upper' endoscopy (esophagogastric-duodenoscopy [EGD]) or a 'lower' endoscopy (colonoscopy); however, some patients will require a nuclear medicine bleeding scan or angiogram (mesenteric catheterization). Bleeding which cannot be controlled by these methods often requires operative intervention.

Gallbladder Disease

The prevalence of gallstones is higher in the older population than in any other age group. Older adults are also at greater risk than younger adults of developing complications from gallstones. The risk of death during surgical removal of the gallbladder (cholecystectomy) increases with age.

Pain from the gallbladder, or biliary pain (also known as **biliary colic**), is the classic symptom of gallstone disease. Patients with biliary colic typically complain of sharp right upper quadrant pain (**Figure 11-8**). Ingestion of fatty food can trigger a painful episode, as the gallbladder contracts in response to fatty particles entering the digestive tract. The pain, which may radiate to the back and the right shoulder, may cause

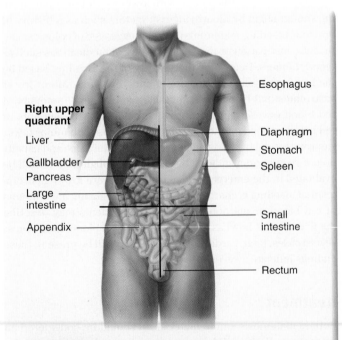

Right upper quadrant

Liver

Gallbladder

Pancreas

Large intestine

Appendix

Esophagus

Diaphragm

Stomach

Spleen

Small intestine

Rectum

Figure 11-8   Older patients with sharp right upper quadrant pain may have biliary colic, which indicates gallbladder disease. Right upper quadrant pain with fever can be a sign of infection of the gallbladder or biliary system.

nausea and vomiting. Episodes of biliary colic are usually separated by several weeks or months.

Management

In assessing older patients with complaints of biliary colic, it is important to determine the presence of fever and jaundice (yellow appearance of the eyes and skin). Right upper quadrant pain with fever is a worrisome combination that could signify an infection of the gallbladder (**cholecystitis**) or the biliary system. Older patients with right upper quadrant pain, fever, and jaundice represent a true medical emergency and need immediate medical evaluation, as they may have ascending **cholangitis**, an overwhelming infection of the biliary system. These patients are very susceptible to having the infection spread to the blood, causing overwhelming sepsis and shock. Physical examination should focus on localizing tenderness to the right upper quadrant. Patients complaining of sharp right upper quadrant pain that radiates to the back and shoulder should have a 12-lead ECG performed to rule out a myocardial infarction.

Colorectal Cancer

The incidence of colorectal cancer doubles each successive decade between the ages of 40 and 80. Consequently, older people are disproportionately affected by colorectal cancer. Individuals over the age of 65 years have an age-adjusted colorectal cancer incidence rate of 254 per 100,000 persons compared with 18 per 100,000 in individuals under the age of 65 years.[36]

Screening for colorectal cancer involves a colonoscopy, which requires proper bowel preparation to be successful. Two types of bowel preparations have been traditionally used for colonoscopy: polyethylene glycol electrolyte lavage solution (PEG) and, to a lesser degree, oral sodium phosphate (OSP). Adverse reaction to bowel preparation solutions may occur; common adverse reactions associated with PEG include dizziness, fecal incontinence, abdominal pain, and nausea.

Problems with Elimination: Constipation and Fecal Incontinence

Chronic constipation, characterized by unsatisfactory defecation due to infrequent stools, difficult stool passage, or both, is a frequent problem in the older population and is even more frequent among older adults residing in long-term care facilities. Contributing factors of constipation in the older adult may include the following:

- Increased use of certain medications (such as anticholinergic agents, opioid analgesics, calcium supplements, calcium-channel blockers, and NSAIDs)
- Dietary changes (such as poor fluid intake, poor nutritional intake, and diets low in fiber and high in protein and fat)

- Impaired mobility
- Neurological or cognitive disorders such as Parkinson's disease
- Stroke
- Spinal cord disease
- Dementia
- Depression
- Metabolic factors[37]

Fecal incontinence is also a common gastrointestinal complaint in people aged 65 years old and older. It is an under recognized problem in both community-dwelling and institutionalized older people. Fecal incontinence is not an inevitable consequence of aging; instead, it may indicate a more serious condition, such as constipation, excessive laxative use, diarrhea, muscle damage, nerve damage, dementia, Alzheimer's disease, rectal cancer, rectal prolapse, and complications resulting from surgery involving the rectum and anus.

EMS providers are often called to transport older patients (especially from long-term care facilities) to the emergency department for issues involving fecal impaction. Recurring constipation and/or fecal incontinence contributes to a lower quality of life for the older person, as well as medical complications such as fecal impaction, rectal bleeding, ulcerations within the colon, and volvulus.

Malnutrition and Dehydration

The term *malnourished* is commonly used, but there is no real uniform definition of malnutrition. The most common form of malnutrition in the Unites States is obesity, although this is generally not how the term is used. More often, it describes a person who is very thin (low weight) or losing weight, is losing or has low muscle or fat mass, is eating poorly, or has abnormal blood "markers" of nutritional status such as cholesterol, albumin, and prealbumin. However, many of these characteristics and markers can also be associated with diseases not related to nutrient intake, further adding to the complexity in defining who is malnourished. What is important for the EMS provider to determine is whether or not the individual may be *undernourished*, a condition in which the provision of extra nutrients would be beneficial.

Many older people have an increased risk for malnutrition compared with other adult populations. It is estimated that between 2% and 16% of community-dwelling older people are nutritionally deficient in protein and calories. If mineral and vitamin deficiencies are added to this estimate, the rate of malnutrition in persons over the age of 65 may be as high as 35%. Additionally, studies suggest that malnutrition deficiencies exist in 20% to 65% of hospitalized older patients and 30% to 60% of older patients in long-term care facilities; up to 55% of older people admitted to the hospital have preexisting evidence of malnutrition.[38]

To understand nutrition and hydration in older people, remember that certain age-related changes can affect fluid and nutrient needs and utilization. For example, with aging, total body water content decreases, and energy requirements drop because of lower muscle mass (**Figure 11-9**). Sedentary behavior can worsen muscle loss, so that even less energy is used. The "drives" to eat and drink may also be weaker in older people due to the diminished senses of taste and smell, and there is some evidence that the perception of thirst lessens even when dehydrated. Additionally, a compromised ability to sense temperature changes can contribute to the older person failing to seek a cooler environment and increase fluid intake during a heat wave; changes in kidney function can result in the inability to concentrate urine and conserve water even with significant dehydration.

Age-related changes in body composition, senses, and water handling predispose an older person to malnutrition and dehydration, particularly when illnesses or injuries that affect the ability to eat and drink are also present. Illness, injury, or medication intake that limits mobility or causes fever, diarrhea, sweating, swallowing disorders, or confusion may adversely affect oral intake of food and fluids.

Although the ideal body weight is somewhat higher in older individuals than in younger individuals, it is well known that very high and very low body weights are associated with higher morbidity and mortality. Similarly, dehydration is associated with a higher morbidity and mortality in the older population, with hospitalized older patients having seven times the mortality rate of patients of the same age with normal water balance.

CASE STUDY 2

© 123dartist/Thinkstock

Mrs. Flowers is an 82-year-old female with Alzheimer's disease who lives alone in her own home and only receives assistance for house work. She sees her family doctor every 6 months and has maintained her weight for 1 year while taking a cholinesterase inhibitor; however, her most recent check-up revealed a weight reduction of 3 kg since her last doctor's visit. Patient height: 160 cm; weight: 48 kg; BMI: 19 kg/m².

1. Should the patient's recent weight loss be a concern to you?
2. What could be some of the causes for the patient's weight loss?
3. What information should be gathered and reported to the emergency department physician?

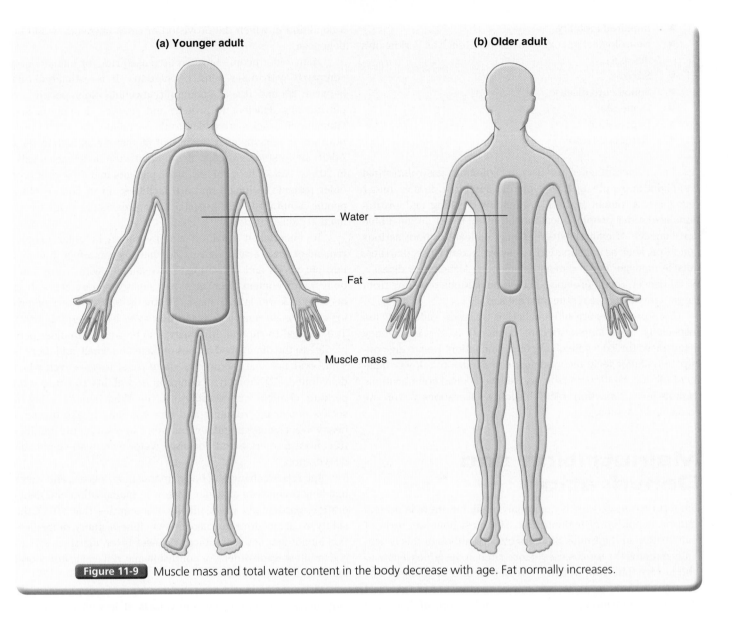

(a) Younger adult **(b) Older adult**

Water

Fat

Muscle mass

Figure 11-9 Muscle mass and total water content in the body decrease with age. Fat normally increases.

Fortunately, hydration problems have been more extensively studied, and there is less debate over what constitutes volume depletion (dehydration).

Assessment

A comprehensive assessment of nutritional status includes **anthropometric** measurements, laboratory values, physical exam, and patient history. The Geriatric Depression Scale, Mini Mental Exam, and Mini-Nutritional Assessment Short-Form (MNA-SF) are tools that can be used to assess areas that affect diet and nutrition. The MNA-SF is a screening tool used to identify older adults who are malnourished or at risk of malnutrition (**Table 11-7**). The exam, which does not require any laboratory data, consists of six questions regarding the person's food intake, weight loss, mobility, psychological stress

or acute disease, dementia or depression, and body mass index (BMI).

Part of ascertaining the older person's nutritional intake is determining whether he or she is able to obtain, prepare, and eat food. Examine the patient and the environment for signs of abuse and neglect. Check if the refrigerator contains food for the person to eat. On examination, note whether the teeth are in poor condition or if dentures are loose-fitting and contributing to weight loss.

The clinical assessment for dehydration is challenging; older people may have some signs of dehydration due simply to their age, and other common signs may not manifest until dehydration is very severe. Thus, determination of dehydration requires quite a bit of detective work and may, at times, be unclear until laboratory values are available. Signs to look for include dry mucous membranes, flat neck veins, increased heart rate or low blood

Table 11-7   Mini-Nutritional Assessment

Screening

A. Has food intake declined over the past 3 months due to loss of appetite, digestive problems, chewing or swallowing difficulties?
0 = Severe decrease in food intake
1 = Moderate decrease in food intake
2 = No decrease in food intake

B. Weight loss during the last 3 months
0 = Weight loss greater than 3 kg (6.6 lb)
1 = Does not know
2 = Weight loss between 1 kg and 3 kg (2.2 lb and 6.6 lb)
3 = No weight loss

C. Mobility
0 = Bed or chair bound
1 = Able to get out of bed/chair but does not go out
2 = Goes out

D. Has suffered psychological stress or acute disease in the last 3 months?
0 = Yes
2 = No

E. Neuropsychological problems
0 = Severe dementia or depression
1 = Mild dementia
2 = No psychological problems

F1. Body Mass Index (BMI) (weight in kg)/(height in m2)
0 = BMI less than 19
1 = BMI 19 to less than 21
2 = BMI 21 to less than 23
3 = BMI 2
3 or greater

If BMI is not available, replace question F1 with question F2. Do not answer question F2 if question F1 is already completed.

F2. Calf circumference (CC) in cm
0 = CC less than 31
3 = CC 31 or greater

Screening Score (maximum 14 points)
12–14 points: Normal nutritional status
8–11 points: At risk of malnutrition
0–7 points: Malnourished

Data from: Mini Nutritional Assement, Nestle Nutritional Institute. www.mna-elderly.com

pressure, absence of urine output, or a weight that is significantly less than the patient's usual weight. Evaluation of skin turgor ("tenting"), though useful in children and younger adults, is very unreliable in older patients. **Table 11-8** summarizes assessment for malnutrition and dehydration.

Management

Malnutrition and dehydration are not generally the main reason EMS is called for an older patient; however, these conditions are important to address to prevent later illness. Dehydration is not

Table 11-8   Assessment for Malnutrition and Dehydration

	Malnutrition	Dehydration
Who is at high risk?	■ People with reduced mobility that affects shopping and/or cooking ■ People who are housebound ■ People living alone ■ People who are showing symptoms of depression ■ People with dementia ■ People recovering from serious illness or a condition likely to affect their ability to eat (i.e. stroke) ■ People with dental and mouth problems that make eating difficult and painful	■ People who are dependent on others for provision or access to fluids ■ People who have swallowing problems ■ People who have a raised temperature or are sweating ■ People with diarrhea and/or vomiting ■ People who have taken part in strenuous physical activities
Signs and symptoms	■ Losing weight unintentionally ■ Eating and/or drinking less than usual ■ Choking or swallowing problems ■ Constipation or diarrhea ■ Inability to keep warm ■ Dizziness or prone to falls ■ Difficulty recovering from an illness ■ Signs of pressure ulcers or dry skin ■ Prone to recurrent infections ■ Difficulty chewing or swallowing ■ A sore mouth or tongue, or bleeding or swollen gums	■ Eating and/or drinking less than usual ■ Strong smelling urine ■ Regular complaints of headaches ■ Feeling of tiredness ■ Dry mouth, lips, or eyes ■ Lack of concentration and/or easily distracted ■ Confusion ■ Constipation ■ Prone to urinary tract infections ■ Regularly thirsty

well tolerated in older people; abnormal vital signs must be treated as soon as possible. If the patient is not mentating well and blood pressure is low, intravenous fluids will be required until the patient is stabilized. Early transport is particularly urgent if your level of certification does not enable you to provide intravenous therapy. At times, establishing intravenous access can be difficult in an older person whose veins tend to roll and may be collapsed because of low blood volume. Because of concern for underlying cardiac, pulmonary, or renal diseases in the older patient, monitor fluid administration closely to avoid overhydration.

The patient's ECG should be monitored as well. Evaluate the patient's glucose; if low, administer dextrose 50% (D50) according to local protocol. Pay special attention to the skin condition of an undernourished or dehydrated person, as it may be very thin and easily subject to tears and pressure ulcers. Treat the skin gently when preparing the patient for transport.

Prevention

The EMS provider can help the older person avoid significant health problems by understanding malnutrition and dehydration, using the appropriate assessment tools, and making referrals. Community-dwelling older people may not know who to call for assistance or may be reluctant to do so themselves, so it is vital that EMS providers understand what resources are available. In-home delivery of meals (Meals on Wheels), adult day care enrollment, or senior center programs can provide the older person with access to nutritional meals.

For older people with difficulty chewing or swallowing, poor appetite, signs of depression, or indications of a medical reason for poor consumption of food or fluid, referral for medical evaluation is warranted. Furthermore, if there is evidence of an increased need for oral hydration, such as for a patient with diarrhea or who has been exposed to a very hot environment, education to promote proper hydration is in order.

Attitude Tip

Pay special attention to gentle handling of the skin in an older patient who may be undernourished or dehydrated; the skin will be particularly vulnerable to tears and pressure ulcers.

Environmental Emergencies

Age-Related Changes in Temperature Regulation

Older people are at increased risk of experiencing life-threatening disturbances of temperature regulation due to a number of normal age-related changes. In order to maintain a constant core body temperature, the **hypothalamus**, the control center for thermoregulation, receives input from **thermoreceptors** throughout the body (**Figure 11-10**). A rise in core body temperature stimulates the anterior hypothalamus, causing blood vessels to dilate and the body to sweat; conversely, a drop in body temperature stimulates the posterior hypothalamus, causing blood vessels to constrict and muscles to shiver. These normal homeostatic mechanisms help individuals regulate body temperature during extremes of cold or heat.

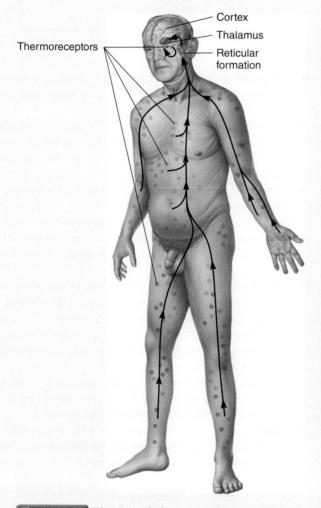

Thermoreceptors

Cortex
Thalamus
Reticular formation

Figure 11-10 The hypothalamus works in conjunction with thermoreceptors throughout the body to minimize changes in body temperature.

In healthy younger people, the body regulates its core temperature to maintain a near-constant level of about 98.6°F (37°C), regardless of environmental conditions; however, with age, the baseline core body temperature decreases and the ability to thermoregulate diminishes.

These changes result in greater temperature variability among the older population, making variation from 98.6°F (37°C) an unreliable indicator of the presence of hypo- or hyperthermia. Additionally, changes in sweat glands cause a progressive decrease in the older person's ability to perspire (**Figure 11-11**). Nutrition, disease states, and the effects of medication may further influence core body temperature. Other environmental conditions and assessment factors also must be taken into consideration.

Hypothermia

Hypothermia, a reduction in the body's core temperature to < 95.0°F (< 35.0°C), is a preventable medical emergency usually caused by prolonged exposure to cold temperatures without adequate protective clothing. Older adults are especially vulnerable to hypothermia because their bodies' response to cold is often diminished by the aging process. For example, a drop in body temperature causes muscles to shiver in order to generate heat, but by the age of 70, 30% of a person's muscle mass is lost, thereby decreasing the amount available to shiver. Another source of heat generation, the release of catecholamines, is also diminished in older people due to the steady decline in normal metabolism. The lack of heat-generating ability is compounded by the older person's tendency to have less insulation (thinner skin, less hair, and less subcutaneous fat).

Chronic medical conditions and certain medications also affect the older person's ability to cope with colder environments. Diabetic patients are six times more likely to suffer from hypothermia, in part due to vascular disease that alters thermoregulatory mechanisms. Patients with impaired heart function are also more susceptible to hypothermia because of common medications used to control their disease (such as beta blockers). Additionally, people with mobility problems may not be able to seek shelter from the cold, and patients with dementia may not know how to make themselves warmer when they are cold.

The signs and symptoms of hypothermia vary. Assessment findings are typically not specific and may suggest other conditions, including metabolic disorders and stroke. Patients may present with confusion, weakness, tachycardia (early sign), hypertension (early sign), lower core body temperature, and shivering (however, this sign may not be present due to the normal aging processes previously described).

Management

Persons 75 years old or older are five times more likely to die than others with hypothermia and can become hypothermic

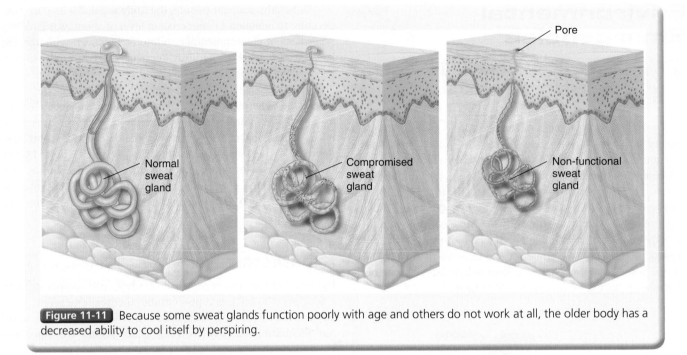

Figure 11-11 Because some sweat glands function poorly with age and others do not work at all, the older body has a decreased ability to cool itself by perspiring.

indoors, even in mildly cool buildings with temperatures from 60 to 65 degrees. To reduce this risk, the home thermostat should be set to at least 68 to 70 degrees. If the older person does become hypothermic, treatment is the same as other age groups. Crucial measures include stabilization of circulation, airway, and breathing and removal from the cold environment. Avoid rough handling of the patient to minimize the chance of triggering abnormal heart rhythms, and when resuscitating cold patients, remember that a patient is not dead until warm. Follow local protocol for resuscitation of hypothermic patients.

Hyperthermia

Hyperthermia is an increase in the body's core temperature due to inadequate thermoregulation that occurs when the body is unable to get rid of heat buildup, often as a result of hot and humid environmental conditions. Three major types of heat illness may occur as a result of hyperthermia: heat cramps, heat exhaustion, and heatstroke. Heatstroke, the most severe form of heat illness, is considered a profound emergency. Patients typically present with confusion, irritability, and combativeness.

The older population is at particular risk for the effects of hyperthermia as the result of a number of factors:

- *Self-care problems.* Frailty, reduced mobility, and mental illness can make it difficult for a person to provide adequate self-care in hot weather.
- *Living alone.* There is no one to take care of the older person if symptoms are ignored.

- *Physical changes.* On hot days, for example, the skin of an older person is not able to produce sweat and cool the body as efficiently as younger skin.
- *Chronic medical problems.* Certain conditions make the body more vulnerable to heat stress, such as cardiovascular disease, pulmonary disease, and diabetes.
- *Medications.* Certain medications can hinder the body's ability to regulate temperature.
  - Antidepressants, antihistamines, phenothiazines, and anticholinergics act on an area of the brain that controls the skin's ability to produce sweat.
  - Beta blockers reduce the ability of the heart and lungs to adapt to stresses, including hot weather.
  - Amphetamines raise body temperature.
  - Diuretics, by acting on the kidneys and encouraging fluid loss, can quickly lead to dehydration in hot weather.
  - Opioids and sedatives can reduce a person's awareness of physical discomfort, which may lead to symptoms of heat stress being ignored.
- *Kidney conditions.* Those persons with chronic kidney problems should consult with their physicians before increasing fluid intake in hot weather.

People over the age of 50 years account for 80% of all deaths from heat stroke, and these emergencies are 12 to 13 times more common in people 65 years and older. **Figure 11-12** summarizes the number of heat-related deaths in the United States from 1999 to 2003 and illustrates the fact that the number of deaths rise exponentially in those over age 65 years. This fact is further strengthened by the following examples:

- In August 2003, a 2-week long heat wave in France resulted in the death of 11,000 people, the majority of which were older adults.
- In the summer of 2010, 1,700 people died from a heat wave that occurred in Japan; of those deaths, 80% were persons over the age of 65 years.
- In 2013, a heat wave rolled through the northeastern United States, killing four people in New York; all of these victims were in their 80s.

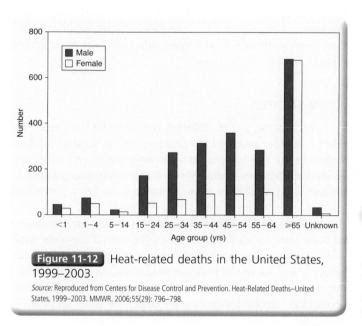

Figure 11-12 Heat-related deaths in the United States, 1999–2003.

Source: Reproduced from Centers for Disease Control and Prevention. Heat-Related Deaths–United States, 1999–2003. MMWR. 2006;55(29): 796–798.

Management

Heat cramps, heat exhaustion, and heatstroke are treated the same in older patients as they are in younger patients. The pulse rate of older patients with heatstroke is most often very slow and thready, and the patient usually presents with hypovolemia.

Prevention

Heat- and cold-related deaths are preventable. EMS providers can help to minimize environmental emergencies in older people by doing the following:

- Provide access information to shelters, during both cold and hot seasons.
- Initiate "well-being checks" for older people known to be living by themselves during cold and hot seasons.
- Partner with local health and aging agencies to provide public information to older people on how to minimize exposure to the elements and ultimately reduce the chances of suffering an environmental emergency.
- When time permits on a call to an older person's residence, check to see that home heating or cooling systems are working.

Burns

According to the National Center for Health Statistics, 3,445 deaths were caused by fire in 2010. Of these deaths, 35% occurred in people age 65 years or older.[39] The risk of death or injury from fire increases with diminished senses (such as seeing, hearing, and smelling) and limited mobility. Older people with infirmities, such as those that confine them

CASE STUDY 3

© 123dartist/Thinkstock

On a fall evening, you are called to the home of a 90-year-old male. You are greeted at the door by the patient's granddaughter. She explains that she lives at the home and is her grandfather's care provider, making sure he takes his medications, has meals served to him, and is generally safe. During the day, she leaves her grandfather to go to work, but he normally manages quite well at home alone; however, today when she got home she found him confused and acting unusual.

The granddaughter takes you to a living room with large windows and beautiful views facing east, south, and west. The room is sunny, bright, and quite warm. A frail older man is sitting on a couch covered with a blanket. He is mumbling to himself. He responds when you use a loud voice and touch, but he does not seem to make sense when he speaks. You note he is wearing multiple layers of clothing: several long-sleeved shirts, long underwear, thick pants, and long socks.

The granddaughter tells you the patient has COPD, CHF, and diabetes; and that he was recently started on a diuretic and diphenhydramine (Benadryl) to help him sleep. His other medications include a beta blocker and antidepressant. His granddaughter sets up his medications and keeps them in a locked cabinet. The patient's vital signs are: BP: 100/50; P: 160; R: 28 with oxygen saturation of 94%; T: 104.6°F. His skin is hot, dry, and flushed. Finger stick glucose is 95, and lungs are clear. Monitoring shows sinus tachycardia and the 12-lead ECG is unremarkable.

- What could be the cause of the patient's unusual behavior?
- How should this patient be treated?

to a wheelchair, may have difficulty reacting to a fire threat. Additionally, older people with Alzheimer's disease, dementia, and other disorders that affect mental functions may be unable to recognize a fire hazard, or they may behave erratically or dangerously when faced with fire.

Use of alcohol and medications that cause drowsiness, affect judgment, or do not combine well with alcohol also increase the risk of fire injury or death. Older adults who combine medications and alcohol, or who abuse alcohol, are at risk of starting a fire, or not responding quickly enough to extinguish or escape from a fire.[40] Additionally, because older people have a diminished sense of pain, they often do not seek timely treatment when injured by fire.

Flame is the main cause of burn injury. Other causes include scalds, thermal contact, steam, and inhalation. Significant determinants of mortality following burn injury include the presence of inhalation injury, burn size, and age, with inhalation injury being the most significant predictor of mortality. The risk of morbidity and mortality from burn injuries increases in older persons that have thin skin, poor circulation, low body mass, malnourishment, comorbid conditions, decreased pulmonary reserve, and/or increased susceptibility or impaired response to infection.

Management

The overall approach to burn management for the older adult is the same as for younger adults. There are, however, some special factors that should be taken into consideration. For example, all older adults with third-degree (full thickness) burns or second-degree (partial thickness) burns greater than 10% of the total body surface area should be referred to a burn center.

Fluid resuscitation is a critical component of the early care of a burn patient and should be administered to older people with burns greater than 5% of the total body surface area.[41] Prehospital care providers can begin this therapy at the scene of the burn. The Consensus formula (formally referred to as the Parkland formula) is preferred for fluid resuscitation. According to this formula, lactated Ringer's solution should be administered 4 mL/kg/% burn, with the first half given over the first 8 hours and the second half given over the next 16 hours. Over the second 24 hours, colloid solution should be administered 0.5 mL/kg/% burn plus 5% dextrose in water 2,000 mL.

A patient with both a large, deep burn and a profound inhalation injury, or a patient in whom resuscitation has been delayed, may require significantly more fluid than predicted by the Consensus formula. Underresuscitation of a burn patient can lead to complications such as hypovolemic shock, renal failure, and the conversion of partial-thickness wounds to full-thickness wounds. Additionally, older burn patients require more fluid to avoid hypovolemia and resuscitate the same burn size of that in a younger patient. To ensure adequate fluid resuscitation, mean arterial pressure (MAP) should be maintained above 60 mm Hg.

A word of caution: overresuscitation of a burn patient can also lead to complications, including compartment syndrome, pulmonary edema, congestive heart failure, acute respiratory distress syndrome, prolonged periods of ventilation, and increased mortality. The older burn patient with underlying disease, lower cardiac output, or impaired renal function will be even less tolerant of fluid overload.[42] Therefore, the EMS provider should consult the closest burn center when beginning fluid resuscitation and must be extremely careful when administering large volumes of crystalloid solution to an older burn patient.

Older persons with inhalation burns require the same aggressive approach used for the treatment of inhalation burns in younger adults. Wound care is also extremely important in older burn patients. Maintaining as sterile an environment as possible is paramount, as the risk of infection is great. Older burn patients are often undertreated for pain, partly due to their decreased pain sensation and the clearance of narcotic analgesics; these patients should receive adequate pain management for their burns.

Prevention

Prevention is the key to reducing fire-related deaths and burn injuries in older people. EMS providers are in an ideal position to discuss fire and burn safety with older people and their caregivers. Safe living environments for the growing older population are necessary for injury prevention. Fire and burn prevention programs are essential in achieving this goal.

Working smoke alarms should be strongly encouraged in all homes and living facilities. However, even if the older adult with a hearing impairment resides in a home with an operable smoke alarm, he or she may not hear the alarm and, therefore, may not respond quickly enough. Smoke alarms with built-in or separate strobe lights may be more beneficial and can be purchased through many home improvement store websites. BRK/First Alert, Gentex, and Kidde brands offer this type of smoke alarm. Additional smoke alarm accessories, such as bed/pillow shakers, transmitters, and receivers, are available through www.lifetonesafety.com, www.safeawake.com and www.silentcall.com (**Figure 11-13**). Make sure any smoke alarm or accessory device in use has been labeled by a recognized testing laboratory.

In addition to smoke alarms, homes should be equipped with carbon monoxide alarms. Heating systems are associated with the largest percentage of non-fire carbon monoxide poisoning fatalities. Smoke and carbon monoxide alarm batteries should be changed twice a year, and smoke and carbon monoxide alarms should be replaced every 10 years. Fire and EMS personnel can replace the batteries or alarms for older people who are not physically able. **Table 11-9** provides resources that can be utilized when discussing burn and fire prevention with older adults.

In addition to ensuring working smoke and carbon monoxide alarms, a complete home safety inspection can ensure the older persons living environment is fire safe. See **Table 11-10** for a home inspection checklist.

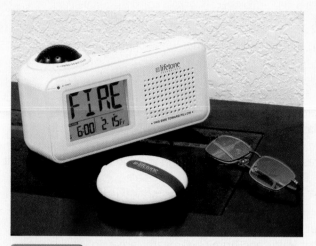

Figure 11-13 A bedside fire alarm with a low-frequency sounder and bed shaker, such as this unit manufactured by Lifetone Technology, can aid the hearing impaired in the event of a fire alarm activation.

Lifetone Technology

Cancer

Cancer is a group of diseases characterized by the uncontrolled growth and spread of abnormal cells. Older adults have a high risk for cancer and other diseases that may affect cancer treatment, care, and recovery. The incidence of cancer development in this age group is 11 times that of younger individuals; in the last 30 years, the incidence has increased 26% in the over-65 years population,

compared to 10% in the younger population. Additionally, while cancer-related mortality has decreased by 5% in the younger population, it has increased by 15% in the older population, with 70% of all cancer deaths occurring in the over-65 years population.[43]

Breast cancer, prostate cancer, colon cancer, lung cancer, and non-Hodgkin's lymphoma are common types of cancer in the older adult. Despite the fact that cancer occurs most often in the older population, older adults often receive less frequent cancer screenings and testing, milder treatments or no treatment at all, and are significantly under-represented in cancer clinical trials.[44]

Older people with cancer often have a different set of concerns than other adults with cancer, and these unique concerns may affect how patients cope with their disease. Co-existing conditions often influence how cancer treatment affects the person's prognosis, ability to deal with side effects, and recovery from treatment:

- Heart conditions, such as congestive heart failure, high blood pressure, arrhythmia, and a decrease in heart function, may reduce the person's ability to deal with the physical effects of treatment. Additionally, medications for these types of conditions may interact with chemotherapy.
- Chronic obstructive pulmonary disease and decreased lung function affect how well the body handles certain medications. Smoking may make chemotherapy less effective, increase the person's risk of developing lung problems after surgery, and increase recovery time.
- Alcohol or drug dependency can interfere with the ability to make treatment decisions and follow through with taking medication and having important screenings or

Table 11-9	Fire and Burn Prevention Resources for Older Adults	
Agency	**Resource/Program**	**Web Address**
American Burn Association	■ Cooking Safety for Older Adults ■ Fire and Burn Safety for Older Adults	http://www.ameriburn.org/preventionEDRes.php
Electrical Safety Foundation International	■ Home Fire Safety for Older Adults: A Safety Awareness Program Toolkit	http://esfi.org/index.cfm/page/Home-Fire-Safety-for-Older-Adults-Safety-Awareness-Program-Toolkit/cdid/12821/pid/11406
National Fire Protection Association	■ Remembering When: A Fire and Fall Prevention Program for Older Adults	http://www.nfpa.org/safety-information/for-public-educators/education-programs/remembering-when
U.S. Consumer Product Safety Commission	■ Safety for Older Consumers: Home Safety Checklist	http://www.cpsc.gov/PageFiles/122038/701.pdf
U.S. Fire Administration	■ Fire-Safe Seniors program ■ Fire Safety Checklist for Older Adults	http://www.usfa.fema.gov/prevention/outreach/older_adults.html

Table 11-10 Home Safety Checklist

Home: General	<ul><li>Install smoke and carbon monoxide alarms throughout the home. Remember: change your clock, change your battery.</li><li>Have an emergency escape plan.</li><li>Post emergency contact information near a telephone for emergency responders.</li><li>If living in an area prone to natural disasters, prepare a disaster kit (water for 3 days, list of medications, copy of insurance policies, flashlight, battery operated radio, extra hearing aid batteries).</li><li>Make sure walking surfaces are flat, slip-resistant, free of objects, and in good condition to prevent falls from occurring.</li><li>Install ground fault circuit interrupters (GFCIs) in potentially damp locations (kitchen, bathroom, garage, outside receptacles).</li><li>Make sure lighting is adequate throughout the home.</li><li>Keep electrical cords out of the flow of foot traffic and from underneath carpeting.</li><li>Do not overload extension cords. (Standard 16-gauge extension cords can carry 1625 watts. Discard older extension cords that use small 18-gauge wires).</li><li>Check for loose rugs, runners, and mats. Double-sided tape may be used to keep them in place.</li><li>Keep all portable space heaters and wood-burning heating equipment at least 3 feet away from walls, furniture, and other flammable or combustible materials. Portable space heaters should be stable and located away from walkways.</li><li>Have a nightlight between the bed and the bathroom for use at night.</li><li>Make sure stairwells are well lit.</li></ul>
Kitchen	<ul><li>Keep a fire extinguisher in the kitchen.</li><li>Do not cook while wearing loose-fitting clothing or clothing with long-hanging sleeves.</li><li>Ensure that the stove area is free of clutter.</li><li>Ensure that stepstools are stable and in good working order.</li></ul>
Living room and family room	<ul><li>Have fuel burning appliances, including furnaces and chimneys, inspected by a professional every year to make sure they are working properly and not leaking carbon monoxide.</li><li>Make sure all candles, smoking materials, and other potential fire sources are located away from curtains, furniture, and other flammable or combustible objects and never left out unattended.</li></ul>
Bathroom	<ul><li>Equip all bathtubs and showers with non-skid mats or surfaces that are not slippery and have at least one secure and easily graspable grab bar.</li><li>Make sure the bathroom floor is slip-resistant or covered with slip-resistant materials.</li><li>If grandchildren are in the home, keep medications out of their reach.</li></ul>
Bedroom	<ul><li>Never smoke in bed.</li><li>Ensure that electrically-heated blankets are not folded, covered by other objects, or "tucked in" when in use. The power cord should not be pinched or crushed and the cord should be removed from the wall outlet when not in use.</li><li>Keep a flashlight within reach of the bed in case of a power outage.</li><li>Keep a telephone within reach of the bed in case of an emergency.</li></ul>
Basement and/or storage area	<ul><li>Make sure the water heater is set to no more than 120°F.</li><li>Do not store containers of flammable and combustible liquids inside the house.</li><li>Do not operate portable generators in the basement, garage, or anywhere near the house.</li></ul>
Entryway	<ul><li>Make sure the porch, entryway, and approach to the entryway are well-lit.</li><li>Make sure outside steps and entryways are in good condition and slip-resistant.</li><li>Make sure outside steps have handrails that are easily graspable.</li></ul>

Data from: U.S. Consumer Product Safety Commission's "Safety for Older Consumers-Home Safety Checklist, Publication 701.

tests. In addition, alcohol or drug use often increases recovery time.

- Depression, anxiety, and other mental health issues also may interfere with the ability to make treatment decisions. Additionally, some antidepressants and anti-anxiety medications interact with chemotherapy.
- Difficulty with pain and immobility caused by conditions such as arthritis can affect the person's ability to get to doctors' appointments or receive certain treatments. Pain and immobility may also increase the risk of side effects.
- Older adults with memory loss, confusion, or a change in thought process may have difficulty keeping track of medications and appointments.[45]

Comorbidities affect the treatment selections for cancer and the type and severity of treatment side effects. Cancer treatments can also worsen existing conditions or cause new conditions in the older person. For example, chemotherapy can worsen heart problems, while radiation therapy given near the heart or in conjunction with chemotherapy can cause heart problems. Aging kidneys may also have difficulty processing some types of chemotherapy, increasing the person's risk of developing kidney problems and preventing some older adults from

receiving intense treatment. Chemotherapy may worsen anemia, potentially resulting in longer recovery times and delays in receiving further treatment. Difficulty absorbing nutrients from food can also be made worse by chemotherapy, especially if treatment causes nausea, vomiting, or diarrhea.

Additionally, older people with cancer may be concerned about being able to take care of themselves and feeling in control of their life. Those who need help accomplishing activities of daily living are even less able to tolerate the stress of cancer treatment. Having to rely on others for care may be overwhelming and, in some cases, impossible, especially if there are no family members or friends around to act as caregivers. By understanding what tasks the older adult can and cannot perform, it is easier to identify which form of treatment is most appropriate and how much supportive care the person will need.

Additional concerns of the older person with cancer may include spiritual and religious issues regarding treatment, limited financial resources to pay for treatment, and resulting limitations on physical abilities and mobility. The EMS provider must take the time to evaluate the needs of the older person with cancer and then make the appropriate referrals. Community resources can be set up so the older adult does not have to deal with these types of issues alone. The time you take may have a profound impact on recovery for the older cancer patient.

Summary

Older people tend to have less body reserves. They may not tolerate medical emergencies and other conditions as well as younger patients, and, therefore, these emergencies can result in life-threatening circumstances for the older patient. An understanding of these conditions and early intervention will have a positive impact on outcome.

References

1. Crossley KB, Peterson PK. Infections in the Elderly. *Clin Infect Dis* 1996:22:209–215.
2. Zenilman, J. Infection and Immunity in *Oxford American Handbook of Geriatric Medicine*. New York, NY: Oxford University Press, 2010. p. 640.
3. Htwe TH, Mushtaq A, Robinson SB, Rosher RB, Khardori N. Infection in the Elderly. *Infect Dis Clin N Am* 2007:21:711–743, p. 713
4. Ibid.
5. Administration on Aging. *Older Adults and HIV/AIDS*. Available at: http://www.aoa.gov/AoARoot/AoA_Programs/HPW/HIV_AIDS/
6. Centers for Disease Control and Prevention. *HIV among Older Americans*. Available at: http://www.cdc.gov/hiv/risk/age/olderamericans/index.html
7. Ibid.
8. Carrion AF, Martin P. Viral Hepatitis in the Elderly. *Am J Gastroenterol* 2012:107:691–697, p. 691.
9. Ibid, p. 692.
10. Ibid.
11. Ibid, p. 693.
12. Ibid, p. 694.
13. National Institutes of Health, National Institute of General Medical Sciences. *Sepsis Fact Sheet*. Available at: http://www.nigms.nih.gov/Education/Pages/factsheet_sepsis.aspx
14. Girard TD, Opal SM, Ely EW. Insights into Severe Sepsis in Older Patients: From Epidemiology to Evidence-Based Management. *Clin Infect Dis* 2005:40:719–727, p.720.
15. Nasa P, Juneja D, Singh O. Severe sepsis and septic shock in the elderly: An overview. *World J Crit Care Med* 2012:1(1): 23–30, p. 25.
16. Girard, Opal, & Ely, pp. 721–722.
17. AgingCare. *Urinary Tract Infections in the Elderly: Why are they different?* Available at: http://www.agingcare.com/Articles/urinary-tract-infections-elderly-146026.htm
18. Ibid.
19. Centers for Disease Control and Prevention. *National Diabetes Statistics Report, 2014*. Available from: http://www.cdc.gov/diabetes/pubs/statsreport14.htm
20. Kirkman SM et al. Diabetes in Older Adults: A Consensus Report. *J Am Geriatr Soc* 2012:60(12):2342–2356.
21. Wallace, JI. Management of Diabetes in the Elderly. *Clinical Diabetes* 1999:17(1).

22. American Thyroid Association. *Thyroid Disease in the Older Patient*, 2012. Available at: http://www.thyroid.org/wp-content/uploads/patients/brochures/ThyroidDisorderOlder_broch.pdf

23. Ibid.

24. Brillhart BB. Preventative Skin Care for Older Adults. *Medscape Multispecialty.* Available at: www.medscape.com/viewarticle/531999

25. Kirman CN. Pressure Ulcers and Wound Care. *Medscape.* Available at: emedicine.medscape.com/article/319284-overview

26. Centers for Disease Control and Prevention, National Center for Immunization and Respiratory Diseases (NCIRD), Division of Viral Diseases. *Shingles (Herpes Zoster).* Available at: http://www.cdc.gov/shingles/hcp/clinical-overview.html

27. Ibid.

28. Grassi M, Petraccia L, Mennuni G, Fontana M, Scarno A, Sabetta S, Fraioli A. Changes, functional disorders, and diseases in the gastrointestinal tract of elderly. *Nutr Hosp* 2011: 26(4):659-68.

29. Ibid.

30. Saljoughian M. Gastrointestinal Bleeding: An Alarming Sign. *US Pharm* 2009:34(12):HS12–HS16.

31. Trivedi CD, Pitchumoni CS. Gastrointestinal Bleeding in Older Adults. *Pract Gastroenterol* March 2006, p. 15.

32. Ibid, p. 16.

33. Ibid, p. 28.

34. Seymour K, Darrell S. Inflammatory Bowel Disease of the Elderly: Frequently Asked Questions (FAQs). *Am J Gastroenterol* 2011:106:1889–1897.

35. Ibid.

36. Day LW, Walter LC, Velayos F. Colorectal Cancer Screening and Surveillance in the Elderly Patient. *Am J Gastroenterol* 2011:106(7):1197–1206.

37. Gallegos-Orozco JF, Foxx-Orenstein AE, Sterler SM, Stoa J M. Chronic Constipation in the Elderly. *Am J Gastroenterol* 2012:107:18–25.

38. Wells JL, Dumbrell AC. Nutrition and Aging: Assessment and Treatment of Compromised Nutritional Status in Frail Elderly Patients. *Clin Interv Aging* 2006:1(1):67–69.

39. United States Fire Administration. Federal Emergency Management Agency. Fire Risk to Older Adults in 2010. *Topical Fire Report Series* 2013:14(9):1–8, p.1.

40. Ibid, p. 6.

41. Uygur F, Noyan N, Ülkür E, Çeliköz B. A Geriatric Patient With Major Burns. *Annals of Burns and Fire Disasters* 2008:XXI(1):43–46.

42. Huang S-B, Chang W-H, Huang C-H, Tsai C-H. Management of Elderly Burn Patients. *Int J Gerontol* 2008:2(3):92–93.

43. Browner I. Applications in Geriatric Oncology. The Johns Hopkins Medicine Geriatric Education Center Consortium. Available at: http://www.hopkinsmedicine.org/gec/series/cancer_aging.html

44. American Society of Clinical Oncology. Aging and Cancer. Available at: http://www.cancer.net/navigating-cancer-care/older-adults/aging-and-cancer

45. Ibid.

CASE STUDY SUMMARIES

© 123dartist/Shutterstock, Inc.

Case Study 1 Summary

This patient's illness could be the result of a number of different causes. You need to obtain a temperature, listen to lung sounds, perform a 12-lead electrocardiogram, get a finger stick glucose, check pupils, and obtain a medical and medication history as quickly as possible. Ask family members when the patient became semiconscious and if there have been any other symptoms, such as vomiting, diarrhea, urinary symptoms, bleeding, seizures, cough, fever, change in behaviors, or complaints of pain. You should also determine if the patient has experienced any recent trauma or change in medications. Additional considerations include:

- Does the patient need a hearing aid to respond to you?
- Did family members notice a deficit on one side of the patient's body or the other?
- Has the patient or a family member recently traveled out of the country?
- Does the patient have any indwelling devices (such as a catheter or PICC line)?
- Has the patient recently had surgery?
- Did the patient miss dialysis?
- Did the patient accidentally or intentionally take the wrong dose of medication?

Perform a thorough head-to-toe survey of the patient, looking for bruising and open wounds (especially pressure sores that are oozing and/or infected). This patient may have an infection, sepsis, dehydration, gastrointestinal bleeding, serosanguineous fluid loss, or an environmental issue. A febrile patient most likely has an infection; however, older adults will not always have a fever with an infection. Other possible causes include late onset diabetes, a thyroid problem, or volume loss. If you can identify a problem to treat, do so; however, cause determination often will require multiple tests in the hospital. The EMS provider should focus on starting an IV, applying oxygen, repeating vitals, obtaining a medication and allergy list, and transporting the patient to the hospital.

Case Study 2 Summary

Mrs. Flowers has lost 6% of her body weight in 6 months. This is a cause for concern. Her physician needs to consider causes for weight loss such as new hyperthyroidism, diabetes, malignancy, depression, or oral problems. These can be ruled out through history taking, physical examination, and laboratory tests. Collateral history from family or caregivers is very important in assessing a person with dementia. Older patients with dementia often have an atypical presentation of many illnesses, especially in cases of depression.

A medication review is also an important part of the assessment for this patient. For example, cholinesterase inhibitors can cause nausea, vomiting, anorexia, or diarrhea and can be associated with weight loss. Because Mrs. Flowers was able to maintain her weight for a year on the medication, other causes of weight loss associated with dementia should also be considered. These causes include the loss of caregiver support, social isolation, limited access to food, inability to cook and prepare food, and inability to recognize hunger. Collateral history from a caregiver and a home visit can provide invaluable insight into these issues. EMS providers can assist in this assessment. A nutritional treatment plan for Mrs. Flowers may include treating any newly diagnosed medical issues and prescribing nutritional supplements. In this case, considering a referral to social and community programs (such as adult day care, home care services, or a delivered meal program) would be appropriate following patient discharge.

Case Study 3 Summary

In this case, there could be a variety of causes for the patient's change in behavior; however, the clues (an elevated temperature, hot room, multiple layers of clothing, and medications that decrease the ability to dissipate heat from the body [diphenhydramine, beta blockers, and antidepressant]) all point toward heat stroke! Older patients do not cool themselves well due to changes in physiology. The patient may also have fever due to illness, but not all high temperatures are due to infection. The EMS provider must consider the environment when assessing patients. Treatment of this patient should focus on cooling the patient, starting an IV, replacing lost fluid (be cautious due to the patient's history of CHF), and transporting to the hospital.

CHAPTER 12

Pharmacology and Medication Toxicity

LEARNING OBJECTIVES

1. Identify the effects of various medications on the older patient population.

2. Recognize the impact of polypharmacy, medication nonadherence, and dosing errors on the older patient population.

3. Identify medications commonly used by older patients, including prescription medications, over-the-counter medications, and supplements.

4. Apply older patient assessment and management principles to pharmacology emergencies.

5. Describe the EMS provider's role in preventing medication errors in older patients.

Introduction

There is no doubt that medications can improve an older person's health, diminish symptoms, and improve quality of life. However, medications can also lead to various complications and unanticipated consequences. This is particularly true in the aging population: One-third of all hospital admissions in older adults are due to adverse drug reactions.[1] Older people frequently have extensive medical problems, take numerous medications (polypharmacy), and have multiple physicians prescribing medications for them. Older people also often have difficulty taking their medications as prescribed. Collectively, these factors significantly increase the risk of adverse drug effects in the older population.

Medications and Age-Related Changes in the Geriatric Patient

Pharmacokinetics is the study of the body's absorption, distribution, metabolism, and elimination of medications. The aging process leads to physiological changes that can affect the pharmacokinetics of all medications, including prescription and over-the-counter (OTC) medications, herbal medications, supplements, and vitamins. EMS providers are often an older person's first contact with the healthcare system when acute problems develop, so it is important for EMS providers to understand age-related changes in the body's function and composition in relation to medication absorption, distribution, metabolism, and elimination.

The term **pharmacodynamics** refers to the effects of medications and their mechanisms of action. Pharmacodynamic changes associated with aging have not been well studied in older populations, and as such are not completely understood. Generally, older patients are considered to have a heightened response to most medications. In other words, many drugs, such as warfarin (Coumadin), opioids, oxycodone/acetaminophen (Percocet), and benzodiazepines such as lorazepam (Ativan), appear to have an increased potency in older people.

Having an understanding of pharmacodynamics is particularly important when a medication that increases the risk of falls is prescribed to an older person. You must gather a thorough medication history for every older patient. This includes a list of all prescription, OTC, and herbal medications. Record the prescribing information of each medication, and make sure to ascertain whether the older person has recently begun a new medication or stopped a current medication.

Attitude Tip

Remember, as older patients mature, they frequently need reductions in the dose or strength of medications.

Passage of Medications Through the Body

Absorption

Absorption is the process of a substance entering the blood circulation. When a medication is taken orally, it needs to be absorbed by the gastrointestinal (GI) tract in order for it to get into the bloodstream. Several age-related changes occur in the GI tract that can potentially affect drug absorption after oral administration: gastric acidity decreases, gastric emptying slows, and the absorptive surface of the intestine is diminished. Older people are also prone to swallowing difficulties, poor nutritional status, erratic meal patterns, and interactions with other prescription and nonprescription medications—all additional factors that can potentially alter absorption. Since older people often take multiple oral medications, EMS providers should be alert for drug interactions that can affect the absorption of medications. For example, taking phenytoin

CASE STUDY 1

You are called to a retirement community for a 78-year-old female who lives alone. The patient is alert and ambulatory, but she is complaining of general weakness and fatigue. During the patient history, she tells you she takes a "few" medications. You also notice a faint odor of alcohol on her breath.

After talking to the patient and collecting the medication bottles from around the house, you determine that she takes the following medication: antacid tablets, Xanax, a calcium supplement, an unknown antibiotic (she cannot remember the name or find the bottle), Dilantin, Coumadin, Echinacea, and Fosamax. You also determine that the patient has four different prescribing physicians and two different pharmacies, and you notice that the bottle of Xanax is almost empty before it should be. The patient mentions she takes all of her medications in the morning with grapefruit juice and a piece of toast.

- What are your concerns about this patient's medications?
- What questions should you ask regarding this patient's medication use?
- What is your management of this patient?

(Dilantin) with calcium affects absorption in such a way that it may decrease serum phenytoin levels. Another drug interaction that can affect absorption is taking the antibiotic levofloxacin (Levaquin) with an oral iron (ferrous sulfate or ferrous gluconate): When taken together, the ferrous sulfate or ferrous gluconate decreases the availability of the antibiotic. Older persons should consider separating the intake of supplements of any kind with the intake of active medications by at least 2 hours.

Distribution

Distribution is the dispersion or dissemination of substances throughout the fluids and tissues of the body. Age-related changes in body composition can alter the distribution of medications; lean body mass and total body water can decrease by 20% while body fat can increase by 40%.[2] These changes have the potential to alter the distribution of both water-soluble and fat-soluble medications.

The drop in total body water can result in higher blood levels of more water-soluble drugs. As a result, the initial dose of some medications (such as digoxin and lithium) may need to be lowered. Fat-soluble drugs, however, tend to have lower blood levels, though the increase in fat tissue means these medications are eliminated more slowly (because fat tissue acts as a reservoir for fat-soluble medications). This can prolong the effects of fat-soluble medications, warranting consideration of lower doses. For example, blood levels of diazepam (Valium) may be lower in older patients following a single dose, but the sedative effects may be prolonged due to slower elimination or metabolism.

Some drugs, such as phenytoin (Dilantin) and warfarin (Coumadin), are carried in the bloodstream attached to proteins (**Figure 12-1**). Older people who have a low blood protein level require a lower dose of these types of drugs. Low blood protein levels can occur as a result of liver disease, malnutrition, or other chronic conditions.

Metabolism and Elimination

Metabolism is the conversion of a drug from its parent compound into metabolites. **Elimination** is the process of removing compounds from the body. Most drugs are eliminated through either the kidneys or the liver. Both of these organs are subject to age-related changes that can have a significant impact on medication usage and complications in older people.

Half-life is the time it takes for the amount of active medication in a person's system to decline by 50%, and can be expressed in seconds, minutes, hours, or days. Examples of half-life for two commonly administered medications include 10 seconds for adenosine (Adenocard) and approximately 58 days for amiodorone (Pacerone).

Kidneys

The kidneys undergo several important changes with aging: renal blood flow declines and the kidneys become less-efficient filters. This leads to a slowdown in renal filtration and decreases the rate of elimination of medications that are excreted by the kidneys. As a result, it is often necessary to decrease the dose or frequency of administration of these drugs.

> ### Medication Tip
>
> The kidneys and the liver are the primary routes of drug elimination. Age-related changes in the function of these organs can have a major impact on drug effects, and may require changes in dosages and frequency.

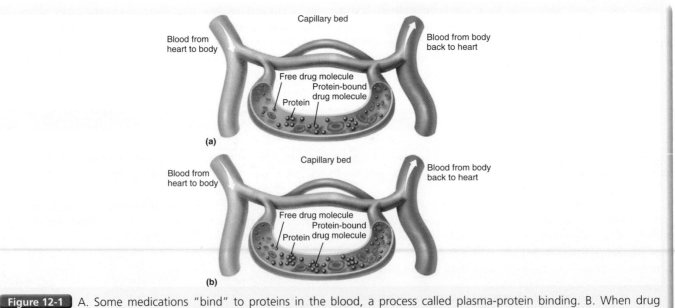

Figure 12-1 A. Some medications "bind" to proteins in the blood, a process called plasma-protein binding. B. When drug elimination is significantly decreased by renal or hepatic disease, changes in protein binding can be important.

It is important to understand the impact active metabolites can have on the older patient. **Active metabolites** are byproducts of drug metabolism that can have their own effects on the body. For example, meperidine (Demerol) undergoes metabolism by the liver into an active compound called normeperidine. Normeperidine has a longer half-life than meperidine, and so it can more quickly accumulate in the body. Its excitatory neurotoxicity can be lethal in patients who abuse medications such as Demerol.[3]

Changes in kidney function can also alter the effect of diuretics on electrolyte balance. For example, the use of potassium-sparing diuretics such as triamterene and spironolactone increase the risk of **hyperkalemia**, while hydrochlorothiazide (HCTZ) and loop diuretics, such as Lasix, raise the risk of **hyponatremia**.

Liver

The primary site of drug metabolism in the body is the liver (**Figure 12-2**). Age-related changes that can alter drug metabolism include a reduction in liver mass, a decrease in blood flow to the liver, and a reduction in the intrinsic activity of drug-metabolizing enzymes. The decrease in liver blood flow essentially decreases the rate at which a drug reaches the liver to be metabolized, while a decrease in the number and activity of metabolic enzymes diminishes the metabolic capacity of the liver. Disease, nutrition, polypharmacy, tobacco or alcohol use, and genetics are also important factors in drug metabolism.

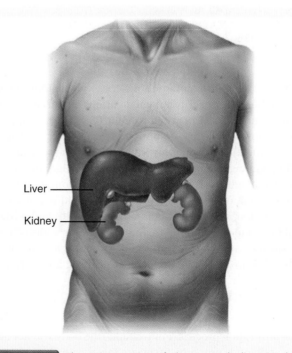

Figure 12-2 The primary site of drug metabolism in the body is the liver. The kidneys and the liver are the main routes of drug elimination.

The clinical effects of age-related changes on hepatic elimination depend on the degree to which medications undergo metabolism. Because nearly all older people have declines in kidney and liver function, it is best to "start low and go slow" with medications in this age group. New medications should be started at the lowest possible dose, and adjusted slowly to account for any build-up of medication that may result from sluggish metabolism or elimination.

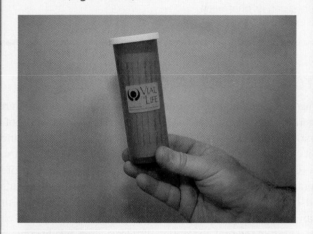

Attitude Tip

You and your EMS agency can support community education and assistance programs to help the older population establish and maintain EMS-accessible medical information and medication containers and storage devices, such as the "OK MedCard/MedFile," "Vial-of-Life," "U.S. MedGear," and others (**Figure 12-3**).

Figure 12-3 Medication containers such as the Vial-of-Life can be distributed to older patients at risk for medication-related emergencies.
© Jones & Bartlett Learning. Courtesy of MIEMSS.

Drug Interactions

A drug interaction can occur between a drug and other medications, foods, or a disease state. The interaction results in a change in the pharmacologic effect or toxicity of the drug. Drug interactions occur more frequently as the number of drugs used increases. Since older patients are the largest consumers of medications (for example, nursing home patients with cognitive impairment, such as dementia, take an average of eight drugs daily[4]), they are at increased risk of drug interactions. Other risk factors associated with drug interactions in older patients include mixing alcohol or over-the-counter medications with prescription drugs, having drugs prescribed by multiple physicians, and purchasing medications from more than one pharmacy (**Figure 12-4**). Also, older people do not tolerate adverse effects of drugs as well as younger patients.

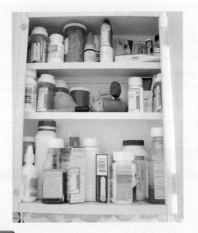

Figure 12-4 Risk factors for harmful drug interactions include use of multiple medications, the combination of alcohol and medications, and prescriptions from more than one physician or pharmacy.
© Jamie Otto-coenen/Dreamstime.com

Table 12-1 Resources to Check for Drug–Drug Interactions

Resource Website	Resource Description
www.epocrates.com	A free or purchasable drug interaction checker that will display any interaction between your chosen drugs. Available online and as an application for smartphone devices.
www.drugs.com/drug_interactions.html	A free drug interaction checker that will display any interactions between your chosen drug(s) and food. Available online only.
naturaldatabase.therapeuticresearch.com	A free herbal drug interaction checker that will display any interaction between your chosen herbal drugs. Available online only.
lexi.com	A purchasable drug interaction checker that will display any interactions between your chosen drugs. Available online and as an application for smartphone devices.

Reproduced from Atkinson, Steven. "*Geriatric Pharmacology: The Principles of Practice and Clinical Recommendations.*" Wisconsin: PHC Publishing Group, 2012, p.38.

Drug–Drug Interactions

Drug–drug interactions occur when two drugs administered together alter the pharmacokinetics or pharmacodynamics of at least one of the medications. The effects can cause a magnification or reduction in pharmacologic actions of the affected drug.

Commonly used OTC medications such as ibuprofen, acetaminophen, and aspirin interfere with warfarin (Coumadin) and can increase the risk of internal bleeding.[5] Antacids and vitamins containing aluminum, calcium, iron, magnesium, and zinc can decrease the oral absorption of tetracycline, bisphosphonate bone medications (e.g., Fosamax or Actonel), and quinolone antibiotics, which can result in therapeutic failure. Patients taking these medications can avoid problems by separating administration of the interacting drugs by at least 2 hours.

Interactions affecting elimination usually involve one drug either enhancing or decreasing the metabolism of another drug. Increased drug metabolism can result in failure of a medication to exert its therapeutic effect, while inhibition of metabolism can result in greater pharmacologic effect or drug toxicity. Patients are at highest risk of complications from metabolic drug interactions when an interacting drug is stopped or started. Even if patients provide a list of medications, you should specifically ask if any new medicines have been started recently or if the dose of any medications has changed.

Pharmacodynamic interactions among two or more drugs occur when one medication directly enhances or inhibits the action of another drug, usually in the same system. For example, alcohol combined with central nervous system depressants such as antidepressants, antihistamines, or benzodiazepines can increase CNS depression.

One study of drug–drug interactions in older patients found that the overall risk of potential drug–drug interactions was 63%, with the risk of major drug–drug interactions at 12%.

The risk of drug–drug interactions goes up considerably when the number of prescription medications is three or more.[6] Cardiac and central nervous system (CNS) drugs appear to account for a majority of potential drug–drug interactions; three medications commonly involved in adverse drug events (ADEs) among older patients are insulin, digoxin, and warfarin (Coumadin).[7] Examples of drug pair combinations that can cause major drug–drug interactions include nortriptyline and clonidine, atenolol and clonidine, atenolol and diltiazem, clonidine and verapamil, digoxin and hydrochlorothiazide, digoxin and amiodarone, and ginkgo biloba and ibuprofen.[8] **Table 12-1** provides resources for drug–drug interactions.

Drug–Nutrient Interactions

Many clinically important drug–nutrient interactions are related to the absorption process. For example, the body will not absorb some antibiotics properly if they are taken with vitamins or supplements that contain calcium, magnesium, or iron. It is important that these medications not be taken with dairy products or other foods containing high levels of these minerals (**Figure 12-5**).

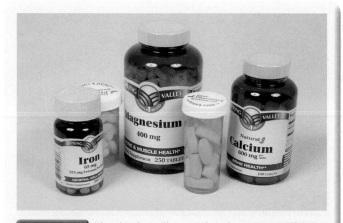

Figure 12-5 The body will not absorb some antibiotics properly if they are taken with vitamins or supplements that contain calcium, magnesium, or iron, or with dairy products or other foods containing high levels of these minerals.
© Jones & Bartlett Learning. Courtesy of MIEMSS.

Nutritional supplements, including those delivered by feeding tube, may also contain minerals that can interfere with drug absorption. For example, tube feedings can impair the absorption of phenytoin, which may result in poor seizure control.

The administration of some medications with grapefruit juice can interfere with the phase of metabolism that occurs in the intestinal wall. This results in higher blood levels of the drug and an overall increase in pharmacologic effect and risk of drug toxicity. These medications include some calcium channel blockers (diltiazem, verapamil), some benzodiazepines (diazepam, triazolam), lovastatin, and astemizole.

There are some circumstances in which drug–nutrient interactions are pharmacodynamic in nature. For example, if the dietary intake of vitamin K increases significantly from food, nutritional supplements, or **enteral** products, it can interfere with the anticoagulant effect of warfarin. Conversely, if vitamin K intake decreases significantly, patients may experience an increase in anticoagulant effect, which can then increase the risk of bleeding. Patients taking warfarin who present either with possible clotting events or with bleeding complications should be questioned about any recent changes in their diet, the use of nutritional supplements, or enteral nutrition.

Drug–Disease Interactions

A drug–disease interaction occurs when one or more medications act to worsen an existing disease. For example, the effect of nonsteroidal anti-inflammatory drugs (NSAIDs) on the kidneys can interfere with blood pressure control or place some patients at risk of developing congestive heart failure.[9] Of particular concern for older patients is the potential for medications to compromise mental function and physical mobility. Both of these complications can increase the risk of fall injuries.

Medication Tip

Grapefruit juice can interfere with the metabolism of some drugs, and several minerals can affect absorption of a number of antibiotics. In addition, vitamin K alters the anticoagulant effect of warfarin.

Drug-induced mental impairment can occur in older patients as a direct result of the effects of medication on the central nervous system, or secondary to metabolic imbalances caused by drugs. Patients with preexisting cognitive problems are at the greatest risk, but drug-induced confusion can occur in any older patient (**Figure 12-6**). In many instances, confusion is not due to a single agent, but to the additive effects of two or more drugs used together.

Fall injuries are a leading cause of hospitalization and death among the older population.[10] Medication usage is a modifiable risk factor for fall injuries. Fall-risk increasing drugs (FRID) include antidysrhythmics, diuretics, benzodiazepines, antidepressants, and narcotics (**Table 12-2**). Benzodiazepines and psychotropic medications appear to be most strongly associated with falls in older people.[11] These drugs, as well as others, can trigger movement disorders or affect balance through a variety of mechanisms.

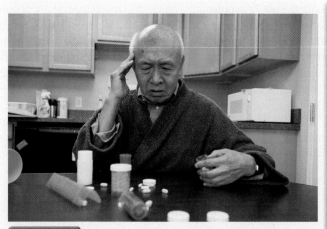

Figure 12-6 Drug toxicity may initially show itself in the form of confusion.
© Jones & Bartlett Learning. Courtesy of MIEMSS.

Attitude Tip

Drug-induced confusion can occur in any older patient. Do not assume dementia or psychiatric problems: Assess the patient for medication problems and other medical causes.

Table 12-2	Fall-Risk Increasing Drugs
Drug Class	**Example**
Benzodiazepines and other hypnotics	Diazepam (Valium)
Tricyclic antidepressants	Amitriptyline
Selective serotonin-reuptake inhibitors (SSRIs)	Sertraline
Antipsychotics	Haloperidol
Anticonvulsants	Phenytoin
Class 1A antiarrhythmics	Procainamide
Diuretics	Furosemide
Digoxin	Lanoxin
Skeletal muscle relaxants	Carisoprodol

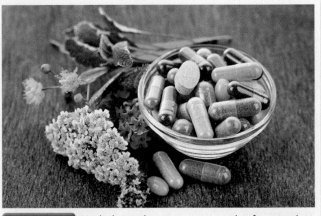

Figure 12-7 Herbal supplements are popular for a variety of purported health effects.
© Elenathewise/iStockphoto.com

Drug–Herb Interactions

The available information on pharmacokinetics is largely dominated by drug–drug interactions, with little data on drug–herb interactions. The occurrence of drug–herb interactions appears to be rare; however, EMS providers should include questions about the use of supplements and herbal medicines. Many people do not think of herbs as supplements, so it is necessary to specify both categories during the patient history. Popular herbal remedies include Echinacea, Ma Huang (Ephedra), Ginkgo biloba, and St. John's Wort (**Figure 12-7**). Because drug–herb interactions are not common, ensure that your assessment covers other possible causes of existing signs and symptoms.

When you suspect a drug–herb interaction, bring the medication(s) and herb(s) with you and obtain the following information:

- Patient diseases and conditions
- Medications being taken: name, dose, timing
- Herb(s) involved
- Brand name, label information
- Dosage and timing, including timing relative to medications

Echinacea

Echinacea is an immune stimulant. It appears to be safe for short-term use by most people; however, there is not enough information to know what the long-term effects may be. Side effects of Echinacea include nausea, vomiting, GI upset, dry mouth, headache, and insomnia. Echinacea can cause allergic reactions, especially in people who are allergic to ragweed and certain flowers.

Echinacea may slow down the body's ability to break down caffeine, which can result in too much caffeine in the bloodstream and increase the risk of side effects, including restlessness, headache, and tachycardia. In addition, taking Echinacea along with some medications, such as Cardizem and estrogens, might increase both their effects and side effects. Echinacea may also slow the metabolism of certain drugs and suppress immune system function.

Ephedra

Ephedra, also known as Ma Huang and Mormon Tea, has been used to treat asthma and other respiratory conditions, with its bronchodilator properties coming from substances such as ephedrine and pseudoephedrine. Ephedra has also been marketed as a dietary supplement under the name Metabolife; it appears Ephedra may help promote weight loss, but the effects typically only last while taking the supplement. Major drug interactions that may occur with Ephedra include medications that can cause an irregular heart beat (QT interval-prolonging drugs), such as amiodarone; methylxanthines like aminophylline; stimulant drugs such as diethylpropion; dexamethasone; medications for depression (MAOIs), such as phenelzine; medications for diabetes, such as glimepiride; and medications used to prevent seizures, such as phenobarbital.

Medication Tip

The use of herbal medications by older patients is growing in popularity despite the lack of adequate medical research describing their benefits, risks, and potential interactions with other medications.

Ginkgo

Ginkgo (*Ginkgo biloba*) is one of the best-selling herbal medicines in the United States, and it is also one of the most prescribed medicines in France and Germany. It is used as a memory enhancer. Ginkgo is contraindicated in patients using anticoagulants and NSAIDs, as the combination inhibits platelet function, and may increase the risk of bleeding problems. Other adverse effects include seizures, headaches, dizziness, and GI upset.

St. John's Wort

St. John's Wort has been used since the time of Hippocrates as a popular treatment for depression, anxiety, and sleep disorders. St. John's Wort is one of the best-selling herbs in Germany, outselling Prozac 20 to 1.[12] St. John's Wort is contraindicated in patients taking selective serotonin-reuptake inhibitors (SSRIs) such as Paxil and Zoloft (**Figure 12-8**); taking St. John's Wort with these medications may increase side effects and potentially lead to a dangerous condition called serotonin syndrome. Symptoms of serotonin syndrome include confusion, agitation or restlessness, dilated pupils, headache, changes in blood pressure and/or temperature, nausea and/or vomiting, diarrhea, rapid heart rate, loss of muscle coordination or twitching

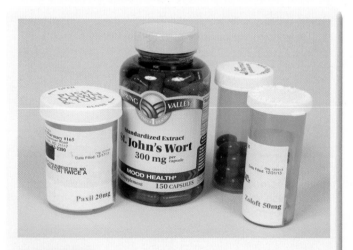

Figure 12-8 St. John's Wort, a popular herbal treatment for depression, is contraindicated in patients taking SSRI-type antidepressants, such as Paxil and Zoloft.
© Jones & Bartlett Learning. Courtesy of MIEMSS.

Attitude Tip

Do not forget to gather related vitamin and mineral supplements, and herbal or other over-the-counter (OTC) remedies being taken by the patient, which could contribute to adverse drug reactions or other polypharmacy complications.

muscles, shivering or goose bumps, and perfuse sweating. Serotonin syndrome can be life threatening in severe cases. Severe symptoms include high fever, seizures, irregular heartbeat, and unconsciousness. St. John's Wort can also increase sensitivity to sunlight and may inhibit the binding of naloxone (Narcan) to opioid receptor sites.

Evidence-Based Research

Evidence-based research (EBR) is the practice of using the growing volume of available research to guide clinical decision making and improve patient care, and is extremely important in the care of older patients. Geriatrician Dr. Mark H. Beers studied medication use by nursing home residents and discovered that prescription medications used by many residents resulted in potentially harmful side effects. This research was used to develop a list of drugs with risks that outweigh the benefits in older patients. For example, psychoactive drugs, including antidepressants, sedative-hypnotics, and anxiolytics, pose several risks, such as high abuse potential, respiratory depression, and altered level of consciousness; thus, these medications have a high severity rating according to the list now known as Beers Criteria. Beers Criteria has led to changes at both Medicare and Medicaid.[13] (A free reference/pocket card showcasing the Beers Criteria is available at www.americangeriatrics.org)

Research has shown that the mean rate of drugs being inappropriately prescribed to older patients was over 20%, with diphenhydramine (Benadryl) and amitriptyline being two of the most common.[14] Current and evolving knowledge is being used to help avoid potentially dangerous prescribing patterns and adverse drug–drug interactions. This knowledge seems to be most effective when used by a physician as part of a multidisciplinary team, including pharmacists and geriatric specialists.[15]

Research also indicates older patients are frequently underrepresented in the randomized controlled trials of the drugs they are likely to be prescribed.[16] Based on the rapid growth of the older population and the inherent complications of drug usage in this age group, the Food and Drug Administration (FDA) has recommended that older patients be adequately represented in clinical drug trials. Despite this recommendation, it appears pharmaceutical companies may be using unfounded exclusion criteria to reduce the presence of older adults in these trials.[17]

Assessing Problems Related to Medication Toxicity or Adverse Effects

Often, the potential benefits of medication usage in older people are outweighed by the potential side effects or complications that may occur. In addition, an older person's physical or mental condition and economic situation may make it more difficult to take medications as prescribed. Common causes of drug-related hospitalizations include adverse drug reactions, medication nonadherence, and withdrawal reactions due to stopping a medication abruptly.

History

In reviewing the medication history, assess the patient's knowledge of his or her current medications (**Table 12-3**). Gather the medication names, doses, and prescribing physicians. Determine if the patient is taking the medications as prescribed. Ask if the patient is experiencing any side effects, or has any problems that may prevent medication adherence. Older patients must possess multiple physical and cognitive abilities in order to manage medications independently, and geriatric assessment and clinical care guidelines often do not include a comprehensive assessment of these abilities.[18] Research indicates behavioral interventions for medication nonadherence, such as simplification of the medication regimen, medication reminders, and administrative aids, are more effective than educational interventions. Information about actual use is important because additional adverse drug events can occur if hospital personnel are not aware of the patient's medication nonadherence.

In addition, ask the patient if he or she is taking any medication that was not prescribed specifically for him or her. Older persons may use family members' medications on a trial basis to see if they are helpful. It is also important to determine if the patient understands what his or her medications are used for. Consider the case of an older patient with asthma who has frequent attacks. Upon interview, the patient reports that when he uses his Flovent inhaler, he finds no acute relief. Confusion about what his medications are for has prevented the patient from picking the right inhaler for immediate relief; if properly informed, he would use the inhaled corticosteroids on a daily basis for prevention of asthma attacks, and a bronchodilating inhaler (such as albuterol) for acute relief.

It is a good idea for EMS providers to familiarize themselves with the most commonly prescribed medications. This knowledge will help EMS providers more quickly spot medication problems in older patients. A current drug reference source is an

Table 12-3	Key Questions in the Medication History of an Older Patient

1. What medications are you taking?
2. What is the purpose of these medications?
3. Do you currently take any medications that you can purchase without a doctor's prescription for any medical condition? Herbal products? Vitamins and nutritional supplements?
4. Have you ever had an allergic reaction to a medication, such as hives or difficulty breathing?
5. Have you ever had a bad reaction to a medication that made you have to stop taking that medication and/or report it to your doctor?
6. Do you use more than one pharmacy or physician?
7. Do you carry a medication list so your pharmacy and physician can review what you are taking?
8. Have you stopped taking any medications recently?
9. Have you added any medications recently?
10. How do you remember to take your medications on a daily basis?
11. Do you smoke or drink alcohol on a daily basis? If so, how much?
12. Do you use any other drugs? If so, how often?

Controversy

Exactly which medications pose the highest risks to older patients is not well established. However, carrying drug information resources may help you spot medication-related problems.

CASE STUDY 2

© 123dartist/Thinkstock

You are called to a residence for a fall injury. Upon arrival, you find an 88-year-old male supine on the floor in the hallway. His daughter tells you he has been staying with her because he has been falling more frequently. You note some minor abrasions and contusions in various stages of healing. The patient is awake, but mildly confused.

Your physical exam indicates the patient did not suffer any serious injuries as a result of the fall. The daughter states her dad has a history of cardiac problems, Type II diabetes, insomnia, and early-onset Parkinson's. He takes Clonidine, digoxin, a potassium supplement, Benadryl, and Levodopa. BP is 102/60, pulse is 60 and irregular, ECG is a borderline sinus bradycardia with occasional PVCs, and the blood glucose is 140 mg/dL.

- What additional information would you like to know?
- What are your concerns about this patient's medications?
- How will you manage this patient?

important tool for EMS providers to carry at all times. This could be a print resource or a mobile electronic application.

Medication Nonadherence

Determine whether the patient is adherent with medication directions. Methods for evaluating adherence include direct patient reporting, as well as counting the number of pills in the bottle to see if the number remaining matches up with the interval since the last time the prescription was refilled (**Figure 12-9**).

Poor adherence is often associated with underuse of a medication. There are also certain medication classes, such as narcotics and benzodiazepines, that have a high abuse potential. Reporting suspected medication nonadherence or abuse to hospital personnel is extremely important, as nonadherence can increase morbidity and mortality in older patients. With an increasing older population and a rising number of prescriptions being written for older patients, there has been an increase in the rate of nonadherence. Many factors can contribute to nonadherence, including:

- Forgetting to take medications on time
- Not remembering the correct amount or dose to take
- Poor technique with medicine administration devices (e.g., metered-dose inhalers [MDIs], insulin syringes)
- Difficulty understanding the label or other directions
- Difficulty opening containers
- Financial problems (cannot afford medications)

Today, there are a number of resources (smart phone apps, software programs, etc.) to help patients follow their medication regime. These resources can help track dosages, monitor

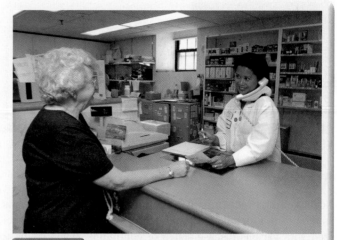

Figure 12-10 Having the patient, pharmacist, and physician work together can help improve adherence by ensuring that dosing schedules fit the patient's lifestyle, and that the patient can afford the prescriptions.
© Jones & Bartlett Learning. Courtesy of MIEMSS.

for possible drug interactions, and remind users when refills are needed. Here are some additional ways to help improve adherence:

- Have the physician modify medication schedules to fit the patient's lifestyle.
- Have the physician and pharmacist work with the patient in selecting medications that are more affordable (**Figure 12-10**).
- Have the pharmacy dispense easy-to-open containers.
- Switch to dosage forms that are easier to swallow.
- If vision impairment is a problem, have the pharmacy provide labels and directions with larger type.
- Provide adherence-enhancing aids such as special blister packaging, pillboxes of various sizes, drug calendars, insulin pens, or dosage-measuring devices.

As the list suggests, it is important to determine the cause of nonadherence before selecting a strategy to address it. Identification of family members who can act as caregivers may assist in improving adherence, especially if the patient is cognitively impaired. If you suspect the patient is nonadherent, inform the hospital staff during the transfer of care report.

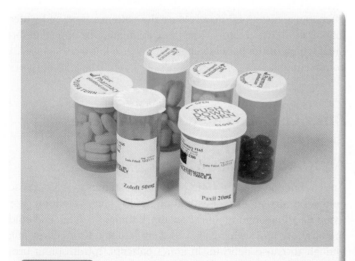

Figure 12-9 You may be able to evaluate medication adherence by comparing information on the container label (total number of pills dispensed, date dispensed, and number of pills to be taken per day) with the number of pills remaining in the container.
© Jones & Bartlett Learning. Courtesy of MIEMSS.

Communication Tip

Any patient may be nonadherent, but intentional nonadherence is more common in the older population. When assessing adherence, look at the patient's prescription bottles to see when it was last filled. Carefully question the patient to obtain a thorough medication history.

Adverse Drug Events

Adverse drug events are often hard to detect in older patients, as medication toxicities can mimic signs and symptoms associated with various disease states or conditions. When trying to determine reasons for functional impairment in the older person, medications should always be a part of the assessment. Specifically, assessing the older person's use of multiple pharmacies and physicians helps identify risk factors for adverse drug interactions. The risk is increased when the patient does not share medication information with his or her different service providers. Additional history information useful for the prevention of prescribing problems includes history of allergies to medications, history of adverse drug events, and smoking or alcohol use. Most drug-related side effects involve the cardiovascular, central nervous, or GI system.

Cardiovascular System Problems

The most frequent adverse effects on the cardiovascular system are orthostatic hypotension and dizziness that can contribute to syncope and falls. Medicines used to treat high blood pressure are the usual causes of these problems.

Central Nervous System Problems

Confusion is a common side effect of numerous medications. Most medications associated with mental confusion or psychiatric symptoms have anticholinergic or fat-soluble properties. Medications that are fat-soluble are more easily absorbed into the brain and therefore increase the risk of these adverse effects in the brain. There are numerous drug reference books and smartphone apps that can help EMS providers quickly determine if a drug is known to cause confusion (**Figure 12-11**).

Gastrointestinal Problems

Nausea, vomiting, constipation, and diarrhea are common side effects of many medications. Taking these medications with food or water, as directed, can help significantly. If your older patient has GI complaints, check his or her medications, then find out which ones should be taken with food or water and if the patient is doing so. Anticholinergic medications and narcotics

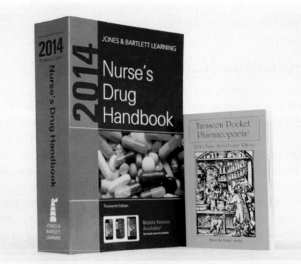

Figure 12-11 A drug handbook or mobile device app will help determine whether a medication has anticholinergic or fat-soluble properties, and thus could be causing confusion or psychiatric symptoms.
© Jones & Bartlett Learning.

Medication Tip

The cause-effect relationships between medications and a patient's signs and symptoms can be complex. When in doubt, treat ABCs, gather as much information as possible about medications, and report thoroughly to receiving personnel.

often cause constipation. Evaluate the patient's food and water intake and bowel history. Use your field guide or app to determine which of the patient's medications are known to cause GI complications.

Other Common Categories of Adverse Events

Anticholinergic Effects

Anticholinergics, often found in antihistamines, can cause confusion, dry mouth, constipation, and urinary retention. For example, diphenhydramine (Benadryl), found in cough and cold preparations and sleeping aids, has anticholinergic effects strong enough to cause delirium in some patients. Iptratropium bromide (Atrovent) also has anticholinergic properties and can lead to the same side effects.

Metabolic Disturbances

Another common adverse drug event is metabolic disturbance, such as low potassium (hypokalemia), low sodium (hyponatremia), or low bicarbonate levels. All of these conditions can contribute to possible cardiac dysrhythmias, mental confusion, and acid-base imbalances. Diuretics can cause these conditions as well (**Figure 12-12**). Hyperkalemia can be produced by potassium-sparing diuretics such as spironolactone, which is often used to treat congestive heart failure. The class of medications known as ACE inhibitors, used to treat high blood pressure, diabetes, and congestive heart failure, may also contribute to hyperkalemia.

Hypoglycemia is another major metabolic disturbance that can be caused by medications. Check blood glucose anytime the patient has an altered level of consciousness. An older patient does not have to be diabetic to be hypoglycemic.

Drug Withdrawal Problems

In order to reduce the risk of side effects and unwanted drug interactions, physicians work to take their patients off of unneeded medications. Unfortunately, many patients intentionally stop a medication on their own, a practice that can lead to an **adverse drug withdrawal event (ADWE)**. An ADWE is a set of clinical signs or symptoms caused by discontinuing use of a drug. ADWEs are most frequently caused by stopping use of cardiovascular and CNS drugs, and are possible for several weeks after use of a medication is discontinued.

A withdrawal event can worsen an underlying disease. For example, withdrawal due to discontinuing use of diuretic medications can aggravate a patient's CHF. When assessing a patient whose condition is worsening, ask if the patient has recently stopped taking a medication (**Figure 12-13**). **Table 12-4** reviews medications older adults should avoid or use with caution.

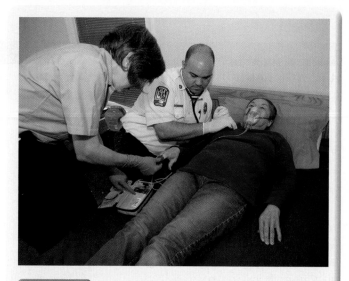

Figure 12-13 When assessing a patient whose condition or disease is worsening, ask if the patient has recently stopped taking a medication.
© Jones & Bartlett Learning. Courtesy of MIEMSS.

Medication Tip

Be sure to ask your older patients, beyond what is prescribed for them, what medications they are actually taking today (and every day, recently), because their physical condition (unwanted side effects, or "I feel fine without it") or economic status ("I can't afford to take all of it!") may force them to be nonadherent with their doctor's orders.

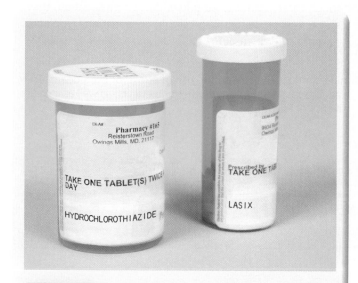

Figure 12-12 Common diuretics, such as hydrochlorothiazide and furosemide (Lasix), can cause metabolic disturbances that may lead to arrhythmias, confusion, or acid-base imbalances.
© Jones & Bartlett Learning. Courtesy of MIEMSS.

Intervention, Management, and Transport

Adverse drug events in older people should be treated symptomatically. Depending on the adverse drug event, administration of a reversal agent may be indicated; use caution, however, as use of some reversal agents can pose serious risks of their own. For example, flumazenil is a drug used to reverse the effects of benzodiazepines, but giving flumazenil to patients who take benzodiazepines for seizures can induce withdrawal seizures.[19] Additionally, diphenhydramine is a drug often used to reverse allergic reactions to medications; however, high doses of diphenhydramine may contribute to delirium, constipation, and urinary retention in the older person. Patients having an anaphylactic reaction to a medication may require high doses of IV corticosteroids, such as methylprednisolone, which can cause psychiatric symptoms. Finally, rapid administration of the narcotic antagonist naloxone (Narcan) can cause vomiting, so older patients must have their airway protected at all times.

Table 12-4 Ten Medications Older Adults Should Avoid or Use with Caution

Medication	Reason
USE WITH CAUTION non-steroidal anti-inflammatory drugs (NSAIDs). **AVOID long-acting NSAIDs** like indomethacin (Indocin) and piroxicam (Feldene).	NSAIDS can increase the risk of indigestion, ulcers, and bleeding in the stomach or colon. They can also increase blood pressure, affect the kidneys, and make heart failure worse.
AVOID digoxin (Lanoxin) in doses greater than 0.125 mg.	Digoxin can be toxic in older adults and people whose kidneys do not function properly.
AVOID certain diabetes medications such as glyburide (Diabeta, Micronase) and chlorpropamide (Diabinese).	These drugs can cause severe hypoglycemia.
AVOID muscle relaxants such as: ■ Cyclobenzaprine (Flexeril) ■ Methocarbamol (Robaxin) ■ Carisoprodol (Soma)	Muscle relaxants can leave the older person feeling groggy and confused, increase the risk of falls, and cause constipation, dry mouth, and problems urinating. Plus, there is little evidence they work well.
AVOID certain medications used for anxiety and/or insomnia such as: ■ Benzodiazepines (diazepam [Valium], alprazolam [Xanax], or chlordiazepoxide [Librium]) ■ Sleeping pills (zaleplon [Sonata] or zolpidem [Ambien]).	These medications can cause confusion and increase the risk of falls. In addition, it takes the body a long time to eliminate these medications, so the older person could feel groggy and sleepy for a while.
AVOID certain anticholinergic medications such as: ■ Antidepressants amitriptyline (Elavil) and imipramine (Tofranil) ■ Anti-Parkinson medication trihexyphenidyl (Artane) ■ Irritable bowel syndrome medication dicyclomine (Bentyl) ■ Overactive bladder medication oxybutynin (Ditropan)	Some anticholinergic can cause confusion, constipation, problems urinating, blurry vision, and low blood pressure. Men with an enlarged prostate should be particularly cautious when taking these medications.
AVOID the pain reliever meperidine (Demerol).	Meperidine can increase the risk of seizures and can cause confusion.
AVOID certain over-the-counter products such as products that contain the antihistamines diphenhydramine (Benadryl, Tylenol PM) and chlorpheniramine (AllerChlor, Chlor-Trimeton).	Although these products are sold without a prescription, they can cause confusion, blurred vision, constipation, problems urinating, and dry mouth.
If the older person is NOT being treated for psychosis, AVOID using antipsychotics such as: ■ Haloperidol (Haldol) ■ Risperidone (Risperdal) ■ Quetiapine (Seroquel)	Antipsychotics can increase the risk of stroke or even death. They can also cause tremors and other side effects, as well as increase the risk of falls.
AVOID estrogen pills and patches.	Estrogen pills and patches can increase the risk of breast cancer, blood clots, and even dementia.

Data from: American Geriatrics Society (AGS) Foundation for Health and Aging. "Ten Medications Older Adults Should Avoid or Use with Caution," April 2012.

Prevention

You have read about a number of ways to reduce adverse drug events and improve medication adherence. A comprehensive prehospital patient history must include a complete medication history, including medication adherence, OTC medication use, nutritional supplements, and herbal medication use.

Other specific ways to prevent adverse medication-related events in older patients include:

- Collect all of the patient's medications, including OTC drugs, and bring them to the emergency department when time does not allow for a detailed medication history.

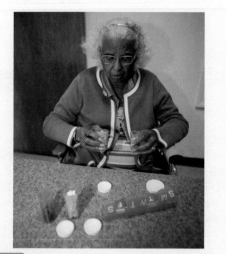

Figure 12-14 Assess whether a patient is taking the medication as prescribed.
© Jones & Bartlett Learning. Courtesy of MIEMSS.

- Assess whether a patient is taking the medication as prescribed (**Figure 12-14**).
- Assess the patient for any known side effects to current medications.
- Encourage the patient to develop a complete and up-to-date medication list to carry at all times.

Medication Tip

The most important contribution that EMS providers can make to improve medication adherence and prevent medication problems in older patients is to get a thorough history of medications, nutritional supplements, and herbal medicines.

Summary

Older people consume the largest proportion of medications and, due to age-related changes, are at increased risk of adverse drug events. As the number of drugs consumed increases, the risk of drug interactions also rises, which makes obtaining a thorough medication history and transporting medications with the patient all the more important.

EMS providers must also take a proactive role in addressing potential problems, such as nonadherence and its causes. There is more information and technology available to help EMS providers than ever before. Drug-related problems can contribute to the functional decline of an older person and to an increase in emergency department visits. Successful treatment of older patients relies on a multidisciplinary team approach. EMS providers should consider themselves a part of that team.

References

1. Berryman SN, Jennings J, Ragsdale S, Lofton T, Huff CD, Rooker SJ. Beers Criteria for potentially inappropriate medication use in older adults. *MEDSURG Nursing* 2012:21.3:129–132.
2. Parker BM, Cusack BJ, Vestal RE. Pharmacokinetic optimization of drug therapy in elderly patients. *Drugs Aging* 1995:7:10–18.
3. Jiraki K. *Lethal effects of normeperedine*, March 1992. National Center for Biotechnology Information, National Library of Medicine, National Institute of Health. PubMed ID 1585886.
4. Colloco G, Tosato M, Vetrano DL, et al. Inappropriate drugs in elderly patients with severe cognitive impairment: Results from the shelter study. *PLoS One* 2012:7(10):e46669.
5. Berryman SN, Jennings J, Ragsdale S, Lofton T, Huff CD, Rooker SJ.
6. Teixeira J, Crozatti M, Santos C, Romano-Lieber NS. Potential drug-drug interactions in prescriptions to patients over 45 years of age in primary care, Southern Brazil. *PLoS One* 2012:7(10):e47062.
7. Berryman SN, Jennings J, Ragsdale S, Lofton T, Huff CD, Rooker SJ.
8. Teixeira J, Crozatti M, Santos C, Romano-Lieber NS.
9. Field TS, Gurwitz JH, Glynn RJ, et al. The renal effects of nonsteroidal anti-inflammatory drugs in older people: findings from the Established Populations for Epidemiologic Studies of the Elderly. *J Am Geriatr Soc* 1999:47:507–511.
10. Huang AR, Mallet L, Rochefort CM, et al. Medication-related falls in the elderly. *Drugs Aging* 2012:29(5):359–376.
11. Ibid.
12. Murray M. Common questions about St. John's Wort extract. *Am J Nat Med* 1991:4(7):14–19.

13. Berryman SN, Jennings J, Ragsdale S, Lofton T, Huff CD, Rooker SJ.

14. Opondo D, Eslami S, Visscher S, et al. Inappropriateness of medication prescriptions to elderly patients in the primary care setting: a systematic review. *PLoS One* 2012:7(8):e43617.

15. Topinkova E, Baeyens JP, Michel JP, Land PO. Evidence-based strategies for the optimization of pharmacotherapy in older people. *Drugs Aging* 2012:29(6):477–494.

16. Konrat C, Boutron I, Trinquart L, Auleley GR, Ricordeau P, Ravaud P. Underrepresentation of elderly people in randomized controlled trials. *PLoS One* 2012:7(3):e33559.

17. Ibid.

18. Topinkova E, Baeyens JP, Michel JP, Land PO.

19. Brierley, J. *Danger of flumazenil use in pediatric patients in pediatric status epilepticus*, March 2006. National Center for Biotechnology Information, National Library of Medicine, National Institute of Health. PubMed ID 16628099.

CASE STUDY SUMMARIES

Case Study 1 Summary

There are indications the patient may be nonadherent with her medications. For example, she cannot find her antibiotic medication, and is therefore probably not taking it. Also, she appears to be taking too much of her Xanax prescription. There are also indications the patient is at risk for dangerous drug interactions. For example, vitamin K alters the anticoagulant effect of Coumadin. The patient may also be drinking alcohol while taking Xanax, and alcohol increases the depressant effects of Xanax. Antibiotics should not be taken with grapefruit juice. Antacids and Fosamax should be taken at least 2 hours apart. The patient uses at least two different pharmacies, which increases the risk of drug–drug interactions. The patient should be asked the following questions:

- What specific medications do you take?
- What is the dose and frequency of each medication?
- Who prescribed each medication?
- Are the medications being taken as prescribed?
- Are any of the medications or dosages new?
- Are all of the medications filled at the same pharmacy?
- Do you take any OTC medications or supplements?
- What time of day is each medication taken?
- Are any of the medications supposed to be taken with food or water? If so, are they?

This patient should be managed as follows:

- The patient should be transported for further evaluation.
- The patient's medications should be brought with her to the hospital.
- The residence should be surveyed for indications of the patient's activities of daily living, including alcohol use.
- Your transfer of care report should include all of your concerns about the patient's medications.

Case Study 2 Summary

The additional information you would like to know includes the following:

- Is the patient's confusion new?
- Has the patient been seen by his physician for the recent falls?
- Does the patient take his medication as prescribed?

The daughter states her dad has been confused off and on for several weeks. He has not seen his doctor for almost one year. The daughter gives her dad his medications as soon as she gets home every afternoon.

The patient's recent falls and confusion could be due to dangerous drug interactions. For example, clonidine and digoxin can cause major drug–drug interactions when used together. Digoxin levels should be carefully monitored in older patients and this patient has not seen his doctor in almost one year. Benadryl can cause significant problems when used by older patients. According to the FDA, Levodopa may increase the risk of cardiac problems.

The patient should be transported for further evaluation of his mentation and recent falls. The patient should also be evaluated for potential drug interactions. All medications should be brought with the patient to the hospital.

CHAPTER 13

Elder Abuse

LEARNING OBJECTIVES

1. Define elder abuse and neglect and discuss their incidence.

2. Discuss the profiles of an at-risk elder and an abuser.

3. Describe the techniques used to assess elder abuse and neglect.

4. Demonstrate sensitivity to the abused older person.

5. Discuss the proper documentation and reporting of elder abuse and neglect cases.

6. Understand the link between animal cruelty and other forms of domestic abuse.

Introduction

With the increasing number of older persons in society, new challenges and, sadly, new problems are being created. Elder abuse and neglect is one such problem. **Elder abuse** is a shocking revelation. It is a full-scale national problem that can occur anywhere, at any time. It is insidious, forcing many older persons to live the end of their lives in fear and deprivation. However, it has not always been viewed as a crime; up until the 1980s, the maltreatment of older adults was considered a mere social problem in the United States. This changed when legislators across the country began developing elder abuse statutes and mandatory reporting laws.

Despite the legislation that has been passed, the phenomenon of elder abuse continues to be coined "the hidden iceberg," as estimates are that many more incidents take place than are reported. According to the House Select Committee on Aging, elder abuse is less likely to be reported than child abuse. But like child abuse and domestic violence a decade ago, it is an issue that is moving toward the front of the nation's social consciousness. With this move, a variety of issues involving the identification and management of elder abuse must be confronted.

Attitude Tip

Acting in the patient's best interest is at the forefront of the prehospital care provider's responsibility. Nowhere is this responsibility more important than in the face of elder abuse and neglect.

Definitions

Elder abuse is defined as any form of mistreatment that results in harm or loss to an older person.[1] The National Center on Elder Abuse uses the following terms to describe the specific types of abuse and neglect:

- **Physical abuse**: the use of physical force that may result in injury, physical pain, or impairment. Examples include direct physical harm, such as shoving, pushing, hitting, shaking, hair-pulling, and unreasonable physical or chemical restraint.
- **Sexual abuse**: nonconsensual sexual contact of any kind.
- **Psychological or emotional abuse**: infliction of anguish, pain, or distress through verbal or nonverbal acts. Examples include verbal assaults, threats, creating fear or isolation, and withholding emotional support.
- **Financial/material exploitation**: illegal or improper use of an older person's funds, property, or assets.
- **Neglect**: failure to provide needed care, services, or supervision. Examples include failure to provide food, clothing, shelter, health and safety, and/or medical care. Two types of neglect have been identified:
  - **Active neglect**: deliberate withholding of companionship, medicine, food, exercise, and/or assistance to the bathroom.[2]
  - **Passive neglect**: ignoring, leaving alone, isolating, or forgetting the older person. Passive neglect can result from inadequate knowledge, laziness, or illness on the part of the care provider (**Figure 13-1**).[3]
- **Self-neglect**: behaviors of an older person that threaten his or her health or safety. Self-neglect can result from the older person being in poor health, having mental

CASE STUDY 1

You are called for a patient assist to the home of Mr. Weinberg, an 82-year-old man who lives with his 52-year-old son. On this date, a neighbor stopped by to see Mr. Weinberg and found him lying in bed with soiled sheets and soiled pajamas. The neighbor asked Mr. Weinberg where his son was, and Mr. Weinberg replied that he had not seen his son the last couple of evenings but that he was at work.

Your scene observation reveals that the bed sheets and the 82-year-old man's pajamas are indeed soiled. Additionally, you note that bed sores are beginning to form on the older man's thigh and buttocks. During your initial interview, Mr. Weinberg states that he and his son are under extreme financial difficulties and that his illnesses are getting worse. Mr. Weinberg's son receives his father's monthly pension check and handles all deposits and withdrawals. His son is also responsible for paying all of his bills, along with purchasing groceries, medications, and personal items for Mr. Weinberg. However, according to Mr. Weinberg, it seems that the worse his illnesses get, the less he sees his son.

- What are your immediate priorities?
- What are your thoughts regarding the son's obligations to his father?

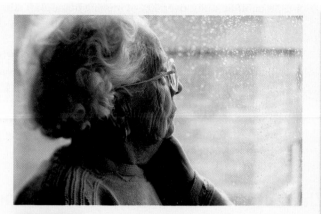

Figure 13-1 Passive neglect occurs when the older person is ignored, left alone, isolated, or forgotten.
© PhotoDisc

decline, or lacking the financial resources to care for him- or herself. Examples of self-neglect include not providing for one's own needs, such as hygiene, food, and medications. Older persons most at risk for self-neglect are those living alone in the community.

- **Abandonment**: the desertion of an older person by an individual who has physical custody of the older person or by a person who has assumed responsibility for providing care to the older person.

These definitions help provide an understanding of the various types of abuse and neglect. However, one of the problems with defining elder abuse and neglect is that there is no national, uniform set of definitions. In addition, more than one form of abuse can be, and often is, occurring at the same time. In fact, more than 50% of abusers tend to commit more than one type of abuse.

A simple way of understanding the manifestations of any type of abuse or neglect is to ascribe to the principle of *inadequate care*. Suspect abuse or neglect if the care of the older person appears inadequate for any reason.

Attitude Tip

The goal of elder abuse detection and reporting is to help the older victim live a life free from abuse, fear, and intimidation.

Incidence

As previously mentioned, incidents of elder abuse often go unreported. This could be due to a number of reasons. The older person may be reluctant to report the incident, fearing retaliation by the abuser or not wanting to get the abuser—who is a family member nearly 90% of the time—in trouble. Another reason for not reporting may be that the older person lacks the ability to

report the incident, perhaps due to a physical or cognitive disability. Additionally, professionals may miss the signs of abuse because of a lack of detection training. Regardless of the reason, it is simply not known exactly how many older people suffer from abuse and neglect.

The National Elder Abuse Incidence Study, reported by the National Center on Elder Abuse (NCEA) in 1998, provides one of the best national estimates of elder abuse incidence. According to the study, an estimated 551,011 persons, aged 60 years and older, experienced some type of abuse and/or neglect in a domestic setting in 1996, with older women being abused at a higher rate than males.[5] Of the total estimate, only 21% of the incidents were reported to Adult Protective Services (APS).

More recently, the NCEA provided additional information regarding the incidence and prevalence of elder abuse and neglect. According to the NCEA, the most recent major studies reported that about 10% of study participants experienced abuse in the prior year. This number does not include financial abuse. Major financial exploitation was self-reported at a rate of about 4%.[6]

Despite the accessibility of APS in all 50 states, as well as the mandatory reporting laws for elder abuse found in most states, an overwhelming number of cases of abuse, neglect, and exploitation still go undetected each year. In fact, one study estimated that only 1 in 14 cases of elder abuse ever come to the attention of authorities. Although these numbers are discouraging, available data from APS agencies shows that there is an increasing trend in the reporting of elder abuse. Still, given the standard error, the importance of recognizing and reporting elder abuse and neglect cannot be overemphasized. Recognition and referral will have a profound impact on the life of the older victim, who may otherwise continue to be subjected to a life of abuse and neglect.

Elder Abuse in Long-Term Care Facilities

The National Elder Abuse Incidence Study did not address abuse in institutional settings. In July 2001, the United States House of Representatives released a study entitled "Abuse of Residents Is a Major Problem in U.S. Nursing Homes." The study investigated the incidence of abuse in nursing homes in the United States by evaluating state inspections and complaint investigations that occurred between January 1, 1999 and January 1, 2001. The study reported that nearly one out of every three nursing homes in the United States was cited for an abuse violation during the study period, with more than 2,500 of those violations being serious enough to cause actual harm to residents (**Figure 13-2**).[7] Many of these violations—which included cases of physical, sexual, and verbal abuse—were only discovered after a formal complaint was filed.

Although only about 5% of the nation's older persons reside in nursing facilities, those who do often suffer multiple chronic and debilitating illnesses. Additionally, many residents of nursing facilities do not receive visits from relatives or close acquaintances. Nursing home residents who receive no visitors have a

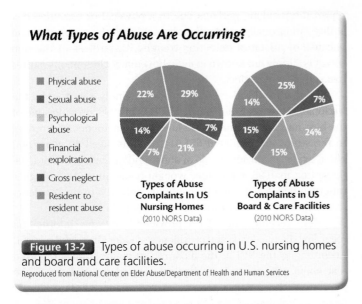

What Types of Abuse Are Occurring?

- Physical abuse
- Sexual abuse
- Psychological abuse
- Financial exploitation
- Gross neglect
- Resident to resident abuse

Types of Abuse Complaints In US Nursing Homes (2010 NORS Data)

Types of Abuse Complaints in US Board & Care Facilities (2010 NORS Data)

Figure 13-2 Types of abuse occurring in U.S. nursing homes and board and care facilities.
Reproduced from National Center on Elder Abuse/Department of Health and Human Services

higher likelihood of abuse and neglect, as there is no outside influence to watch over the resident's care. The NCEA provides the following additional statistics regarding elder abuse in long-term care facilities:

- In one study, 44% of nursing home residents said they had been abused and 95% said they had been neglected or seen another resident neglected.

- In another study, over 50% of nursing home staff admitted to abusing or neglecting older patients within the prior year.
- In a survey of certified nursing assistants, 17% of participants admitted to physically abusing a nursing home resident, 51% admitted to yelling at a resident, and 23% admitted to insulting or swearing at a resident.
- In another survey, 7% of all complaints reported to long-term care ombudsmen regarding long-term care facilities pertained to abuse, neglect, or exploitation.[8]

Characteristics of Elder Mistreatment in Long-Term Care Facilities

As in the domestic setting, many cases of elder abuse and neglect in nursing homes go unreported. Victims may not have a way to report the abuse, may not know how to report it, or may fear retaliation for reporting it. Additionally, older people are at an increased risk for abuse if they reside in nursing facilities that have a history of providing inadequate care, being understaffed, and providing poor training to employees. The National Institute of Justice provides four categories of characteristics that can be used to determine whether mistreatment of an older adult is occurring or has occurred in the long-term care facility (**Table 13-1**).

Table 13-1	Characteristics of Abuse and Neglect in Long-Term Care Facilities
Category	**Specific Characteristics**
Physical condition and quality of care	■ Documented but untreated injuries ■ Undocumented injuries ■ Multiple, untreated, or undocumented pressure sores ■ Medical orders not followed ■ Poor oral care, poor hygiene, and lack of cleanliness of residents ■ Malnourished residents that have no documentation for low weight ■ Bruising on nonambulatory residents or bruising that occurs in unusual locations ■ Family statements and facts concerning poor care ■ Level of care for residents with non-attentive family members
Facility characteristics	■ Unchanged linens ■ Strong odors (such as urine or feces) ■ Trash cans that have not been emptied ■ Food issues (such as smells that come from the cafeteria at all hours, or food that has been left on trays) ■ Past problems
Inconsistencies	■ Between medical records, statements made by staff members, or what is viewed by the investigator ■ Between statements given by different groups ■ Between the reported time of death and condition of the body
Staff behaviors	■ Staff members who follow the investigator too closely ■ Lack of knowledge or concern about a resident ■ Evasiveness, unintended or purposeful, verbal or nonverbal ■ Facility's unwillingness to release medical records

Reproduced from National Institute of Justice. "Potential Markers for Elder Mistreatment." January 8, 2008.

The Nursing Home Reform Act

In response to the estimated incidence of elder abuse, the Nursing Home Reform Act was passed as part of the Omnibus Budget Reconciliation Act of 1987. To ensure that nursing home residents receive quality care, the Act addresses the services and standards that nursing home facilities must provide for their patients. Specifically, the Nursing Home Reform Act requires that all nursing home facilities must "promote and protect the rights of each patient" (**Table 13-2**).

Table 13-2   Rights of Nursing Home Residents

Quality of Life: The law requires nursing homes to "care for the residents in such a manner and in such an environment as will promote maintenance or enhancement of the quality of life of each resident." A new emphasis is placed on dignity, choice, and self-determination for nursing home residents.

Provision of Services and Activities: The law requires each nursing home to "provide services and activities to attain or maintain the highest practicable physical, mental, and psychological well-being of each resident in accordance with a written plan of care which …is initially prepared, with participation to the extent practicable of the resident or the resident's legal representative."

Participation in Facility Administration: The law makes "resident and advocacy participation" a criterion for assessing a facility's compliance with administration requirements.

Assuring Access to the Ombudsman Program: The law grants immediate access by ombudsmen to residents and reasonable access, in accordance with state law, to records. It requires facilities to inform residents how to contact an ombudsman to voice complaints or in the event of a transfer or discharge from the facility and requires state agencies to share inspection results with ombudsman.

Specific nursing home residents' rights include:

Rights to Self-Determination: Nursing home residents have the right:

- to choose their personal physician;
- to full information, in advance, and participation in planning and making any changes in their care and treatment;
- to reside and receive services with reasonable accommodation by the facility of individual needs and preferences;
- to voice grievances about the care and trweatment they do or do not receive without discrimination or reprisal, and to receive prompt response from the facility;
- to organize and participate in resident groups (and their families have the right to organize family groups) in the facility.

Personal and Privacy Rights: Nursing home residents have the right:

- to participate in social, religious, and community activities as they choose;
- to privacy in medical treatment, accommodations, personal visits, written and telephone conversations;
- to confidentiality of personal and clinical residents.

Rights Regarding Abuse and Restraints: Nursing home residents have the right:

- to be free from physical and mental abuse, corporal punishment, involuntary seclusion or disciplinary use of restraints;
- to be free of restraints used for the convenience of the staff rather than the well-being of the residents;
- to have restraints used only under written physician's orders to treat a resident's medical symptoms and ensure the resident's safety and the safety of others;
- to be given psychopharmacologic medication only as ordered by a physician as part of a written plan of care for a specific medical symptom, with annual review for appropriateness by an independent, external expert.

Rights to Information: Nursing homes must:

- upon request provide residents with the latest inspection results and any plan of correction submitted by the facility;
- notify residents in advance of any plans to change their rooms or roommate;
- inform residents of their rights upon admission and provide them with a written copy of the rights, including their rights regarding personal funds and their right to file a complaint with the state survey agency;
- inform residents in writing, at admission and throughout their stay, of the services available under the basic rate and of any extra charges for extra services, including, for Medicaid residents, a list of services covered by Medicaid, and for those for which there is an extra charge;

(Continued)

Table 13-2   Rights of Nursing Home Residents (*Continued*)

- prominently display and provide oral and written information for residents about how to apply for and use Medicaid benefits and how to receive a refund for previous private payments that Medicaid will pay retroactively.

Rights to Visits: Nursing homes must:

- permit immediate visits by a resident's personal physician and by representatives of the licensing agency and the Ombudsman program;
- permit immediate visits by a resident's relatives, with the resident's consent;
- permit visits "subject to reasonable restriction" for others who visit with the resident's consent;
- permit an ombudsman to review resident's clinical records if a resident grants permission.

Transfer and Discharge Rights: Nursing homes "must permit each resident to remain in the facility and must not transfer or discharge the resident unless":

- the transfer or discharge is necessary to meet the resident's welfare and the resident's welfare cannot be met by the facility;
- appropriate because the resident's health has improved such that the resident no longer needs nursing home care;
- the health or safety of other residents is endangered;
- the resident has failed, after reasonable notice, to pay an allowable facility charge for an item or service provided upon the resident request;
- the facility ceases to operate.

Notice must be given to residents and their representatives before transfer:

- Timing: at least 30 days in advance, or as soon as possible if more immediate changes in health require more immediate transfer;
- Content: reasons for transfer, the resident's right to appeal the transfer, and the name, address, and phone number of the Ombudsman Program and protection and advocacy programs for the mentally ill and developmentally disabled;
- Returning to the Facility: the right to request that a resident's bed be held, including information about how many days Medicaid will pay for the bed to be held and the facility's bed-hold policies, and the right to return to the next available bed if Medicaid bed-holding coverage lapses.

Orientation: A facility must prepare and orient to ensure safe and orderly transfer or discharge from the facility.

Protection of Personal Funds: Nursing homes must:

- not require residents to deposit their personal funds with the facility;
- if it accepts written responsibility for resident's funds:
  - keep funds over $50 in an interest bearing account, separate from the facility account;
  - keep other funds available in a separate account or petty cash fund;
  - keep a complete and separate accounting of each resident's funds, with a written record of all transactions, available for review by residents and their representatives;
  - notify Medicaid residents when their balance account comes within $200 of the Medicaid limit and the effect of this on their eligibility;
  - upon the resident's death, turn funds over to the resident's trustee;
  - purchase a surety bond to secure residents' funds in its keeping;
  - not charge a resident for any item or service covered by Medicaid, specifically including routine personal hygiene items and services.

Protection Against Medicaid Discrimination: Nursing homes must:

- establish and maintain identical policies and practices regarding transfer, discharge and the provision of services required under Medicaid for all individuals regardless of source payment;
- not require residents to waive their rights to Medicaid, and must provide information about how to apply for Medicaid;
- not require a third party to guarantee payment as a condition of admission or continued stay;
- not "charge, solicit, accept or receive" gifts, money, donations or "other consideration" as a precondition for admission or for continued stay for persons eligible for Medicare.

Reproduced from Title 42 Code of Federal Regulations, Part 483.

Long-Term Care Ombudsman

As noted, the Nursing Home Reform Act acknowledged the right of residents to have access to the Long-Term Care Ombudsman Program. A long-term care **ombudsman** is a resident advocate who can be a valuable resource for the EMS provider. The purpose of the Ombudsman Program is to respond to the needs of residents facing problems in long-term care facilities and intervene when necessary. The ombudsman is also a direct link to the long-term care administrator.

Specific responsibilities of a long-term care ombudsman include:

- Resolving complaints made by or for residents (**Table 13-3**)
- Educating consumers and providers about the rights of residents and good care practices
- Promoting community and volunteer involvement
- Providing information to the public regarding long-term care facilities and their services, residents' rights, and legislative and policy issues
- Advocating for residents' rights and quality care in long-term care facilities
- Promoting the development of citizen organizations, family councils, and resident councils

State Long-Term Care Ombudsman Programs operate in all 50 states, the District of Columbia, Guam, and Puerto Rico. As of 2010, there are an additional 578 local programs.[9] The EMS provider should learn if there is an ombudsman in the long-term care facility they serve. EMS agencies can arrange to train with the ombudsman on topics such as elder abuse and other issues that affect the health, safety, welfare, or rights of long-term care facility residents. Establishing these relationships will lead to improved patient care.

Table 13-3	Top Complaints of Residents in Nursing Homes
1. Unheeded requests for assistance
2. Problems with discharge planning or eviction notification and procedures
3. Lack of dignity or respect for residents by staff
4. Problems with organization or administration of medications
5. Resident conflict, including roommate conflict

Data from Congressional Research Service: Older Americans Act: Long-Term Care Ombudsman Program, July 1, 2009.

Risk Factors

Older people who are at risk for abuse and neglect include those with chronic, progressive, disabling illnesses that impair function and create care needs that exceed or will exceed their caregivers' ability to meet them, such as:

- Dementia
- Parkinson's disease
- Severe arthritis
- Severe cardiac disease
- Severe chronic obstructive pulmonary disease (COPD)
- Severe non-insulin dependent diabetes
- Recurrent strokes[10]

According to a study reported by the NCEA, abuse and neglect of dementia patients was detected in 47.3% of surveyed caregivers in the United States.[11] Of those caregivers, verbal abuse was the most reported type of abuse of patients with dementia, with 60% of caregivers reporting that they had been verbally abusive with the person for whom they were providing care. Another 5% to 10% of caregivers reported that they were physically abusive, and 14% reported that they were neglectful.

Those with progressive impairments who are without informal support from family or neighbors, or whose caregivers manifest signs of burnout, are also at increased risk for abuse. According to the NCEA, 1 in 3 adults aged 65 years or older has a disability. In a review of literature published from 2000 to 2010, lifetime prevalence of abuse against adults with disabilities was found to be 26% to 90% for women and 28.7% to 86.7% for men. As is demonstrated by these numbers, abuse and neglect occurs at disproportionate rates among men and women with disabilities. Sometimes this abuse comes from the disabled adult's care provider. In one study, institutionalized adult women with disabilities reported a 33% prevalence of having ever experienced abuse, versus 21% for institutionalized adult women without disabilities. In another study, 30% of disabled adults receiving some form of personal assistance services for support with activities of daily living reported that they received one or more types of abuse or neglect from their primary provider.[12]

Additional older adults who are at risk for abuse and neglect include:

- Those with a personal history of substance abuse or violent behavior or a family member with a similar history
- Those who live with a family in which there is a history of child or spousal abuse
- Those with family members who are financially dependent on them
- Those residing in institutions that have a history of providing substandard care

■ Those whose caregivers are under sudden increased stress due, for example, to loss of a job, spouse, or other family member; diminishing health; or other financial concerns

If assigned to the same location for a period of time, or in a small community, many EMS providers know the people they serve. This can be helpful for identifying abuse in older patients (**Table 13-4**). Suspicion should be aroused if an older person repeatedly presents with injuries that are inconsistent with the history stated, has experienced recurring multiple injuries, or has symptoms that cannot be explained medically. When an older person is injured, any delay in accessing emergency medical care should be noted. EMS providers should also take note of a caregiver who will not allow the patient to provide his or her own history, as well as frail or cognitively impaired older people who are alone (**Table 13-5**). Careful questioning and detailed observations will help yield clues as to the presence of elder abuse and/or neglect.

Theories of Abuse and Neglect

There are many theories that attempt to explain abuse and neglect. Among the most prominent theories are the social learning or transgenerational theory, the stressed caregiver theory, isolation theory, dependency theory, and the psychopathology of the abuser theory.

Table 13-4 Profiles of the Abused
While elder abuse can occur anywhere, and at any time, profiles of potential victims (i.e., those that are most at risk) can be drawn. Abused older people are more likely to:
■ Be women
■ Be over age 75 years
■ Have one or more chronic physical or mental impairment(s) placing them in a care-dependent position
■ Live with their abusers
■ Be socially isolated
■ Exhibit problematic behavior (such as incontinence or shouting in the middle of the night)
Data from National Center for Victims of Crime. (n.d.) *Focus on the future: A systems approach to prosecution and victim assistance, a training and resource manual*. Washington, DC: U.S. Department of Justice, Office for Victims of Crime.

Table 13-5 Profiles of the Abuser
As with the abused, profiles of abusers can be drawn. Abusers tend to:
■ Live with their victim, as most abusers are adult children and spouses
■ Be over 50
■ Be dependent on the victim for financial support
■ Be poor at impulse control
■ Be ill-prepared or reluctant to provide care
■ Have a history of domestic violence
■ Have drug or alcohol dependency problems
Data from National Center for Victims of Crime. (n.d.) *Focus on the future: A systems approach to prosecution and victim assistance, a training and resource manual*. Washington, DC: U.S. Department of Justice, Office for Victims of Crime.

The **social learning theory** or **transgenerational theory** maintains that violence is learned. It states that if children are abused, they will abuse their own children. If this theory is extended to elder abuse, the theory holds that these same children will abuse their parents as well. The **stressed caregiver theory** contends that when the caregiver reaches a certain stress level, abuse and neglect situations will occur. **Isolation theory** maintains that a diminishing social network is a major risk factor in elder abuse. The **dependency theory** maintains that frailty and medical illness set up the older person for abuse and neglect. Finally, the **psychopathology of the abuser theory** states that the abuser has problems (such as personality or substance abuse) that lead to abuse and neglect.[13]

Observing for Clues to Elder Abuse

Elder abuse can be very subtle and may be overlooked in a crisis or emergency setting. Prehospital care professionals can be of valuable assistance in evaluating the potential victim of elder abuse. The EMS provider is one of the first responders on the scene and performs the initial medical evaluation of the patient. In addition, the EMS provider is able to provide information regarding the patient's environment that may otherwise be unknown to social services and other health care providers.

The EMS provider should evaluate each incident involving an older person with a critical eye toward the potential for elder abuse and/or neglect. Awareness and a high index of suspicion are extremely important. If the environment, care, and attitudes of those surrounding the older patient are anything but adequate, *suspect that something may be wrong.*

Environmental Assessment

Many of the risk factors associated with elder abuse—alcohol/substance abuse by the caregiver, family violence, ineffective coping strategies of the caregiver, and dependency between caregiver and victim—will, in most circumstances, be unknown to the EMS provider. Given these unknowns and the sometimes subtle nature of neglect, the assessment phase should begin with a scene survey of the patient's environment (**Figure 13-3**). When performing the environmental assessment, consider the following:

- What is the physical condition of the patient's residence? Is the exterior of the home in need of repair? Is the home secure?
- Are hazardous conditions present (i.e., poor wiring, rotten floors, unventilated gas heaters, broken window glass, or clutter that prevents adequate egress)?
- Is the home too hot or too cold?
- Are the utilities (electricity, heat, water, sewer) working and adequate?
- Is there a fecal or urine odor in the home?
- Is food present in the home? Is it adequate and unspoiled?
- Are liquor bottles present (lying empty)?
- Is bedding soiled or urine soaked?

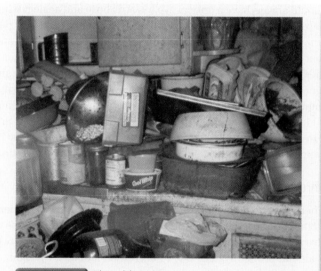

Figure 13-3 The older person's environment can provide clues to abuse and neglect.
Courtesy of Baltimore County Police Department, Baltimore, Maryland

CASE STUDY 2

You are called to the home of an 84-year-old female. When you arrive at the residence, you are greeted by the patient's daughter who tells you that she called 911 after she arrived to visit her mother and found her in bed barely arousable. The patient, although typically alert and fairly active, requires supervision for wandering. The family recently hired a 24/7 live-in home care provider through an agency; however, when the daughter arrived to her mother's house, the care provider was not present. Upon contacting the provider's agency, she was told that the regular care provider had a family emergency and they had sent a substitute to cover the shift.

The patient mumbles when shaken. She is warm and dry, and her color is good. Her vital signs are: BP: 160/70; P: 92, R: 10 and oxygen saturation of 89%. As you assess the patient's environment, you notice a bottle of 50 mg diphenhydramine on the nightstand next to her bed. The daughter was unaware her mother was on this drug, and the name on the bottle has been scratched off, so you are not sure who the medication was prescribed to. You note the prescription was filled yesterday evening and ten pills are missing.

- How should you manage this patient?
- What are your concerns regarding this patient?

- If the older person has a disability, are appropriate assistive devices (such as a walker or wheelchair) present?
- Are there restraints in the home?
- Does the older person have adequate access to a telephone (near the bed or other location where the older person spends time)?
- Are medications out of date, unmarked, or prescribed by many different doctors?
- Are smoke detectors present and working?
- If the older person is living with others, is he or she confined to one part of the home?
- If the older person is residing in a nursing facility, does the care appear to be adequate to his or her needs?

Clinical Assessment

When performing the physical examination of an older person, the EMS provider must be sure to preserve the older person's dignity. In addition, the EMS provider should always have a critical eye toward abuse and neglect when performing an assessment or clinical evaluation of an older person. There are, however, clinical syndromes and disease states that can mimic elder abuse and neglect. (For example, some medications cause changes in the older person's clotting and bleeding mechanisms, placing them at risk to bruise more easily.) Important elder abuse clues can be yielded from environmental and social indicators, the interaction between the patient and caregiver, and the physical assessment, but these factors must be weighed together. Context is the key in making a determination.

Hygiene

There may be many factors that contribute to improper hygiene in the older person. Some older people, for example, choose to live an eccentric lifestyle; others may be limited in their ability to maintain proper hygiene due to decreased mobility, eyesight, or underlying disease processes. When assessing the older individual, look at his or her overall hygiene and consider the following: Is the older person's clothing clean? Is the older person dressed appropriately for the season? Are there cigarette burns on clothing? Are undergarments torn, soiled, or bloody? Does the older person have poor hygiene?

Age alone does not bring about changes to one's hygiene. In the face of neglect, the EMS provider should attempt to determine if there is someone responsible for the older person's care. If so, an investigation is warranted as to why proper hygiene is not being maintained for the older person.

Malnutrition and Dehydration

Malnutrition generally describes a person who is very thin or losing weight, has a low muscle or fat mass, is eating poorly, and/or has abnormal blood markers of nutritional status. Malnutrition can be the result of caregiver neglect, such as if a caregiver fails to maintain proper oral hygiene of a patient or if an institution's staff-to-patient ratio is inadequate and they fail to assist residents who require assistance with eating. Additionally, inappropriate prescribing of certain medications, such as anticholinergic drugs, psychotropic drugs, and other medications that impair mentation or appetite, may lead to malnutrition.[14]

Dehydration can also occur in cases of neglect, such as if food or liquid is withheld from the older person. Dehydration is defined as an inadequate level of water in the body. A loss of fluid from the body can lead to a variety of clinical manifestations in older people, including death. In cases of neglect from malnutrition and dehydration, a medical investigator will need to review the victim's medical records in order to document (or show lack of documentation for) weight loss, fluid intake/output, and appropriately prescribed medications. Evidence of recent weight loss may have to be obtained through an interview with the patient or caregiver.

Skin

Skin tears are common in older persons due to the loss of elasticity and collagen that occurs in the skin with age (**Figure 13-4**). However, suspicion should be aroused if skin tears appear in areas other than the arms or legs, or if the patient has multiple skin tears.

Recall that a pressure ulcer (as described in the *Changes with Age* chapter) is a sore, initially of the skin, that is caused by prolonged pressure, usually in a person who is lying down. The formation of a pressure ulcer is possible at any site but most

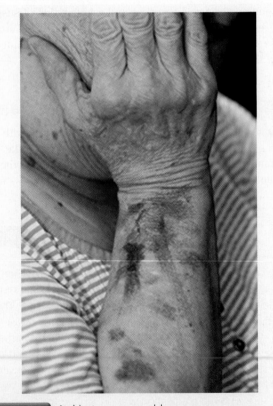

Figure 13-4 A skin tear on an older person.

commonly occurs over bony prominences, such as the sacrum, heels, trochanter, lateral malleoli, and ischial areas. The combination of pressure, shearing forces, friction, and moisture cause a lack of blood supply to the area, leading to tissue death. It is often difficult to distinguish pressure ulcers that result from illness from those that result from neglect. In the presence of pressure ulcers, the EMS provider should ask, were the ulcers preventable and how are they being cared for?

Urine burns may be suggestive that a person has been allowed to remain unchanged for long periods of time. **Excoriations** or chaffing may also suggest poor attention to continence (bladder control). Additionally, **infestations** may be present. Assess skin turgor for signs of dehydration. Other pertinent integumentary findings relevant to elder abuse include traumatic **alopecia** (as opposed to hair loss suggestive of normal aging); ecchymosis; burns; lacerations; skin disorders such as rash, impetigo, and eczema; and undiagnosed and untreated fractures (**Figure 13-5**).

Abrasions and Lacerations

An abrasion is a superficial injury involving the outer layer of the skin, and a laceration is full-thickness splitting of the skin (**Figure 13-6** and **Figure 13-7**). The patient should be evaluated for abrasions and/or lacerations. When evaluating an abrasion or laceration, identifying the mode of injury is the most important factor.[15] The victim or care provider may be able to provide information regarding the mechanism of injury. Suspicion should be aroused for an implausible explanation or injury patterns inconsistent with the description of how the laceration or abrasion was caused. Lacerations found on the palms of the hand or on the underside of the forearm may indicate that the victim was defending himself or herself from being stabbed. Additionally, EMS providers should be aware that abrasions often heal with scarring.[16]

Bruises

A bruise is the result of blunt force trauma with concomitant rupture of small blood vessels under the skin (**Figure 13-8**).[17] The

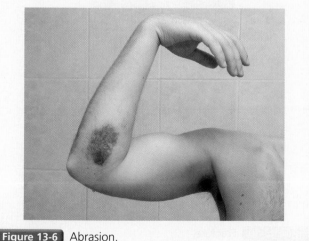

Figure 13-5 Knife wounds can also suggest abuse; this wound was inflicted by a husband during elder domestic violence.
Courtesy of Daniel J. Sheridan, PhD, RN

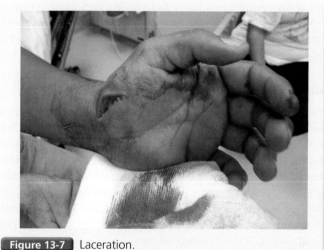

Figure 13-7 Laceration.
© E.M. Singletary, M.D. Used with permission.

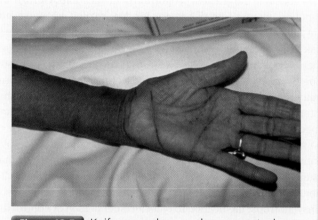

Figure 13-6 Abrasion.
© Kondor83/Shutterstock, Inc.

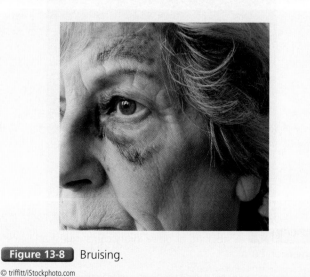

Figure 13-8 Bruising.
© triffitt/iStockphoto.com

eyelids, neck, and scrotum are very susceptible to bruising.[18] The evaluation of bruising on an older person must be taken in context. For example, blood-thinning medications taken by older people (such as Coumadin and Plavix) can cause bruising to occur more easily from non-assault-related causes. Additionally, older people are more prone to fall-related injuries that may cause bruising.

The most common locations for non-accidental bruising are the face and neck, chest wall, abdomen, and buttocks.[19] Bruising on the palms and soles may also indicate abuse, as these areas are not usually injured.[20] Bilateral bruising on soft parts of the body (such as the inner arm or thigh) also should be thought of as suspicious, as well as bruising that is clustered.

The pattern of a bruise may suggest its cause. Look for bruising that is in the shape of familiar objects (such as a belt buckle). Bruises will also retain the shape of fingers or knuckles. Parallel marks, called **tramline** bruising, indicate injury from a stick.[21] Multiple bruises and bruises in various stages of healing may indicate abuse.

Medical research and data indicate that bruising can be dated by its color. However, the dating of bruises is very problematic and is dependent upon many factors that vary from person to person, such as age, overall health, and medications. It is best to simply describe the location and size of bruises that are found on the victim's body.

Burns

The age group at greatest risk for experiencing a burn injury is those older than 75 years of age. Unlike other age groups, this population is most commonly burned by space heaters, cookers, and flammable liquids. Burns to older people should be evaluated as to their cause. For example, immersion burns (stocking or glove injuries) may be the result of a caregiver placing the older person in water that is too hot (**Figure 13-9**). Cigarette burns can result from a self-neglecting situation or from an intentional burn inflicted by someone else.

Fractures

Unfortunately, there is little data on fracture resolution in older people.[22] Fractures in older people often result from falls; however, falls alone may not be the sole indicator of abuse or neglect (**Figure 13-10**). There are certain fracture locations that should arouse suspicion and warrant further investigation as to their origin. Fractured, subluxed, or avulsed teeth or fractures of the zygomatic arch or the mandible and maxilla may indicate abuse.[23] Research also indicates that fractures of the head, spine, and trunk are more likely to be assault injuries than are limb fractures, sprains or strains, or musculoskeletal injuries.[24] Additionally, a spiral fracture of a long bone with no history of gross injury is diagnostic of abuse, as are fractures with a rotational component. Fractures at sites other than the hip, wrist, or vertebrae should raise suspicion of abuse in non-alcoholics.[25]

Medication Use and Misuse

Although older people represent only 12% of the U.S. population, they consume the greatest proportion of medications. Old age itself is not an independent risk factor for drug-related adverse events, but the number of medications used may significantly increase the risk of drug-related complications. Regarding abuse and neglect, there are many instances related to medication use and misuse. For example, drug interactions (drug–drug interactions, drug–nutrient interactions, drug–disease interactions, and drug–herb interactions) may result from a practitioner failing to understand specific precautions in older people. Furthermore, a caregiver can be guilty of intentional neglect by failure to administer an older patient's medications. Undermedication could also be a sign that a family member or caregiver is stealing the older person's medication. Conversely, the caregiver who overmedicates or administers a psychotropic medication to quiet an older person or control their behavior for the caregiver's comfort also can be guilty of abuse.

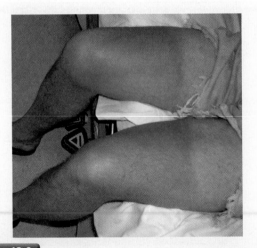

Figure 13-9 A stocking or glove injury can suggest an immersion burn.
© E. M. Singletary, M.D. Used with permission.

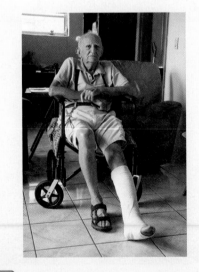

Figure 13-10 Fracture.
© Rauluminate/iStock/Thinkstock

Additionally, older patients who suffer any form of confusion or dementia who are dependent upon a caregiver for medication assistance may over- or undermedicate themselves if the caregiver does not regulate medication administration. This situation will be extremely difficult for the EMS provider to discern. Gathering a thorough medication history, including dosages and prescribed quantity, will aid a medical investigator in determining (through blood sampling) therapeutic levels and appropriate prescribing dosages.

Restraints

Restraints can be a way of controlling the behavior of an older person. However, older people do have rights regarding abuse and restraints. The previously mentioned Nursing Home Reform Act states that nursing home residents have the right to be free from disciplinary use of restraints or restraints used for the convenience of staff rather than the well-being of the resident. Restraints should only be used under a physician's written orders and only to "treat a resident's medical symptoms and ensure the resident's safety and the safety of others."[26] These rules apply to the use of chemical restraints (medications) as well. Additionally, physical restraints should not be so tight as to restrict movement completely, or cause injury to the skin and underlying tissues. Abuse occurs whenever the older person is restrained in a noncritical manner.[27]

Financial Exploitation and Fraud

Financial and material exploitation, as previously defined, is the illegal or improper use of an older person's funds, property, or assets. Financial exploitation can include credit card and telemarketing fraud, predatory lending, and theft or exploitation.

Additional Assessment Pearls

When observing an older person with a head injury listed as resulting from a fall, observe for other associated injuries (such as to the extremities or trunk). A head injury ascribed to a fall with no other associated injuries may be the result of an assault. Observe for additional signs of abuse and/or neglect, such as the presence of facial bruises, lacerations, or abrasions; tooth fractures; ill-fitting dentures (secondary in some cases to weight loss); mandibular and maxillary fractures; poor dental hygiene; oral venereal lesions; uvula ecchymosis (indicating possible forced oral copulation); and cigarette burns on the lips (this may signal either a neglect situation or a functional decline of the person).

Ophthalmologic assessment may indicate recent or chronic trauma. Examination of the eyes and periorbital area should be limited to assessing the pupils for size, reactivity, and extraocular movements, and observing for signs of orbital fractures. Findings indicative of recent trauma include subconjunctival or vitreous hemorrhage. If the victim is deceased, observe for signs of petechial hemorrhage.

When examining the nasal area, observe for signs of a deviated septum, which may indicate repeated trauma. When examining the anterior and posterior neck, observe for signs of circumscribed rope burns or handprints, or fingertip bruising (indicative of recent strangulation attempts or inappropriate restraint). If strangulation is suspected, patency of the trachea and an adequate airway must be confirmed. Bruising of the tracheal rings can result in gradual swelling that may lead to hypoxia and death. In persons with arthritis, the risk of paralysis or death increases with the worsening of atlantoaxial cervical subluxation (partial or incomplete dislocation of the atlas and the axis [the first and second cervical vertebrae]). In older persons with severe osteoporosis, cervical fractures or spinal cord injuries may result.

Blunt trauma to the thorax and abdomen may result in rib fractures and a **pneumothorax** or **hemothorax**. Serious abdominal trauma can lead to life-threatening conditions such as splenic rupture and intra-abdominal hemorrhage. **Grey Turner's sign** and **Cullen's sign** are suggestive of extravasation of intra-abdominal hemolyzed blood to the flank and periumbilical region, respectively. These forms of ecchymosis may not be immediately apparent, and context is the key to discovery. Abdominal bruising ascribed to a fall without other associated trauma to the older person should be viewed as suspicious.

Vaginal or rectal bleeding in the older person requires the differential diagnosis of sexual abuse or malignancy. Injuries to either the vagina or rectum should be treated accordingly. If sexual abuse is suspected, the preservation of evidence should be performed, as with all other sexual assault victims.

A neurological examination in the older person may prove difficult due to preexisting neurological conditions. The person's level of orientation upon presenting to EMS should be weighed against the person's normal level of orientation; however, this may be difficult to determine unless someone well known to the older person is present who can provide information regarding subtle cognitive changes. Focal neurologic signs and symptoms may be the result of spinal cord injury or head trauma with development of concussion or subdural or epidural hematoma. Note the person's orientation to person, place, and time, and his or her recollection of the present circumstances. More appropriate mental status examinations and neurologic testing can be performed at the hospital.

Social Assessment

Social assessment of an older person or caregiver is usually not solicited by the EMS provider. However, when considering cases of elder abuse and neglect, a social assessment can prove valuable if taken in context with other information. Some of the most important social assessment indicators are activities of daily living (ADLs). ADLs include self-care activities that people must accomplish to survive, such as eating, dressing, bathing, transferring, and toileting. Persons who are unable to perform these activities usually require a caregiver. If, during your observations, you find that an older person is unable to perform one or several of these functions, ask the following:

- Are these activities being provided for the older person? If so, by whom?
- Are there any delays in obtaining food, medication, or toileting? The older person may complain of this, or the environment may be suggestive of this. For example, there may not be food in the home.
- If the older person resides in an institutional setting, is the person able to feed himself or herself? If not, is food sitting out on a food tray? Has the person been lying in his or her own urine or feces for long periods of time?
- Does the person lack assistive devices (such as glasses, a hearing aid, dentures, a walker, or a wheelchair) when it is obvious he or she requires them?

Emotional suffering is one of the most important clues pointing to psychological abuse, but it is also very difficult for the EMS provider to assess. Examples of psychological abuse include harassment, intimidation, manipulation, belittling, and isolation. Victim responses and the observed interaction between the older person and the family or caregiver may yield clues as to the presence of abuse or neglect. For example, a victim who has been psychologically abused may appear to be ambivalent, deferent, passive, withdrawn, resigned, depressed, helpless, or hopeless. He or she may also seem to fear the caregiver or EMS provider. Fearfulness may be expressed in the eyes (in some cultures it is considered rude to look a person directly in the eye; be careful not to confuse deference with fear).

Sexual Assault in the Elderly

Being the victim of a sexual crime will be emotionally devastating for the older person, and is often seen as a loss of dignity. The majority of older victims are female and highly dependent, with dementia often being a factor. Older people with any degree of cognitive impairment or dementia are unable to consent to sex, unable to defend themselves, and often delay reporting a rape. In addition, these victims will be difficult to interview (refer to the *Communication* chapter for a review of communication challenges).

Many older victims are sexually assaulted in their own homes, and by those they know; in some cases, the perpetrator is even a family member. Three types of individuals who perpetrate rape against older victims have been identified. The first type is known as a **gerophile**—a sexual predator targeting older people. These individuals often seek jobs in nursing homes. A second type is the sexually aggressive older person, who also resides in the nursing home. The last type is a stranger or person who is known to the victim. Behaviors common in older sexual assault victims include withdrawal, fear, depression, anger, insomnia, increased interest in sexual matters, or increased sexual or aggressive behavior.

A 2005 study of forensic markers in female sexual abuse cases reported that the offender's hand was the primary mechanism of physical injury to nongenital areas of the older victim's body, and the offender's hands, fingers, mouth, or penis, or a foreign object, caused injury to the genital area.[28] Over half of the older victims in the study had at least one part of their body injured, and nearly half had signs of vaginal injury.[29] Age-related changes in older women make them more prone to injury after a sexual assault than younger women. Vaginal linings are not as elastic due to hormonal changes, increasing the risk of bleeding, pain, infections, or tears that may never fully heal. Brittle bones such as the pelvis and hips can be more easily broken or crushed by friction and weight of the rapist.[30] Victims of sexual abuse may also present with oral venereal legions. Additionally, bruising of the uvula and bruising of the palate and the junction of the hard palate may indicate forced oral copulation. Bleeding and bruising of the anogenital area, as well as difficulty in sitting and walking, may also indicate sexual abuse.

If sexual assault is encountered in a nursing home facility, the EMS provider should inquire about any new cases of sexually transmitted diseases or clustered cases of urinary tract infections.[31] When encountering sexual crimes against an older person, the prehospital professional must keep in mind the intergenerational difference that exists. Most older people were raised in a time when sexual matters were not discussed; victims may wish to not discuss the crime with medical personnel or law enforcement. The older female victim may also be reluctant to submit to a pelvic exam, or physical limitations (such as lower extremity contractures) may make examination difficult.[32]

Interviewing the Patient

As we learned in the *Communication* chapter, interviewing older people requires more time than interviewing younger people (**Figure 13-11**). Although the urgency of the situation will

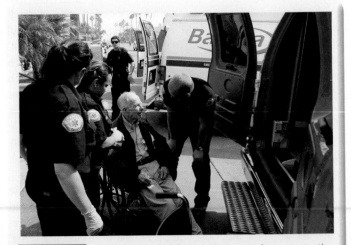

Figure 13-11 Interviewing older victims requires more time and must be done with compassion and respect.
© Joshua Lott/Bloomberg/Getty Images

determine the time that can be spent, the EMS provider should try not to rush through the interview. Some aging persons tend to integrate past events with the present.

When interviewing the older person, observe for the following:

- Does the older person appear fearful of a family member?
- Does the older person appear reluctant to respond when questioned?
- Does the older person appear depressed? Recall that the symptoms of depression include:
  - Dissatisfaction, restlessness, malaise
  - Sleep disturbance
  - Poor concentration, slowed thoughts
  - Change in appetite or weight
  - Loss of interest in usual activities
  - Psychomotor agitation or retardation
  - Suicidal ideations, recurrent thoughts of death
  - Sense of worthlessness, self-reproach, excessive guilt
  - Loss of energy
  (*Note*: Symptoms of depression are present for at least 2 weeks with no other major psychiatric or organic disorder present and are not due to bereavement.)
- Do the older person and caregiver provide conflicting accounts of the situation?
- Does the caregiver seem indifferent or hostile toward the older person?
- Does the caregiver "hover" around, not allowing the EMS provider privacy with the older person?
- Does the caregiver seem concerned about the problem at hand but not with the older person's overall health?
- Does the caregiver answer for the older person even when that person can provide a verbal history?
- Does the older person look to the caregiver before answering?
- Does the older person sound like he or she is reciting a "script" to explain injuries?
- Does the caregiver refer to the older person as "accident-prone"? Remember, injuries that do not fit medically or differ from the stated history should arouse suspicion.

If abuse or neglect is suspected, the following questions may help the EMS provider elicit a history from the older person:

- Are you afraid of anyone at home?
- Has anyone ever made you do things you did not want to do?
- Are you in fear of your caregiver?
- Have you ever been threatened or scolded by your caregiver?
- Has anyone ever touched you without your consent?
- Has anyone at home ever hurt, beaten, or struck you?

- Has anyone ever taken anything that was yours without asking?
- Have you ever signed any documents you didn't understand?
- Have you ever been left alone?
- Have you ever been restrained?
- Has anyone ever failed to help you take care of yourself when you needed help?

These are difficult questions to ask, and it may be best to save them for the end of the interview. If the perpetrator is a family member or the older person's care provider, the victim may be reluctant to identify them as the abuser. If the suspected perpetrator is on the scene, ask these questions when you are alone with the victim. You may have to wait until the patient has been removed to the ambulance. It is essential to document the patient's response in quotes.

Interviewing Suspected Abusers

With suspected cases of abuse or neglect, it may be necessary to interview family members or the older person's caregiver. The abused or neglected older person must always be the EMS provider's first responsibility. If it is necessary to interview the suspected abuser, use the following basic principles:

- Do not be accusatory, as this will put the suspected abuser on the defensive and limit the amount of information that will be offered.
- Interview the suspected abuser alone; discrepancies between the victim's account and the suspected abuser's account of the situation may be revealed.
- Focus initially on the present situation, and then move to broader questions regarding the victim's general condition. For example:
  - What happened to the older person (victim) today?
  - What is the older person's medical history?
  - What kind of care does the older person require?
  - Who provides this care?
  - Is there anything else I should know about the older person?
- If the suspected abuser is cooperative and calm during the interview, and a strong index of suspicion is present, consider asking more direct questions, such as:
  - Can you tell me how the older person received those bruises (lacerations, abrasions, etc.)?
  - The older person appears undernourished. Can you tell me how he/she got that way?
  - Have you ever threatened or struck the older person?

When interviewing a suspected abuser, note whether he or she offers an implausible explanation for the older person's injuries, or is uncooperative and disinterested or dominant and overly protective. If the suspected abuser admits to abuse or neglect during the interview, ask him or her to specify the abusive or neglectful event(s). Record exactly what the abuser states (in quotes). While the suspected abuser may be arrested, and ultimately convicted, for their admission, the victim is not always removed permanently from their residence or caregiver in cases of documented abuse or neglect. Often, counseling and effective coping strategies or resources will allow the relationship between the family/caregiver and the patient to improve. In these cases, APS will monitor the victim and abuser for a period of time.

Putting It All Together

As stated, context is the key to discovery in elder abuse and neglect cases. You must weigh your findings from the environmental and social assessments with the patient's physical condition, as well as with your observations of the patient/caregiver interaction. For example, does the caregiver dominate the situation or show a marked lack of concern? Or, does the caregiver blame the older person for his or her condition? Evaluate the caregiver for the presence of drug or alcohol intoxication. If the caregiver is absent, note whether the older person presents as someone who should be left alone, or if he or she speaks of the caregiver in a negative way. Additionally, assess the older person's affect and nonverbal behavior. Is the older person fearful or overly quiet?

Abuse should be suspected whenever the older person presents with multiple injuries in various stages of healing. Neglect should be suspected whenever a dependent person (who has adequate resources and a caregiver) presents with deficiencies in hygiene, nutrition, and medical needs. If one type of abuse is present, look for other types. Are there previous reports of similar injuries? Does the older person express fear of intervention? After you have made your assessment and conducted patient and caregiver interviews, if your intuition tells you all is not well between the older person and the caregiver, it probably is not.

Evidence of abuse can be determined, in part, by a physical examination. Evidence of neglect can be determined, in part, by the failure of the caregiver to:

- Assist with personal hygiene, or with the provision of food, clothing, shelter;
- Provide medical care for physical and mental health needs;
- Protect from health and safety hazards; and/or
- Prevent malnutrition.

Many hospitals set aside "safe beds" where victims needing immediate removal can be transported and housed until more suitable living arrangements can be made. If the older person is not being transported to the hospital, determine whether he or she is receptive to assistance from local APS. If the older person is receptive to assistance, notify the appropriate agency. There

may be circumstances where referral to APS may be necessary and may be the only action that can be immediately undertaken.

Some older persons choose to remain in an abusive or neglectful situation, despite offers of assistance and/or where a lack of criminal evidence exists. If the older person is competent, often times there is little that can be done since, unlike cases involving children, competent adults' rights must be honored. A report should still be initiated and documented and the case referred to APS.

Documentation

Documentation is crucial. Detailed descriptions of the patient's environment, injuries, social assessment, and interactions between the victim and the caregiver must be described. Specifically, you should document the following:

- Physical environment in which the patient is living
- Injuries (type, location, size, and shape)
- Complete past medical history
- Social history
- Name of the patient's physician and any health insurance the patient may have
- Patient's current prescribed medications (Attempt to determine if these medications are being taken by the patient. This will be important later in determining whether therapeutic levels are present.)
- Name of the patient's caregiver (if appropriate)
- Any statements made by the patient and/or caregiver (These statements must be written in quotes. If specific questions are asked relative to elder abuse, document the question that was asked, as well as the response.)
- Observation of interactions between the patient and the caregiver

Elder Abuse, Domestic Violence, and Animal Cruelty

A discussion of elder abuse would be remiss if it did not include the link among animal cruelty, domestic violence, child abuse, and elder abuse. Over the last decade, social service and law enforcement agencies have begun to examine cruelty to animals as a serious *human* problem closely linked to domestic violence, child abuse, elder abuse, and violent crimes.[33] Case histories of serial killers and mass murderers reveal an early history of abusing animals. Additionally, research has revealed a strong connection between animal cruelty and family violence.

Perpetrators of domestic violence often use the family pet to silence, coerce, and further intimidate other vulnerable family members. In many cases, pets are harmed or killed by the abuser. Several studies that included interviews of domestic violence victims reported that victims were reluctant to leave the home or the relationship for fear that the abuser would harm the family pet.[34]

Child abusers also often abuse animals to exert their power and control over children, animals, and other vulnerable family members. In some cases, abusers will force children to engage in sexual acts with animals or demand that they hurt or kill a favorite pet to coerce them into keeping a family secret. Even the threat of animal abuse may intimidate children into maintaining silence about ongoing family violence or other criminal behavior. Unfortunately, many abused children go on to become animal abusers themselves. These children begin abusing animals for a variety of reasons, including imitation of the violence they have seen or experienced; belief that animals' lives are expendable, having seen a parent kill a pet; or in an effort to control what they feel to be the inevitable end for the pet. These children are at risk for future aggressive and antisocial behavior as well.[35]

For many older people, a pet represents a source of companionship, as well as a support system (**Figure 13-12**). Perpetrators of elder abuse may manipulate this relationship to intimidate or threaten the older victim, or out of retaliation. Frequently, as in cases of elder abuse and neglect, the perpetrator is a child or grandchild.

The relationship between animal cruelty and other forms of domestic abuse warrants further investigation. Animal abuse is often one symptom of a dysfunctional or abusive family. There exists an opportunity to perhaps intervene on behalf of other vulnerable family members in the case of animal cruelty. Developing relationships with animal activist organizations, veterinarians, animal control agencies, and mental health organizations can lead to cross-reporting to law enforcement so that other possible forms of family violence may be identified. Additionally, multi-agency training can be initiated regarding the link between animal cruelty and other forms of family violence.

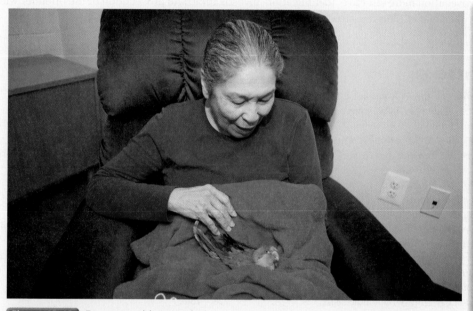

Figure 13-12 For many older people, a pet represents a source of companionship as well as a support system.
© Jones & Bartlett Learning. Courtesy of MIEMSS

CASE STUDY 3

You are called to a nursing home for a female with abdominal pain and bleeding. This is the third shift in a row that you have been called to the facility for a female patient with these symptoms. With the other two patients, it was difficult to determine during your exam whether the bleeding was vaginal, urinary, or rectal; and the hospital where they were transported has not provided feedback.

Upon assessing the patient today, you note more similarities between her and the previous two female patients: (1) each patient has a history of dementia; (2) each patient became very agitated when a male approached and seemed calmer when interactions were with another female; (3) each patient wore adult incontinent pads that were noted to be stained with bright red blood, although bleeding was not active at the time of transport; and (4) each patient had stable vitals and no history of urinary or bowel problems. In addition to these assessment findings, the patient you are assessing today has bruising on both of her upper arms.

- What do you suspect to be the cause of the patient's bleeding?
- What should you do?

Summary

Elder abuse is one of the most overlooked public health hazards in the United States and is a multifaceted societal problem. Unlike other cases of abuse and neglect, the response to elder abuse and neglect involves the coordination of key organizations and individuals. These organizations and individuals include Adult Protective Services, case management services, district attorneys, state attorney general, state ombudsman, mental health organizations, departments of aging (local and state), state nursing home licensing agencies, the police, and health care organizations (such as local hospitals and outreach health screening services). In addition, the EMS provider's role in elder abuse and neglect cases is crucial. EMS agencies should have written protocols in place that address the response to elder abuse and neglect cases. The development of such protocols should be a collaborative effort involving the above-mentioned organizations and individuals. Such protocols should reflect local, regional, and state laws and policies governing elder abuse cases.

Additionally, local municipalities should form a consortium of key organizations so that each is aware of the others' role in elder abuse response, investigation, prosecution, and prevention. This consortium should meet a minimum of four times a year to discuss progress and problem areas. This will lead to a coordinated effort in elder abuse awareness, prosecution, and prevention. Elder abuse awareness programs should be incorporated into continuing education programs to help open the lines of communication and make identification, investigation, and prosecution more effective. Identification, investigation, and prosecution of the offender will help the older victim live the end of their lives free of fear and deprivation.

References

1. National Committee for the Prevention of Elder Abuse. *Physical abuse*, 2008. Available at: http://www.preventelderabuse.org/elderabuse/physical.html.
2. Fulmer TM & O'Malley TA. *Inadequate Care of the Elderly: A Healthcare Perspective on Abuse and Neglect.* New York, Springer, 1987, pp. 17–18.
3. Ibid.
4. National Center on Elder Abuse. *Elder Abuse Informational Series no. 1.* Washington, DC, Author, 1997. Available at: http://www.ncea.aoa.gov/Main_Site/pdf/basics/fact1.pdf
5. National Center on Elder Abuse. *National elder abuse incidence study,* 1998. Available at: http://aoa.gov/AoA_Programs/Elder_Rights/Elder_Abuse/docs/AbuseReport_Full.pdf
6. National Center on Elder Abuse. *Statistics/Data,* n.d. Available at: http://www.ncea.aoa.gov/Library/Data/index.aspx
7. U.S. House of Representatives. *Abuse of residents is a major problem in U.S. Nursing Homes,* (2001, July). Available at: http://www.hospicepatients.org/ilaswan/nursinghomesabuse.pdf
8. National Center on Elder Abuse (n.d.)
9. Congressional Research Service: Older Americans Act: Long-Term Care Ombudsman Program, February 15, 2012.
10. Fulmer & O'Malley, pp. 29–30.
11. National Center on Elder Abuse. *Research Brief: How at Risk for Abuse Are People with Dementia?,* 2013. Available at: http://www.ncea.aoa.gov/Resources/Publication/docs/NCEA_Dementia_ResearchBrief_2013.pdf
12. National Center on Elder Abuse (n.d.)
13. Lachs MS & Fulmer T. Recognizing elder abuse and neglect. *Clin Geriatr Med* 1993:9(3):665–675.
14. National Research Council. *Elder Mistreatment: Abuse, Neglect, and Exploitation in an Aging America.* Washington, DC: The National Academies Press, 2003, p. 350.
15. Ibid., p.344.
16. Ibid., p. 345

17. Ibid., p. 345.
18. Ibid., p. 346.
19. Ibid., p. 346.
20. Ibid., p. 347.
21. Ibid., p. 346.
22. Ibid., p. 347.
23. Ibid., p. 348.
24. Ibid., p. 348.
25. Ibid., p. 348.
26. The Nursing Home Reform Amendments of OBRA 1987. *Volume 42, Code of Federal Regulations, Part 483.*
27. Burgess AW, Hanrahan, NP & Baker T. (2005). Forensic markers in elder female sexual abuse cases. *Clin Geriatr Med* 2005:21(2): 399–412.
28. Ibid.
29. Brown KM & Muscari ME. *Quick reference to adult and older adult forensics, a guide for nurses and other health care professionals.* New York, Springer, 2010, p. 192.
30. Illinois State TRIAD. *Responding to elder crime victims.* Springfield, IL, Author, 1998, p. 6.
31. National Research Council, p. 359.
32. Burgess AW, Dowdell EB, & Brown K. Sexual assault: Clinical issues. *Journal of Emergency Nursing* 2000:26:516-518.
33. Ponder C, & Lockwood R. *Cruelty to animals and family violence, Training key #526.* Alexandria, VA, International Association of Chiefs of Police, 2000, p. 1.
34. Ibid., p.2.
35. Ibid., p. 3

Additional Resources

Humane Society of the United States (www.hsus.org)

The National Long-Term Care Ombudsman Resource Center (www.ltcombudsman.org)

CASE STUDY SUMMARIES

Case Study 1 Summary

There are several issues involved in this case. Your immediate issue is the care, safety, and health of Mr. Weinberg. This is a patient who must be transported to the emergency department for evaluation. You note the pressure ulcers beginning to form on the victim. If left untreated, these ulcers will continue to become worse and eventually infected. Medical documentation of the patient can be initiated early (and in the victim's surroundings, as the soiled bed linens will contribute to the pressure ulcers becoming infected). Documentation should include the condition of the home and any statements the patient makes regarding his relationship with his son (particularly the care that the son provides to the patient). The police should be called immediately, as the neighbor is a potential witness. The neighbor may attest to the relationship between the victim and his son. Additionally, the neighbor may also be able to relate when she last saw the victim and the victim's overall appearance at that time.

A major concern in this case is the care that the son is providing to the patient. You know that the son assumes responsibility for Mr. Weinberg's finances, as well as for food shopping, picking up medicines, and acquiring other personal items for the victim. Mr. Weinberg stated that he and his son were suffering financial difficulties, and that he has not seen his son for the last several evenings. Part of your scene assessment is a comparison of the conditions of the father's bedroom with respect to the remainder of the home.

There are several possible outcomes to this case. One is that the son is spending his father's money on other things and simply neglecting his father's care. In this case, the son can be charged with neglect. The other scenario is that the son may be trying his best to care for his father, perhaps working a second job at night for additional income. In this scenario, there may be the opportunity for monetary and other support services to aid in the father's care, and the case should be referred to Adult Protective Services. The state's attorney will also need to review the victim's and son's financial records. In this case, the victim may be returned to the residence under the son's care if support services can be obtained. The son may be referred to a caregiver's support program and the victim's care monitored for a period of time.

As in most cases of abuse and neglect, the EMS provider is often the first health care professional that the victim will encounter. Knowing what to look for, requesting law enforcement early, making an Adult Protective Service referral, and completing thorough documentation are all keys to ensuring a positive outcome for the victim.

Case Study 2 Summary

The patient is showing signs of hypoxemia and is at risk of a poor outcome. First, you must stabilize the patient, applying oxygen and making sure she is breathing adequately. You should perform a finger-stick glucose test and consider all the potential causes of the decreased level of consciousness. The 10 missing pills of diphenhydramine are a concern, as even 50 mg could cause drowsiness, especially when combined with the other medications the patient is taking. It is fortunate that the patient did not try to get out of bed, fall, and become injured, or become so sleepy that she stopped breathing.

Maintaining a high index of suspicion, you suspect the care provider may be guilty of intentionally overmedicated the patient so that he or she could go out and not have to monitor the patient. The situation needs to be reported and investigated, as abuse is suspected. The patient will need to be taken to a safe location until she improves and the situation is sorted out.

Case Study 3 Summary

The similarities between the findings in this case and the previous two cases should be red flags to the EMS provider. Although a vaginal exam and evidence collection is required for positive determination, sexual assault must be considered. It would be unusual (although not impossible) for three women from the same nursing home to present with bleeding from the perineal area in the same week. Additional clues to abuse include the patient's anxiety, history of dementia, and bruising. If the possibility of sexual assault occurs to you prior to leaving the nursing home, remember to stay nonjudgmental with the staff currently on duty, as their involvement may only have been calling for help. Additionally, do not forget that the patient takes first priority and other injuries may need to be treated. Age-related changes in older women make them prone to injury after sexual assault, and vaginal tearing can lead to shock.

Generally, it is not the EMS provider's duty to gather evidence, interrogate suspects, or prove or disprove the abuse; however, it is important to not contaminate or destroy evidence if at all possible. For example, the incontinence pad may contain evidence, so try to handle it as little as possible and do not throw it away or clean the patient's perineum. Additionally, the EMS provider is responsible for reporting any reasonable suspicions, so make sure to let the emergency department physician know of your suspicions and follow your department policy related to contacting social services, adult protection services, and/or the police.

CHAPTER 14

Mobile Integrated Healthcare

LEARNING OBJECTIVES

1. Define mobile integrated healthcare (MIH).

2. Discuss the role of MIH programs in caring for older patients.

3. Describe the types of MIH programs that may benefit older persons.

4. Discuss the role of the primary care physician in MIH.

5. Discuss the responsibilities of MIH providers to improve the quality of life for older patients.

6. Discuss the role of MIH in an older person's emotional and physical health, social connections, economic security, and safety.

7. Discuss ways to incorporate MIH into your EMS system.

Introduction

An older patient's quality of life can be improved through the holistic, patient-centered approach to health care delivery known as **mobile integrated healthcare (MIH)**. In its basic form, MIH transforms the EMS provider from a provider of critical and life-sustaining interventions and transport to a fully integrated partner in the delivery of health care services. In some cases, this entails bringing *the care to patients* in the comfort of their own homes, rather than bringing *patients to receive care* in an emergency department.

Mobile Integrated Healthcare Defined

In its simplest definition, MIH is the provision of health care using patient-centered, mobile resources in the out-of-hospital environment that are integrated with the entire spectrum of health care and social service resources available in the local community. MIH may include, but is not limited to, providing services such as:

- Telephone advice to 911 callers instead of resource dispatch
- Follow-up visits after hospital discharge
- Patient education for chronic disease management
- Medication inventory and compliance
- Assessment of depression and anxiety
- Feedback to the patient's primary care network
- Assessment and possible mitigation of the patient's living environment
- Patient navigation to health care resources other than a hospital emergency department
- Care coordination with multiple health care and social resources
- Assurance of adequate nutrition

There is also discussion in EMS circles about use of the terms *community paramedicine*, or *community paramedic*, versus the term *mobile integrated healthcare*. To provide the MIH services previously listed, the MIH program could incorporate the use of community paramedics. However, MIH programs may also use practitioners other than paramedics in this role. They may use EMTs, registered nurses, nurse practitioners, physician assistants, or even physicians. These programs may also incorporate services that go beyond the point of care services in the field, such as programs based in a 911 call center that provide callers with health care advice from nurses.

For these reasons, the term *mobile integrated healthcare* is used to refer to the services provided; and in many, but not all cases, these services may be provided by community paramedics.

Health Care Reform and Mobile Integrated Healthcare

Health care reform, also known as the Affordable Care Act, has changed the health care environment and opened up opportunities for EMS to play an important role. For years, EMS providers have considered themselves providers of only emergency care. All levels of training focus on treating acute illnesses and injuries and transporting patients to the hospital emergency department. Health care reform continually drives changes in the industry, and everyone is struggling to understand where the industry is headed and how EMS providers will need to adapt.

MIH is often centered on reducing health care costs and hospital readmission and in training EMTs and paramedics in the skills most needed in the community. The goals of MIH are the same as the goals of health care reform:

- Improving the patient experience of care (including quality and satisfaction)
- Improving the health of populations
- Reducing the per capita cost of health care

CASE STUDY

An older patient is being considered for your MIH program because of his frequent calls to 911 that are not considered emergencies. As an MIH provider in the EMS agency in your community, you visit the patient's home to discuss whether the patient would be willing to enroll in your MIH program. Your goal is to connect your patient to the health care resources he needs, educate him about the medications he's taking, and therefore reduce his use of 911.

As part of this initial visit, you closely review the patient's medication bottles. Of the 21 different medications you find, you note that three are blood thinners. The patient tells you that he routinely takes *all* of his prescribed medications, including these three prescriptions. Each blood thinner (Coumadin, warfarin, and Jantoven) was prescribed by a different doctor. The patient did not realize the prescriptions were for the same drug. After you explain this to the patient, you contact each of the prescribing physicians and help coordinate which prescription the patient should be taking.

- What is the role of the MIH provider in patient education and improving this patient's quality of life?
- Without the intervention of an MIH provider, what might have happened to this patient?

MIH Program Development

There are two basic models for MIH programs. One is the primary care replacement model, and the other is the urban model. The primary care replacement model may include the provision of primary care such as suturing, medication administration, wound care, and long-term in-home care management if home health care is unavailable. The urban model is essentially patient navigation that involves directing patients to the most appropriate health care resources already available in the community.

To be truly successful, MIH programs must be mobile (focused on navigating patients, even those in remote areas, to the appropriate health care resources), integrated (with hospitals and others in the community), and patient centered (focusing on providing health care). The development of an MIH program should be based on a needs assessment of the community and involves working with all stakeholders (hospitals, physician groups, community service organizations, patients, community leaders, and even elected officials) to create a program that fills those health care needs in the community.

EMS Providers Versus MIH Providers

When the traditional EMS provider transitions to an MIH program, he or she must keep in mind several points. First, the MIH provider should have the clinician and practitioner personality—the skills and abilities to nurture people, communicate effectively, and perform follow up. The MIH provider educates patients to take care of themselves and teaches them, through patient and practical advice, how to manage their disease and thereby reduce the potential for hospital readmission (**Figure 14-1**). The

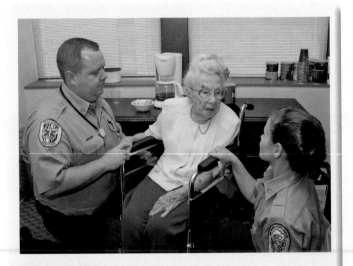

Figure 14-1 The MIH provider must effectively communicate with patients in order to educate them to take care of themselves and teach them how to manage their disease.

© Jones & Bartlett Learning. Courtesy of MIEMSS.

MIH role is different than the traditional role of the EMS provider because it establishes long-term relationships within the community. MIH providers connect with patients to effectively communicate and strategize about their health care. The MIH provider takes 30 to 45 minutes on the scene of a call to educate the patient and family. They are nurturing during on-site visits, strengthening relationships, and understanding patient needs and then fulfilling them.

The Importance of Collaboration with Stakeholders

A coordinated, unified approach to patient care that involves close communication with stakeholders is essential to a successful MIH program. The MIH approach to the older patient involves collaboration between multiple agencies and care providers, including medical providers (such as EMS medical control, primary and specialty care providers, hospitals, and pharmacies) and social providers (such as "Meals on Wheels," senior centers, and faith-based organizations). It is common for older patients to have multiple comorbidities, which makes the integrated approach to managing their health care needs more necessary and more valuable. Services as simple as a thorough medication inventory can help patients not only manage their illnesses more effectively but perhaps even prevent a catastrophe (such as an overdose or adverse drug event) from occurring. In all communities, especially those with large older populations, MIH can play an integral part in addressing gaps in health care needs.

The MIH approach may also be part of an overall strategy focusing on older patients and their disease processes based on a community health needs assessment or a particular goal of local stakeholders. For example, a local stakeholder group may want to reduce preventable injuries resulting from falls, or a hospital may wish to prevent avoidable admissions for chronic obstructive pulmonary disease (COPD) patients at risk for readmission. The goals and desired outcomes should be clearly established prior to the start of the MIH program. Without committed stakeholders and a well-developed plan based on a community needs assessment, attempting to provide integrated care to the older patient will be extremely difficult, if not impossible.

Engaging stakeholders helps them feel that they are part of the solution. When stakeholders are engaged and believe they are a part of the MIH process, they take ownership in the program and will come up with innovative ideas, suggestions, and recommendations. They become advocates and supporters of the MIH programs that are implemented.

The concept of MIH is gaining attention across the nation. Several EMS agencies that have implemented MIH programs have demonstrated its positive impact on patient outcome, patient experience of care, and health care costs. Not all EMS agencies may embrace MIH as part of their services, but it is important to be aware of changes that have already occurred and those likely to happen in the future in the EMS profession and the entire health care system.

Types of MIH Programs that Benefit Older Persons

The number of MIH programs continues to grow. The programs described in this text are only a sample of the programs that have been implemented in communities throughout the country. Other programs are currently being developed and evaluated based on the needs of each community.

Frequent Users of 911 Program

Older patients who are frequent users of 911 calls and emergency department visits (more than 15 calls or visits in 90 days) may be called by an MIH provider and asked whether they would be interested in enrolling in a program designed to help them find better resources for their medical care to reduce the number of 911 calls and emergency department visits. Patients who agree to enroll in the program have MIH providers working with them on a regular basis. Providers schedule proactive home visits with patients, but also are provided HIPAA authorization to share the patients' information with other providers to coordinate care in an effort to reduce the reliance on 911 and the emergency department system for primary medical care.

Congestive Heart Failure Program

Congestive heart failure (CHF) is one of the top killers in the United States and, due to the nature of the disease, is responsible for chronic emergency department visits and hospital admissions. Older patients with CHF who participate in this program receive care from an MIH provider to determine whether the 30-day hospital readmission rate can be reduced. Providers make home visits to CHF patients to educate them on their discharge instruction and discuss managing their disease. A medication inventory is taken, and a home environmental assessment is performed to determine whether there are risks of falling or other dangers that require resources.

Observation Admission Avoidance Program

An observational admission is an admission that occurs in the emergency department when patients are admitted as inpatients, but not discharged from the emergency department. These patients are typically held for 24 to 48 hours in the emergency room or some other department in the hospital in an outpatient status because they are awaiting lab results or other tests or require general observation. A typical scenario for an observational admission is an older patient who enters the emergency department after a fall. Even if the patient's laboratory work and other test results are normal, the emergency department physician may not feel comfortable sending the patient home without

knowing more about the patient's clinical condition or home environment. To keep a patient in the hospital for observation is very costly to the health care system because these admissions are billed at higher rates than other inpatient stays.

Enrollment of an older patient under the observational admission avoidance program may be requested by a hospital case manager and emergency department physician, who meet with the MIH provider to discuss the patient who is being sent home and determine the focus of the patient's care during the 24- to 48-hour enrollment. After the patient returns home, an MIH provider visits within a few hours to review discharge instructions and provide a home assessment. Suggestions are given to make the home safer to help the patient avoid another fall. Patients in the program are given a nonemergency number to contact the MIH call center 24/7 if they feel uncomfortable or if they would like to have an episodic visit before their follow-up appointment with their physician.

Other MIH Programs

MIH providers are able to provide older patients with care in other programs, such as partnering with hospice agencies to assist in providing patients with care if for any reason they are unable to reach their hospice nurse. A 911 nurse triage program helps navigate callers for very low-acuity medical or trauma conditions to settings such as a primary care physician office, dental office, urgent care facility, or even self-care at home, therefore avoiding an unnecessary trip to the emergency department.

Because the health care needs in each community are different, the types of MIH programs may vary. There is no one-size-fits-all MIH program.

The Role of the Primary Care Physician in MIH

One of the critical components of an MIH approach to patient care is the connection and continual involvement of the patient's primary care physician (PCP). The PCP often serves the role of patient advocate and navigator; however, because the PCP does not typically see patients in the home environment, they may find it challenging to effectively fulfill this role. The MIH provider can be the in-home eyes and ears for the PCP, relaying environmental living conditions that may be having an impact on the patient's medical conditions. Furthermore, the MIH provider can also help the PCP by educating patients on how to be "better patients"—for example, teaching patients to write down questions they would like their PCP to answer during the next appointment, learning how to relay specific signs and symptoms to help the PCP determine treatment courses, or helping patients understand the right time to call the PCP for an appointment to prevent an exacerbation of a medical condition.

In many cases, the PCP may be contacted by the MIH provider for medical consultation and treatment recommendations while on scene with the patient. If authorized by the EMS medical director and local regulations, the PCP can instruct the on-scene MIH provider to administer recommended treatments with a follow-up PCP appointment. This type of care coordination is exceptionally valuable for the patient's long-term medical care.

> ## Attitude Tip
>
> By improving your attitudes and the attitudes of other EMS and health care providers toward the older population, you will positively affect the quality of life enjoyed by the older patients in your community.

MIH and Quality of Life

Quality of life for older people includes living with as much choice, independence, and dignity as possible. Quality of life can be viewed as having five interrelated factors: emotional health, physical health, social connections, economic security, and safety. The goal of the MIH program is to empower older patients to manage their own health care and teach them how to live a healthier lifestyle with their medical conditions. MIH providers do not tell patients what they cannot do; they educate patients about what they *can* do. They teach patients how to ask questions and how to report on conditions or situations that might be occurring at home. Patients become more informed and are able to identify early on when they begin to decompensate and warrant care. Collaboration and communication are key to maintaining quality of life for older people.

Emotional Health

The overall health of an older person includes the person's physical, mental, and spiritual well-being. MIH providers, because they often have an established relationship with the patient through in-home care, are able to improve the patient's quality of life by making appropriate referrals based on the patient's described health problems. With communication, the MIH provider may develop a good sense of the older person's mental health and ability to care for himself or herself. If the patient needs behavioral counseling, the MIH provider will ensure that the patient is referred to an appropriate resource for care.

 ## Physical Health: Nutrition and Hydration

Adequate nutrition is imperative for older individuals, as undernutrition and dehydration can cause both physical illnesses and an altered mental status. Poor nutritional intake among the older population may be fairly common, regardless of a person's income. An MIH provider will be able to assess the patient's living situation during an initial visit, especially if he or she lives alone. An older person's decrease in food intake may be caused by the deterioration of smell and taste, as well as the gastrointestinal side effects of the medications the patient is taking. If you suspect that the patient is not eating well or is not drinking enough fluids, ask what the patient had for breakfast, lunch, or dinner. Additional factors in poor eating habits include poverty, difficulty getting to the store, difficulty preparing meals, and poor dental care.

An MIH provider should refer patients who are not receiving proper nutrition to a local "Meals on Wheels" program or a congregate meal site. Arranging for the delivery of free or low-cost nutritious meals can help prevent both short- and long-term medical issues for the patient. Having regular meals delivered also helps bring a "touch point" to the patient—providing them with the opportunity to interact with other people. Furthermore, if the meal delivery person arrives and no one answers the door, or if the patient answers the door but seems to be acting out of norm, the delivery person can notify the MIH provider. Congregate meal sites not only provide patients with adequate meals, but also serve as a social setting, helping them interact with others.

 ## Social Connections

Isolation and loneliness have an adverse impact on quality of life for many older people. Connections with social groups are important factors for the MIH provider to look for when assessing the older patient. If transport is indicated, the family/friend/neighbor network can be of major assistance to the person and to the MIH provider. It is important to know if someone will be there with the person at the hospital and, if necessary, provide transportation home if admission is not planned. MIH providers can arrange for patient transportation and are even able to educate patients in using public transportation for follow-up visits with their PCP.

If there is no one with the patient when you arrive, ask about his or her social network, starting with immediate friends and family and then looking at a broader social system. Find people who the patient can rely on and call for help, and determine whether the person is socially isolated. The following questions will help the MIH provider determine the type of assistance and level of care the patient may need:

- Does someone live here at the house with you? (If yes, who is it?)
- Do you have family nearby?
- Is there someone you would like me to call?
- Does someone come in to help you?
- Do you have friends you can call on if you need help?

If possible, you should also obtain names and phone numbers, either for you to call or to give to the hospital for follow-up.

The patient's responses to your questions will also tell you about his or her relationships. Warm responses indicate warm relationships. Angry responses, such as "I have a daughter who never comes to see me," may indicate relationship difficulties within the family. If the answers provided suggest social isolation, the MIH provider may refer the patient to an appropriate social services agency.

Other questions that may help determine if the patient is socially isolated include, "How do you spend your time? Do you go to church, synagogue, or other religious meetings?" If the person says he or she used to but cannot go anymore, ask if anyone from the religious group visits and how often. "What do you do for fun? What hobbies do you have? Do you do any volunteer work? Do you belong to any clubs?" can also provide information about how the older patient spends his or her time. Depending on the answers to these questions, the MIH provider can suggest other appropriate agencies or activities to enhance the patient's quality of life. For instance, an isolated person who says he or she enjoys playing cards might significantly benefit from joining a local senior center.

Economic Security

Economic security is also an element of quality of life. Older people in poverty are predominantly women, especially those who are living alone or are members of a minority. When an MIH provider is on an initial enrollment visit, he or she should observe the patient's living conditions. Does the person's house appear to be in good condition or does it need significant repair? Do the lights work? Does the phone work? Are there obvious potential dangers (frayed cords or a broken oven or refrigerator door)? Is the house adequately heated or cooled? Is there adequate food in the house? Is the smoke detector working?

Questioning the person about these matters requires sensitivity. You may encounter defensiveness or resistance, but asking questions such as, "Do you like living here? If you had your choice, where would you like to live?" may be more successful.

Many people are not aware that economic assistance and other resources are available to help people maintain independence in their homes. An MIH referral to the **Area Agency on Aging (AAA)** can help older persons find solutions to economic problems.

Safety

When MIH providers enter a patient's home, they sometimes find additional problems that need to be addressed. The MIH provider may recognize issues in the patient's environment that could contribute to health-related problems. MIH providers who help patients find solutions to tough problems can make a big contribution toward improving the patient's quality of life.

It should first be acknowledged that some home environments occur as the result of choice. Different people have different standards with respect to housekeeping and personal hygiene. The key issues that the MIH provider must consider are whether the conditions create health or safety hazards. With regard to safety, the MIH provider must recognize that different people have different tolerance of risk. The provider should avoid a strict "better safe than sorry" approach, and should avoid being judgmental. Providers may assume that the wishes of most people will be to maintain independence in their own homes as long as possible, and are encouraged to confirm this assumption through dialogue with the patient and the patient's family. The assessment of the patient's environment is done to support the patient's quality-of-life choices.

In addition, an environmental assessment may be the only clear indicator of abuse or neglect (**Figure 14-2**). Less obvious but also problematic are the situations that represent self-neglect (problems of abuse and self-neglect are covered in the *Elder Abuse* chapter). MIH providers should also note situations

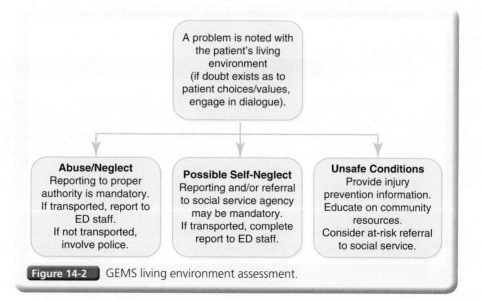

Figure 14-2 GEMS living environment assessment.

that represent potential health and safety problems, such as an absence of food in the home, moldy remnants of old meals, and stacks of unwashed dishes. Additional signs of health and safety problems include improper waste disposal, the presence of vermin, copious amounts of pet urine and feces, inadequate toilet facilities, and mismanagement of incontinence. Such conditions may be the result of inadequate education, sloppy habits, or a psychiatric-behavioral disorder. The problem may also be due to a functional decline that prevents the patient from performing the activities of daily living.

In cases where the problem results from a psychiatric disorder, such as compulsive/obsessive "hoarding" syndrome, a referral to the mental health system is indicated. When there is doubt whether the patient is mentally or legally competent, a referral to an appropriate agency should be made as well.

Attitude Tip

In addition to participating in injury prevention, home safety evaluation, and medical information access programs in your community, you should support programs that promote MIH provider drop-in visits (between calls) to older patients living alone, at risk for health decline, or who are frequent consumers of EMS in your area.

If the basis of the problem is functional disability, an MIH program may be able to assist the patient in finding access to home care, chore services, or home-delivered meals. A great variety of state-sponsored and local volunteer services are also available to assist older persons who want to stay in their own homes but need assistance. Innovative programs in MIH are being adopted to connect older persons with other health care and social service agencies that help older people maintain independence and dignity.

Where unsafe conditions exist because of behavioral choice, education by the MIH provider may promote change. The MIH provider can help the patient better understand the probable consequences of risky choices and suggest modifications of the living environment to help maintain independence.

For example, fall prevention is an excellent opportunity for the MIH provider to facilitate health care system integration to improve patient outcome. Often, the PCP is not aware of the patient's living environment and is therefore unable to assist with referrals to mitigate fall risk. The MIH provider that communicates their findings to the patient's PCP, as well as to other community-based resources, may help in making the home environment safer for the patient. For example, the AAA may be able to provide funding for the installation of grab rails, securing of carpeting or area rugs, and other home safety initiatives to reduce fall risk at home. Programs such as A Matter of Balance, designed to reduce the fear of falling and increase activity levels of older adults who have concerns about falling, may also be provided. A Matter of Balance is conducted over a series of classes that include group discussion, problem solving, skill building, assertiveness training, videotapes, practical solutions, and exercise training. Much of this training can also be conducted in the patient's home.

When injury prevention education is delivered at the time and place of a recent injury, it is said to be a "teachable moment." In addition to providing care for any immediate problem or need, remember that as an advocate for your older patients, providing resource referral is a valuable support service with which you should assist.

Resources

A basic and universal resource for older people is the State Agency on Aging or AAA. Under the Older Americans Act, all state and local agencies provide information services that can lead to public and private resources close to where the person resides. Telephone numbers usually are found under the government or organizational listing for the state or local jurisdiction, under Aging Services; Aging: Area Agency; Office on or Bureau of Aging; or there may be

CASE STUDY 2

You are asked by the emergency department's medical director to perform a follow-up visit with a 63-year-old female patient who was recently discharged from the hospital. After falling in her home, the patient, who had a bump on her head and a fractured dominant proximal humerus, was placed in a shoulder immobilizer and instructed to follow up with an orthopedic doctor. The medical director wants to be sure there is not "more to the story," as the patient was insistent on not being admitted to the hospital. He also wants to confirm that the home is safe for the patient and that she will not need additional assistance.

As you arrive at the residence, you are met at the front door by the patient. She is wearing tattered and stained clothing, and her arms and legs are covered with dirt. She lets you into the house and you immediately trip over a pair of sneakers on the floor. As you follow her into the dining room, you look around and are overwhelmed by the sight. Bags filled with newspapers, bottles, boxes, and plastic containers cover the floor; dishes are piled in the sink; baking sheets and cake pans are piled on the stove top and kitchen counter; and the dining table is covered with papers, books, and 3-ring binders. You notice that the doorways are covered with dust and only one of the light bulbs in the light fixture on the ceiling appears to work.

- What assessments are needed in this case?
- Does the patient need to be sent back to the hospital or a care facility? Should she be reported to a social services agency?

a listing for Senior Information. The national Eldercare Locator is a toll-free number (1-800-677-1116) that can lead you to your state unit on aging or local AAA as well as other services.

When looking for resources, the AAA is a good place to start. They have senior information programs, such as Information and Referral (I&R) or Information and Assistance (I&A), that track all resources in the community. AAAs also sponsor nutrition programs, senior centers (locations where seniors can gather for meals, physical and social activities, and educational and volunteer opportunities), and transportation services.

The Long-Term Care Ombudsman at each local AAA reviews complaints in nursing homes and other long-term care facilities and tries to resolve them before crises occurs, calling on the licensing agency or law enforcement if abuse is suspected. Some area agencies serve as public guardians of last resort if assigned by the Court, some have employment services, and some provide geriatric care management. Some AAAs provide services directly and some contract out the services; regardless, the information program staff will have knowledge about local available resources, public or private.

Senior centers welcome talks by community resources such as MIH providers (**Figure 14-3**). Other groups that may welcome presentations include resident councils in senior living communities, senior citizen clubs, and service organizations. The AAA can be of assistance in connecting you to such groups.

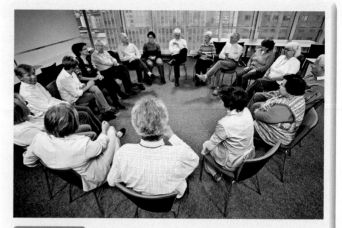

Figure 14-3 Talking with older people in the community can help prevent emergencies and provides a social connection.
© vm/iStockphoto

Attitude Tip

To increase your awareness, understanding, and appreciation of the mobility problems and other sensory deficits faced by the older population, consider participating in geriatric-empathy training programs and workshops.

Summary

MIH providers have an important role to play in improving the quality of life for older people. With a holistic, patient-centered approach to health care delivery, MIH programs can positively affect an older patient's outcome and experience of care, as well as improve health care costs. Several communities that have implemented effective MIH programs have seen incredible clinical, operational, and community relations results since program inception.

CASE STUDY SUMMARIES

Case Study 1 Summary

A major aspect of MIH is reducing health care costs and hospital readmission. In order to accomplish these goals, the MIH provider must understand the needs of the patients and then educate the patients to take care of themselves and manage their disease. The MIH provider should take 30 to 45 minutes on the scene of a call to connect with the patient and family to effectively communicate and strategize about the patient's health care. In this case, after learning that the patient is taking three different blood thinners prescribed by three different doctors, you take the time to educate the patient about the medications he's taking and you find out the patient did not even realize the prescriptions were for the same drug.

It is common for older patients, such as the one encountered on this call, to have multiple comorbidities and to see multiple care providers. The MIH approach to the older patient involves collaboration between these care providers. By contacting each of the prescribing physicians, you are able to help coordinate which prescription the patient should be taking. Your intervention helped the patient not only to manage his illnesses more effectively, but also to prevent a possible overdose from occurring.

Case Study 2 Summary

Getting the full history of the patient's injury and performing a home assessment will be very helpful in determining if the patient's home is safe and if the patient is capable of taking care of herself. As you talk with the patient, you learn that she spent the morning doing a load of laundry, cleaning the garage, mowing the lawn, and preparing her garden for the winter. She had then hosed down her back deck before slipping on the wet boards, crashing into the corner of the house, and injuring herself. She goes on to tell you additional information about herself: She was widowed a few years ago, lives about 30 miles away from her family (who is returning from vacation tomorrow), and is newly retired from an emergency nursing job. The patient explains to you that she and her sister are having a garage sale next week and most of the boxes in the living room and kitchen area are headed to her sister's.

As you look around again, you begin to realize the items in the boxes are actually high-end knick-knacks and collectables, the papers on the dining table are actually paperwork and bills, and the dishes in the sink are actually clean and draining. You ask to see the rest of the home and the patient willingly takes you on a tour. You notice that her bed is made, there are clean towels in the bathroom, and the upper level of the home is generally much less cluttered than the main level. You realize that first impressions are not always what they seem and not all people are the best housekeepers. A messy and/or cluttered house is not a reason to call social services; however, if the bags had been filled with actual trash or there was not a valid reason for all the boxes and bags in the living room and kitchen, your management of the situation would need to be different. Instead, the patient is highly functioning and knowledgeable. She assures you that one of her family members will come over tomorrow upon returning from vacation and that she has an appointment scheduled with a nearby orthopedic clinic.

CHAPTER 15

Disasters and Older People

LEARNING OBJECTIVES

1. Describe the four phases of emergency management.

2. Discuss preparedness strategies for older people.

3. Understand preparedness planning for assisted living and long-term care facilities.

4. Discuss the issues involved in sheltering older people in time of disaster.

5. Discuss recommendations necessary to ensure the needs of older people are met in time of disaster.

Introduction

Age alone does not make an older person vulnerable during a disaster; however, older persons are more likely to experience certain limitations that can increase vulnerability, such as chronic illnesses; functional deficiencies; or sensory, physical, or cognitive disabilities (**Figure 15-1**). Also at increased vulnerability are those who take multiple medications, rely on formal or informal caregivers for assistance, and experience general "frailty."[1] In the context of emergency management, frailty is defined as the physical, cognitive, social, psychological, and/or economic circumstances that limit the ability of individuals aged 65 years or older to perform, or have performed for them, one or more activities of daily living (ADL) or instrumental activities of daily living (IADL) during and after a disaster.[2] An older person's vulnerability is also increased during a disaster if he or she lives alone and/or in an isolated rural area.[3] Those least able to recover from a disaster are often the most vulnerable and least likely to receive assistance.

Recent examples of the tragic consequences that have befallen older people in times of disaster include the events of the Chicago heat wave in 1995, Hurricane Katrina in 2005, and Hurricane Sandy in 2012. The Chicago heat wave is an example of a "silent disaster," as the effects of this disaster were delayed and less apparent than those associated with more violent disasters, such as tornadoes or hurricanes. Nevertheless, over 600 people died as a result of the extreme temperatures, with 65% of those victims being older than age 65 years.[4] At the time, Chicago lacked many basic services for the city's older population, such as medical services, social services, and police protection; this lack of assistance left older persons, particularly those who lived alone, extremely vulnerable.

Hurricane Katrina was also responsible for a number of elderly deaths: An estimated 1330 people died as a result of the storm; approximately 71% of the Louisiana victims were older than 60 years of age, and 47% were older than 77 years of age. Of those victims residing in nursing homes, 22 succumbed to heat conditions, 35 drowned during the storm surge, and at least 140 residents perished during evacuation procedures.[5] Some of these residents died while waiting for transportation, some were simply abandoned, and many others died at the New Orleans Superdome and Convention Center while awaiting further evacuation instructions. Due to the disastrous conditions resulting from the storm, many of those older persons who were evacuated encountered extreme pain, hardship, and "transfer trauma," with existing illnesses often being exacerbated to the point of death.

Although Hurricane Sandy resulted in fewer deaths than Hurricane Katrina, more than one-half of those who died as a result of Sandy were aged 65 years or older.[6] During the storm, many high-rises in New York City became surrounded by flood water. Additionally, most buildings experienced power outages, causing elevators to be inoperable. These circumstances were particularly difficult for those who were older and less mobile, but they were also very challenging for the emergency responders and providers of services such as "Meals on Wheels."

Proper disaster planning is critical to ensuring the results of these three disasters are not repeated. Prehospital care providers see older people in the community every day and have a thorough understanding of this population's unique needs. The provider's knowledge can be a tremendous asset to emergency planners when considering the needs of older people in times of disaster. Disaster planning for the older population should take into account the needs of the following three groups:

1. Community-dwelling older people who are mobile
2. Community-dwelling older people who are frail, home-bound, and immobile
3. Older people residing in assisted-living and long-term care facilities

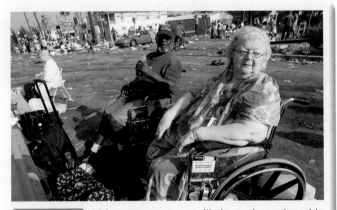

Figure 15-1 Older persons most likely to be vulnerable during disasters are those who have chronic illnesses; functional limitations; or sensory, physical, or cognitive disabilities.

© Mario Tama/Getty Images News/Getty Images

CASE STUDY 1

A fire is consuming thousands of acres in your community, with flames fueled by drought, high winds, and hot summer temperatures. Firefighters are struggling to contain the flames, but the wildfires quickly spread throughout multiple communities. A mandatory evacuation order is issued for a 20-square-mile area, which encompasses numerous private residences and two long-term-care facilities in your service area.

- How should you assist in the evacuation effort?
- What considerations are needed when evacuating older residents?

Emergency Management Phases

Emergencies may be relatively localized (such as tornadoes), or they may be widespread, affecting multiple geographic areas (such as wildfires). The speed at which these events unfold can also vary greatly.[7] For example, Hurricane Katrina was tracked for a few days before it hit land, but other emergencies, such as the terrorist attacks in New York City on September 11, 2001, occur abruptly and can catch providers completely by surprise. Although a full discussion on the different types of hazards or disasters is beyond the scope of this text, communities are typically aware of the types they are likely to face.

In order to better prevent or reduce the impact of the various emergencies that may occur, the United States Department of Homeland Security's **Federal Emergency Management Agency (FEMA)** institutionalized the concept of emergency management in 1979. The functions of emergency management are generally grouped into four phases:

- **Mitigation phase.** The mitigation phase of emergency management includes actions aimed at avoiding or lessening the impact of a disaster, such as choosing not to build a nursing home facility in a flood zone. Assessing risk, as well as developing strategies to manage it, is an essential aspect of the mitigation phase.
- **Preparedness phase.** This phase includes actions taken before the emergency occurs, in order to prepare for the disaster. Preparedness activities include developing and exercising plans, acquiring resources, and training.
- **Response phase.** The response phase includes actions to address the acute and short-term effects of an emergency or disaster that is in progress. Response activities include immediate actions to save lives, protect property, and meet basic human needs. Long-term-care facilities may also be interested in initiating a response outward to support other organizations and the community, such as by serving as a host facility when other facilities are overloaded.
- **Recovery phase.** Recovery occurs after the disaster has subsided. Activities in this phase are designed to help a community return to a pre-disaster level of function.[8]

The primary focus of this chapter is on the preparedness phase of emergency management. This phase should include an "all-hazards" approach to planning, meaning plans must take into account all of the different types of disasters. Emergency medical services providers and agencies must broaden the scope of their authority and include themselves in operational planning for disasters, particularly as they relate to older people.

Preparedness Strategies for Older People

The typical emergency management model for the progression of disaster assistance responsibility is City→State→Federal. According to this model, local emergency services agencies are responsible for providing the initial response activities following a disaster. If additional assistance is needed, the local government may request help from nearby municipalities and the state. If the disaster is catastrophic and requires more assistance than can be provided by the state, federal resources can then be mobilized through FEMA.

With respect to older people, a similar emergency management model should be adapted at the micro level: Personal→Agency→Community.[9]

Personal

The personal level of preparedness responsibility represents the responsibility of older individuals and their families. Because many older people maintain the responsibility of caring for themselves, it is important to promote self-reliance and self-preparation among the older population. For example, if relocation is necessary, it is vital for older people to know to take their medications and assistive devices with them, as well as spare batteries for hearing aids.

Frail older people have less ability than others to prepare for and respond to disasters. For this group, encouraging family responsibility is the next level of attention. Disaster checklists and other educational material can be distributed to older people and their families. During a disaster, public service announcements can encourage people in the community to check in on their older neighbors; it may also be beneficial to set up a hotline for older people to call to obtain information.[10]

There are many ways prehospital care providers can assist with the effort towards personal responsibility. For example, providers can schedule disaster preparation seminars through local senior centers and senior apartment complexes. Large groups of seniors can be accessed and educated through this forum, and literature can be prepared and distributed (**Figure 15-2**). Large numbers of older people can also be reached through community churches, synagogues, and mosques—clergy are usually very receptive and willing to help with such endeavors. Congregations also often have access to shut-ins who are regularly visited by congregational members. If willing, these members can be trained on how to educate older people in disaster preparedness. Additional outreach sources include banks, hair salons, barbershops, and small local eateries where older people frequent. Staff members in these businesses can be trained to distribute literature and educate older people about disaster preparation.

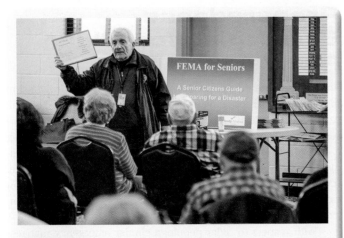

Figure 15-2 Self-preparation is one of the greatest forms of assistance for older people in times of disaster.

Courtesy of K.C.Wilsey/FEMA

Agency

It is not necessary to create new agencies or services dedicated to reducing the vulnerability of older people in times of disaster; instead, emergency managers should focus on leveraging the services of existing agencies. For the purpose of this discussion, the term *agency* is used to denote a broad range of relationships between individuals and larger entities. There exist a number of agencies that provide care for older people: Some agencies are only responsible for a small segment of the older person's care (such as meal services), while others provide 24-hour in-home care that includes a custodial relationship with the older client. Regardless of the relationship, agencies should be educated about disaster issues and encouraged to incorporate disaster planning into their operations.

An example of an agency that has incorporated disaster planning into their operations is the National Association for Home Care and Hospice (NAHC), a nonprofit agency that represents the nation's numerous home care and hospice organizations. The NAHC has prepared a document entitled *Emergency Preparedness Packet for Home Health Agencies*, which outlines an all-hazards emergency preparedness plan to be used by home care and hospice providers. Other agencies—such as utility companies that have a list of customers who utilize life support equipment, or property management companies and retirement communities that have lists of special needs residents—can provide assistance during the preparedness phase of disaster operations by identifying at-risk older people. A database (or registry) can then be created to maintain identification and track these at-risk individuals. Once identified, the older person's needs can be assessed and the individual can be connected with agencies that can provide direct services during the response and recovery phases of a disaster.

Traditionally, local and state governments have provided disaster-planning efforts in a vacuum. However, this model is not effective when considering the comprehensive needs of older people in disasters. Emergency managers must broaden the scope of agencies that are involved in disaster-planning efforts and assist agencies that provide services to older people by helping them to:

- Identify and address their own hazard vulnerabilities
- Better ensure their capability to continue services throughout the disaster
- Receive technical, financial, and other assistance from public agencies to maintain operation and possibly maximize surge capacity
- Develop procedures to enhance the organization's recovery from the incident[11]

To implement this strategy, the four phases of emergency management should be reviewed with agencies that provide services to older people. The following is an example of what might be included in this review:

- *Mitigation.* Determine whether the agency's office or base of operations should be relocated before the disaster in case of flooding, or reinforced against potential wind damage.
- *Preparedness.* Provide education that allows the agency's staff to coordinate more effectively with emergency managers and local government when a disaster occurs.
- *Response.* Integrate the agency into the community incident management system. Provide communications equipment and technical assistance before the precipitating disaster and during the immediate post-impact phase to allow the agency to provide maximal services to their older clients.
- *Recovery.* Help the organization identify technical expertise, volunteer staff, and additional funding sources that will aid them in providing services during their recovery activities.[12]

Assisting agencies that provide services to older people is a crucial aspect of preparedness that emergency managers and local government officials must take into consideration. During the response phase of any disaster, the local government will not be able to provide the array of services that are necessary for vulnerable populations to sustain themselves.

Community

Community strategies for emergency preparedness must include incorporating the needs of older people into the emergency management system.[13] Nontraditional groups and organizations, such as gerontologists; geriatricians; emergency department physicians; home health nurses; nursing home administrators; and area agencies on aging, nursing, pharmacy, and hospice care, should be brought into the planning process. One of the first steps in this process is identifying *who* the older people are that reside in the community. What are the demographics of the older people? How many nursing homes and assisted-living facilities are there? Is there a mechanism already in place to identify older shut-ins?

Emergency planners should have a comprehensive profile of the community's composition, including the cultural and religious affiliations of the older adults in the community. Developing this cultural competence requires a concerted effort, but this information can help emergency planners better understand the beliefs and strategies that will affect disaster preparedness functions. For example, depending on their degree of acculturation, older adults within a particular culture may react to imminent danger or seek assistance in different ways. Understanding these important considerations when interacting with older adults can help ensure that misunderstandings and miscommunication will not occur in times of emergency.[14]

Another critical step in disaster planning is partnering with the community's assisted-living and long-term-care facilities in their disaster planning efforts. Many natural disasters—including hurricanes, wildfires, tornadoes, and extreme heat waves—can be life-threatening to nursing home patients, yet few nursing home facilities have adequate evacuation plans (**Figure 15-3**). For example, only 44 of 130 nursing homes located around the Texas Gulf Coast had evacuation plans at the time of Hurricane Katrina. In addition, only 21 of approximately 60 of the nursing homes that were affected by Katrina evacuated their residents before the storm hit.[15]

There are a few aspects of a community's emergency response that that have been specifically identified as needing enhancement in order to address the needs of the older population. These include transportation, healthcare access, and the design of warning systems.[16]

Transportation

Transportation is one of the greatest limitations for older people during a disaster. Many older people experience high functional capacity inside the home, but are dependent on assistive services to function outside of the home. These homebound patients may not be able to get to an evacuation site or sheltering location without assistance (**Figure 15-4**). Shut-ins will also require assistance during an evacuation. It is vital to identify these groups of older people *prior* to the evacuation order.

During the preparedness phase, emergency planners must help facilities identify modes of transportation that can be utilized during a disaster. The staff at assisted-living or long-term care facilities may be under the impression that if an evacuation is ordered, EMS will provide the necessary transportation to the evacuation site. Although EMS providers will aid in the evacuation of these types of facilities by assisting with the movement of ventilator-dependent patients and those who require special monitoring, providing transportation will likely be impossible, as resources will be strained. As such, other modes of transportation must be identified. For example, many large assisted-living facilities have their own vans or buses. In areas where commercial ambulance services are not integrated into the primary 911 system, a **memorandum of understanding (MOU)** can be arranged to have these ambulances provide transportation assistance during an evacuation. Bus companies that have handicapped-accessible vans are another option. An evaluation of transportation resources in the community should be a priority for emergency planners.[17]

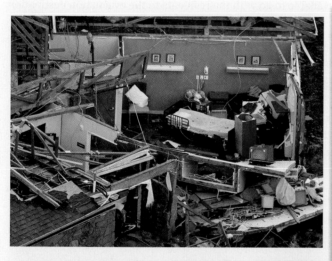

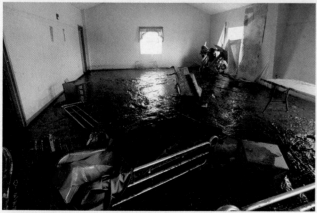

Figure 15-3 Many natural disasters, including hurricanes, wildfires, tornadoes, and extreme heat waves, can be devastating to nursing homes and their residents.

© Khampha Bouaphanh/The Fort Worth Star-Telegram/AP Images; © Anja Niedringhaus/AP Images

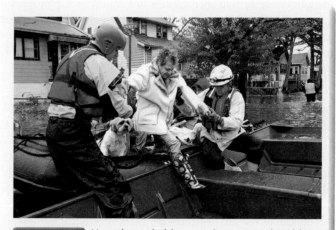

Figure 15-4 Homebound older people may not be able to get to an evacuation site or sheltering location by themselves and may require rescue.

© Adam Hunger/Reuters/Landov

Healthcare Access

In short-duration disasters, chronic disease rarely becomes a public health or medical priority; however, the September 11, 2001, terrorist attack in New York City created a greater awareness of the needs of the chronically ill population during disasters. At the time of the attack, about 6300 older persons lived in the immediate area surrounding the World Trade Center's Twin Towers, and nearly 19,000 lived within a three-block radius.[18] In the days that followed the attack, many frail older adults and persons with disabilities were confined to their apartments without electricity, supplies, medication refills, or communication with the outside world. Home care workers could not get to their clients, and community service providers could not get to their offices or access client information. In addition, many frail adults who were in need of help had never applied for services and were, therefore, unknown to community workers.[19]

Still, it was not until Hurricane Katrina struck the Gulf Coast in 2005 that public health and other response professionals fully began to grasp the importance and urgency of addressing the chronic health needs of vulnerable populations during disasters. Following the hurricane, an estimated 200,000 people with chronic medical conditions lacked access to their medications and usual sources of care.[20] Even those evacuees who had brought with them the recommended 3-day supply of prescriptions eventually ran out.

As shown, the need to care for the chronically ill after a disaster can overwhelm community resources. The vulnerable population's inability to access pharmacies or medical care during 9/11 and Hurricane Katrina contributed to the emergence of chronic diseases as a critical concern for emergency management. Public health personnel, emergency responders, and aging services professionals have begun working together to plan for the needs of frail older adults following a disaster, so that this vulnerable population can be rescued, sheltered, and provided with the routine health care that they require.[21] Plans may include ensuring that medications are available if pharmacies are destroyed or damaged, that transportation will be provided to patients who need to be brought to dialysis sites, and that medical care infrastructure is relocated if a hospital is heavily damaged.

Warning Systems

Emergency warning systems and preparedness materials must be designed with age-related changes in mind. For example, visual, auditory, and cognitive impairments are more commonly present in the older population, so material with larger print is desirable. Service providers and agencies that have regular contact with older people can be used to distribute information. While it is not feasible in every community, going door to door is an effective method to warn inhabitants of an impending disaster. This method may also help to identify an older person requiring assistance who has not been previously identified.[22]

Responsibilities of Assisted Living and Long-Term Care Facilities During Disaster

Assisted living and long-term care facilities that care for vulnerable older persons are responsible for preparing thorough emergency plans and following through on those plans when conditions warrant. The evacuation of these types of facilities is a substantial operation that is associated with many risks and health implications for the facility's residents (**Figure 15-5**). Moving persons who are frail, bed-ridden, comatose, cognitively impaired, and/or dependent upon medical equipment may require the support of the entire community. In addition to moving these residents to safety, the evacuation of assisted-living and long-term care facilities also often includes transporting medical records, medications, medical equipment, disposable products, and food and water.[23] Once these efforts are underway, staff must then be available to go with the residents to the evacuation destination.

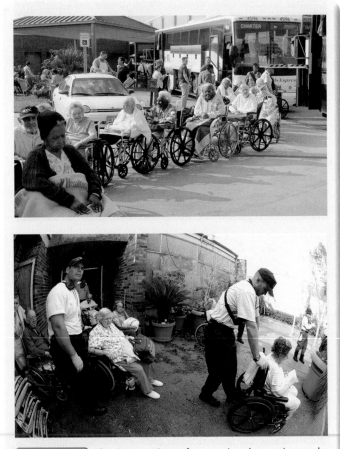

Figure 15-5 The evacuation of a nursing home is a substantial operation that is associated with many risks to the facility's residents.

Due to the responsibilities of assisted-living and long-term care facilities during times of disaster, staff should have an understanding of the national emergency preparedness efforts currently in place. The **National Incident Management System (NIMS)** was rolled out in 2004 by the Department of Homeland Security as a means of enabling all levels of government, nongovernmental organizations, and the private sector to work together during an emergency incident. An essential aspect of NIMS is the **Incident Command System (ICS)**, which is a standardized, all-hazards incident management concept that provides all users with a common organizational structure. The system is structured to support five major incident command functions: command, finance, logistics, operations, and planning. Through the establishment of well-defined roles and responsibilities, responders at the scene of an incident can more efficiently and effectively communicate, make critical decisions, and respond in a coordinated fashion.

While fire and EMS agencies are well versed with the concepts of ICS, key staff members of assisted-living and long-term care facilities will also have to assume positions within the system in the event of a disaster. In these positions, staff may find themselves interacting with emergency services personnel at a higher level than they are used to. During the preparedness and exercise phase of a facility's disaster plan, EMS personnel can instruct facility personnel on ICS and their integration into the overall community response plan. Additionally, assisted-living and long-term care facilities should not be expected to create their disaster plans independently. Emergency services personnel must be ready to assist in these planning efforts. It is imperative that local government organizations, particularly fire and EMS, be knowledgeable of a facility's emergency plan in order to ensure the plan will be executed efficiently when a disaster strikes. These plans must be fluid and reevaluated and exercised on a frequent basis. EMS personnel should also be involved in these exercises and evaluations.

Shelters

Shelters provide temporary emergency relief to disaster victims by providing a range of services, such as food, shelter, health care, and mental health support. Potential shelter sites include:

- *Public and private school buildings.* School gymnasiums and large multipurpose rooms are ideal for sleeping areas.
- *City-owned facilities.* Examples of city-owned facilities that may be used as shelter sites include community centers, senior centers, recreational facilities, and auditoriums.
- *Congregations.* Churches, temples, synagogues, and other privately owned facilities may be utilized during emergencies.

While sheltering operations are not the primary responsibility of EMS agencies, prehospital providers may be requested to assist with these operations, particularly with the assessment and emergent health care of shelter victims. This need may be greatest at the onset of shelter operations. EMS providers can also lend their expertise regarding the sheltering needs of older people. Ideally, older people should be housed in a shelter devoted specifically for them. A suitable site for older people is one that is easily accessible, provides privacy, and has kitchen and showering capabilities. If a location lacks one or more of these characteristics, a mechanism should be in place to have these services provided on-site. Security of the site must also be considered. For those older persons who are cared for by family members or paid caregivers, being accompanied to the shelter by these providers will ensure continuity of care, as well as ease the responsibility of shelter personnel. Supplies that will be needed should be allocated to these shelter sites *before* an impending disaster (**Figure 15-6**).

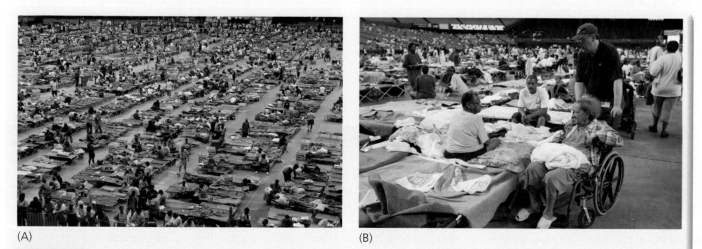

(A)   (B)

Figure 15-6   (A) Evacuation centers are often large and not conducive to older people. (B) If older people are to be housed with other evacuees, a separate area should be provided.

(A) Courtesy of Andrea Booher/FEMA; (B) Courtesy of Andrea Booher/FEMA

Determining Needs of Older Persons in Shelters

Following Hurricane Katrina, many older people were evacuated to makeshift shelters, such as the Reliant Astrodome Complex (RAC) in Houston, Texas. Of the 10,435 people served in the RAC medical unit, 56% were older than 65 years; however, the shelter had no formal mechanisms in place to ensure that older persons were assisted with bathing, eating, or receiving their daily medications.[24] Some older persons were able to voice their own needs or were accompanied by family and friends who were able to advocate for them. In these circumstances, Red Cross personnel were able to provide assistance; however, this help was random and not based on the severity of the older person's condition. There were other older persons at the shelter who were not accompanied by family or friends and were unable to advocate for themselves, and many of these older patients had acute medical conditions that required relocation for treatment at nursing home facilities or hospitals.

It is essential that older people who are brought to a shelter be assessed and triaged based on their needs. The three most important evaluations are the medical assessment (which includes assessment of the older person's daily needs, such as medication requirements and therapies the person is currently receiving), functional assessment, and mental status evaluation. Evaluating these three areas will allow shelter personnel to determine the needs of older people.

SWiFT Assessment Instrument

In the aftermath of Hurricane Katrina, a group of individuals serving the elderly community in Houston, Texas met to come up with ways to serve the special needs of the older population in times of disaster. The Seniors Without Families Triage (SWiFT) assessment tool was devised to rapidly screen for those most in need of help by assessing cognition, medical and social services needs, and the ability to perform ADLs (**Figure 15-7**).[25] Once assessed, the older adult may be assigned to one of three SWiFT levels (**Table 15-1**). SWiFT Level 1 identifies those older persons who cannot perform ADLs, such as bathing, toileting, and remembering to take medications. These persons must be immediately moved to a more suitable environment, such as a nursing home or assisted-living facility. SWiFT Level 2 identifies those older persons who have trouble performing IADLs and cannot easily access health care or other federally offered benefits or manage money. Level 2 patients should be referred to an on-site social worker. Persons who fall into SWiFT Level 3 need to be connected to family, Red Cross, or other volunteers in order to receive assistance for a minor issue.

The SWiFT instrument is ideally suited for EMS providers to utilize. EMS personnel are skilled in assessment and understand the issues that will affect the older person brought to a shelter. It is important that a system be in place so that once evaluations are made, interventions and referrals can be initiated. For example, if an older person evaluated as a SWiFT Level 1 patient must be transferred off-site for a higher level of care, agreements should be in place prior to the disaster so that a seamless transfer can take place. Additionally, a database should be instituted to track all older people who enter the shelter, as well as those who are transferred to another location. Agreements must also be in place with area social services for those falling into the SWiFT Level 2 category, and workers in the shelter must be prepared to respond to the needs of older people identified as a SWiFT Level 3. If the SWiFT instrument is utilized, all personnel involved must be educated in its use and meaning.

Recommendations

In December 2005, the American Association of Retired Persons (AARP) held a conference entitled *We Can Do Better: Lessons Learned for Protecting Older Persons in Disasters*. The recommendations that resulted from that conference are summarized in **Table 15-2**. These recommendations should be provided to community and state emergency planners, as they serve as a template for the planning needs of older people in time of disaster.

CASE STUDY 2

A tornado has left widespread destruction in your service area. One of the buildings partially destroyed was a nursing home facility for residents with care needs that range from independent to total care – including: assisted ventilation, severe Alzheimer's/dementia, assisted living, and transition care after surgery (i.e. recovery after total hip replacement). All injured persons were evacuated and non-injured persons were triaged to an undamaged area of the building; however, the building is not habitable and, therefore, the individuals in the latter group require re-triage and placement. You are responsible for triaging them to appropriate destinations. The local hospital is already overwhelmed with injured patients, but your town has a disaster preparedness plan that includes mutual aid agreements with other agencies and nearby towns.

- What considerations should you keep in mind as you assign triage decisions?
- What additional data or info do you need?

Current date:		Worker's Name:	
Name:		DOB:	

DO YOU HAVE FAMILY OR FRIENDS WITH YOU HERE? ☐ Y ☐ N | **Confirmed?** ☐ Y ☐ N

Level 1: **Health/Mental** **Health Priority** **GOES TO SOCIAL** **WORK BOOTH IN** **MEDICAL CLINIC**	**A.** Do you have any of the following medical problems: ☐ Y ☐ N Diabetes ☐ Y ☐ N Heart disease ☐ Y ☐ N High blood pressure ☐ Y ☐ N Memory ☐ Other Note: **B.** Do you take medicine? ☐ Y ☐ N Do you have your medicine? ☐ Y or ☐ N **If "No," treat as Level 1**		**C.** Do you need someone to help you with: ☐ Y ☐ N Walking ☐ Y ☐ N Eating ☐ Y ☐ N Bathing ☐ Y ☐ N Dressing ☐ Y ☐ N Toileting ☐ Y ☐ N Medication administration **Any checks, treat as Level 1** Do you use something to help you get around: ☐ Cane ☐ Walker ☐ Wheel chair ☐ Bath Bench
D. Where are you right now? **If senior cannot or does not answer correctly treat as Level 1**	**E.** Name 3 ordinary items and have them repeat them; for example, "apple, table, penny."	**F.** What year is it? **If senior cannot/ does not answer correctly treat as Level 1**	**G.** Ask them to repeat the three items you previously mentioned. **If more than one item is missed, treat as Level 1.**
Level 2: **Case Management** **Needs** **IS REFERRED TO A** **CASE MANAGER**	**A.** Ask them what their major need is right now.	**B.** Do you have a plan for where you will go when you leave here? ☐ Yes ☐ No	**C.** *Income/Entitlement* Are you on: ☐ Y ☐ N Medicare ☐ Y ☐ N Medicaid ☐ Y ☐ N SSI ☐ Y ☐ N Social Security ☐ Y ☐ N Food Stamps ☐ Y ☐ N VA Benefits ☐ Y ☐ N Section 8 housing funds **Do you have your documents?** ☐ Yes ☐ No
Level 3: Only needs to be linked to family or friends **DIRECTED TO RED CROSS VOLUNTEER**	**A.** Family Do you need help to find your family/friends? ☐ *Yes* ☐ *No*	**B.** Names: Relationship: Location:	*WHERE IS THE SENIOR LOCATED?*

Figure 15-7 SWiFT Assessment Tool.

Source: Recommendations for Best Practices in the Management of Elderly Disaster Victims, p. 11. Baylor College of Medicine and the American Medical Association.

Table 15-1   SWiFT Level Tool in the Post-Disaster Phase

SWiFT Level	Explanation	Post-Disaster Actions
1	Cannot perform at least one ADL without assistance	Immediate transfer to a location that can provide skilled or personal care (i.e. assisted-living facility, nursing home, hospital)
2	Trouble with IADLs	Needs to be connected with a local aging services case manager
3	Minimal assistance with ADLs and IADLs	Needs to be connected with a rescue organization (i.e. Red Cross)

Source: Recommendations for Best Practices in the Management of Elderly Disaster Victims. Baylor College of Medicine and the American Medical Association.

Table 15-2   Results of the *We Can Do Better* Conference

Planning and Communications

- Establish clear lines of authority among federal, local, and state governments as well as with private sector entities, including nursing homes, with regard to emergency management, especially evacuations of older persons.
- Engage in integrated/coordinated planning that begins at the neighborhood/facility and community levels but reaches to the state, regional, or even national level. Develop strong relationships and partnerships before disaster strikes.
- Provide public information on emergency preparedness to older persons and persons with disabilities that is appropriate to their needs and in accessible formats. As part of these focused education efforts, include information about the need to evacuate if an order to evacuate is given and what can happen if one does not do so.
- Explore the psychological as well as other barriers to heeding orders to evacuate, and ways to overcome them.
- Educate older persons and others to have emergency supplies ready to "shelter in place" for 3 to 6 days without power or being able to go out for food, water, or medicines, and to make a personal plan to meet their "special needs," such as temporary back-up power for home dialysis.
- Train emergency management personnel in the needs of older persons and train aging network personnel in emergency management procedures.
- Practice plans regularly and include older persons and persons with disabilities in emergency drills and training exercises.
- Make better use of aging and disability experts in planning for and responding to disasters, including making better use of "aging network" resources and expertise.
- Ensure that the federal Interagency Coordinating Council on Emergency Preparedness and Individuals with Disabilities also addresses the needs of vulnerable older persons who do not have disabilities.
- Create a team that mirrors the management structure of the federal National Response Plan to support the needs of older persons and persons with disabilities. One component of this team would be a permanent, designated liaison who would report directly to the principal federal officer (PFO).
- Provide more funding to the U.S. Administration on Aging (AoA) to develop and implement its emergency management responsibilities on behalf of older persons.
- Use a combination of methods for public emergency notifications in alternative formats, such as both audible and visual cues to reach populations with sensory and cognitive disabilities, and develop close working relationships with the media to publicize the availability of hotlines in alternative formats.
- Have at least three backup communication plans and test at least one of them regularly.

Table 15-2   Results of the *We Can Do Better* Conference (*Continued*)

Identifying Who Needs Help and What Kind of Help

- Make identifying, registering, and tracking older persons who cannot evacuate on their own a high priority in local communities.

- Have aging services staff work with clients to develop individualized emergency plans and coordinate this work with local emergency management personnel and those responsible for "special needs" registries.

- Encourage voluntary use of "special needs" registries.

- Pay special attention to the needs of persons with dementia and take advantage of special programs, such as the Alzheimer's Association Safe Return Program.

- Use special tools being developed to quickly assess the needs of frail older adults who have been evacuated to settings in the community.

- When preparing for disasters in nursing homes, ensure that residents and their medical information, including medications, can be identified during and after evacuation.

- Move toward a national electronic health record that protects individual privacy, learning from experiences of the U.S. Department of Veterans Affairs, which has a consolidated records system that uses bar codes and captures medical history, medications, and the like.

- In the interim, encourage individuals to write down their medications, including dosage, allergies, and conditions, on an index card and keep it with them at all times.

- Encourage consumers to take advantage of their local pharmacy's computer tracking system by filling out a medication profile that lists all current medications, and to take a waterproof bag with their current medications, even if the bottle is empty, if they have to evacuate.

- Invest in better technology to track individuals during emergencies, such as using "smartcard" chips, while protecting individuals' privacy and confidentiality.

Evacuating Older Persons: How and to Where?

- Plan at the community level to provide accessible transportation for persons with mobility limitations or low vision or for others unable to transport themselves.

- Provide a notification hotline or other mechanism to alert hospitals, nursing homes, and other residential facilities to begin early evacuations, and contact previously identified older persons and persons with disabilities in the community who will take longer to evacuate.

- Identify older persons and persons with disabilities who will need emergency transportation.

- Include plans for transporting emergency supplies and appropriate labeling of medications when evacuating nursing home residents.

- Coordinate plans with transportation vendors for nursing homes residents with other facilities and community groups to avoid having too many providers relying upon too few vendors.

- Plan for transportation for long-term care facility staff as well as truck rentals to get water, food, and medical supplies to facilities.

- Require long-term care facilities, under federal and state licensing standards, to have well-developed, feasible, and practiced emergency plans for residents that are on file with the state; these plans should include evacuating residents, transporting medical records and properly labeled medications and supplies, and providing for care outside the facility.

- Plan for evacuating the families of long-term care facility staff and providing for their care.

- Adopt "special needs" shelter legislation at the state level that provides for appropriate registration, transportation, staffing, and discharge policies. In addition, "special needs" shelter policies should provide for coordination with community-based aging and disability organizations.

(*Continued*)

Table 15-2 **Results of the *We Can Do Better* Conference (*Continued*)**
■ Address barriers to the accessibility of public shelters by persons with disabilities, and the credentialing of health personnel so they can gain access to shelters and other evacuation sites.
■ Provide for a sufficient number of shelters that have backup generators to power life-sustaining medical devices.
Source: We Can Do Better: Lessons Learned for protecting Older Persons in Disasters. Gibson, Mary J. and Hayunga, Michele, pp. 7–10. Reprinted from May 2006 AARP. Copyright 2006. All rights reserved.

Summary

As the size of the older population increases, it becomes progressively more important to understand the vulnerabilities that exist for older adults before, during, and after a disaster. These vulnerabilities, which can prevent the older adult from taking the appropriate response actions, may result from limited mobility, diminished senses, chronic health conditions, or social and economic problems. In order for older adults to be able to appropriately respond to emergencies and disasters, communities must teach these individuals (and their families or caregivers, if applicable) how to shelter in place, develop response and evacuation plans that take their needs into account, provide training for emergency officials on these needs, and arrange the necessary emergency equipment.

Older adults are most likely to follow instructions given by someone they trust. Having confidence in emergency officials and the media are the best predictors of an older person's future willingness to evacuate.[26] Levels of public trust are likely to be higher if emergency officials appear dedicated to the health and well-being of the public. By devoting time to understanding the needs of the older population, you—the EMS provider—will show that you care.

Another critical component of emergency response in a disaster situation is effectively communicating with and providing the necessary disaster information to the general public, particularly the older population.[27] Additional aspects of emergency planning for older people include:

- Defining vulnerable and special needs communities
- Conducting preevent planning with community partners
- Coordinating with agencies that care for vulnerable older patients
- Incorporating the special needs of older people in emergency management plans, and exercising those plans
- Preparing educational materials
- Identifying available resources to support the sheltering of older people
- Designing plans to allow for maximum flexibility

The U.S. Administration on Aging has concluded, "Special efforts are necessary in each disaster if older persons are to be served on a comparable basis."[28] EMS providers are the *front line* of contact for many community-dwelling older people. It is therefore impetrative that providers participate in preparedness efforts to assure that the needs of older people are met when a disaster occurs. These efforts may make the difference between life and death.

References

1. Gibson MJ, Hayunga M. *We Can Do Better: Lessons Learned for Protecting Older Persons in Disasters*. Washington, DC, American Association of Retired Persons, 2006, p. 6.

2. Fernandez, LS, Byard, D, Lin, CC, Barbera, JA. Frail elderly as disaster victims: Emergency management strategies. *Prehosp Disaster Med*, 2002:17(2):71.

3. Gibson and Hayunga, p. 6.

4. Klein, K. *In The Wake of a Natural Disaster: The Elderly Left Behind in Natural Disasters and the Law Seminar*. California Western School of Law: San Diego, 2009, p. 2.

5. Ibid, pp. 4–5.

6. "Hurricane Sandy's Deadly Toll." *New York Times*. November 17, 2012. Available at: http://www.nytimes.com/2012/11/18/nyregion/hurricane-sandys-deadly-toll.html

7. Florida Health Care Education and Development Foundation, 2008, *National Criteria for Evacuation Decision-Making in Nursing Homes*, developed through a project funded by the John A. Hartford Foundation.

8. Vermont Agency of Human Services, Department of Disabilities, Aging and Independent Living. *Emergency Preparedness Planning for Nursing Homes and Residential Care Settings in Vermont*, 2010, pp. 2–3.

9. Fernandez, Byard, Lin, Benson, & Barbera, p. 71.

10. Ibid.

11. Ibid, p. 72.

12. Ibid, pp. 71–72.

13. Ibid, p. 72.

14. Gray-Graves A, Turner K, Swan JH. Sustainability of seniors: Disaster risk reduction management. *The Journal of Aging in Emerging Economies* 2010:2(2). Available at: http://www2.kent.edu/sociology/resources/jaee/upload/article_1.pdf

15. Klein, p. 5.

16. Fernandez, Byard, Lin, Benson, & Barbera, p. 72.

17. Ibid, pp. 72–73.

18. Aldrich N, Benson WF. Disaster preparedness and the chronic disease needs of vulnerable older adults. *Prev Chronic Dis* 2008:5(1), p. 2. Available at: http://www.cdc.gov/pcd//issues/2008/jan/07_0135.htm

19. Ibid, pp. 2–3.

20. Ibid, p. 3.

21. Ibid, pp. 2–3.

22. Fernandez, Byard, Lin, Benson, & Barbera, p. 73.

23. Florida Health Care Education and Development Foundation

24. Klein, p. 6.

25. Baylor College of Medicine, The American Medical Association. *Recommendations for Best Practices in the Management of Elderly Disaster Victims*, p. 8.

26. Gray-Graves, Turner, & Swan.

27. Ibid.

28. Administration on Aging: *Actions by the Administration on Aging to Strengthen the Disaster Response Capability to Serve Older People*. July 1995.

Additional Resources

A Guide for Local Jurisdictions In Care and Shelter Planning. Prepared by the Alameda County Operational Area Emergency Management Organization. September 2003.

Caring for Vulnerable Elders During a Disaster: National Findings of the 2007 Nursing Home Hurricane Summit. Prepared by The Florida Health Care Association.

Disaster Preparedness, For Seniors By Seniors. Prepared by The Greater Rochester Chapter of the American Red Cross.

Emergency Preparedness Packet for Home Health Agencies. 2008. Prepared by The National Association for Home Care & Hospice. 2008.

National Criteria for Evacuation Decision-Making in Nursing Homes. 2008. Prepared by the Florida Health Care Education and Development Foundation.

CASE STUDY SUMMARIES

Case Study 1 Summary

Assistance with the evacuation effort must begin prior to the evacuation order. When an evacuation order is given, many individuals and families will be able to quickly heed the order; however, often this is not the case for the older people in the community. A successful evacuation effort begins with the preparedness phase of disaster planning. Knowing the demographic profile of community-dwelling older people will aid in this effort. Not only is it important to identify *who* the older people are in the community, but also *where* they reside. Once these key pieces of information are identified, targeted preparedness efforts can commence.

Self-preparedness is paramount. Older people must be educated about disaster preparedness efforts. Evacuation planning for assisted living and long-term care facilities must be coordinated between the facilities' owners and operators, emergency planners, and emergency medical services agencies. These plans must be updated and exercised on a regular basis. Evacuation centers that are conducive for housing older people must be identified. These centers must also be staffed by professionals who understand the needs of older people. EMS agencies are an integral component of any successful evacuation effort. If disaster-planning efforts that encompass the needs of older people are undertaken, an evacuation effort will undoubtedly save the lives of those older people who are most vulnerable during a disaster.

Case Study 2 Summary

You pull out the SWIFT assessment tool and begin to apply the tool's concepts. Determine if the patient is independent with daily living, requires assistance with daily living, or is independent but needs to be set up with services.

Considerations to keep in mind include the older person's usual medical condition, number of medications, type of care needed, equipment required to provide usual care, and type of monitoring needed. Issues that need to be considered include: dialysis schedules, dietary issues, obtaining medications, confusion that occurs as result of being removed from usual environ and faces, usual ambulatory, hearing, seeing appliances that may have been lost in process of evacuation. Based on SWIFT title – there is no family, but this could simple be they are not immediately available. Can you find them? It would also be helpful to know what the receiving resource is capable of doing. If they are highly functioning, a level 1 patient might be able to go there. If the community outreach groups can actually reach out to the patient in a timely manner, then perhaps a level 3 will work. Closing the loop of the patient getting the care needed will be extremely important.

Also keep in mind that gathering information, being calm; gaining trust, taking time will help you make the best choices for these patients. It will be important to continue to monitor for signs of physical decompensation, as older adults may not initially show signs /symptoms of injuries. This is not an area that one person should be doing alone, but requires enough help to thoroughly assess both physically, emotionally, and historically.

The answers provided below could be different if the situation or assessment is not clear cut, based on additional information gathered, or just on intuition, but here would be the starting points for each. It also assumes that a community shelter has been set up so the patient has a place to stay. It has been found that older adults do better if separated from the mass confusion of an all aged population community shelter if that is a triage option. (less noise, stimuli, better regulation of schedules, as opposed to living in general population)

PROCEDURES AND HOME HEALTH DEVICES

CONTENTS

1. Urinary Catheters   254

2. Ureterostomy   257

3. Colostomy/Ileostomy   258

4. Tracheostomy   259

5. Respirators/Ventilators   262

6. Patient-Controlled Analgesic Pumps   264

7. Enteral Feeding   266

8. Vascular Access Devices   268

9. Dialysis   273

10. Ventricular Shunts   278

11. Automatic Implantable Cardioverter Defibrillators   280

12. Ventricular Assist Devices   282

Urinary Catheters

Introduction

Catheterization of the bladder involves introducing a rubber or plastic tube through the urethra and into the bladder. Bladder catheterization is an invasive procedure that carries some associated risks. Special training and authorization from medical control is required to perform bladder catheterization.

Rationale

The urinary catheter provides a continuous flow of urine for patients unable to control the bladder, for patients with an obstruction, or for patients who are unable to ambulate. It usually remains in place until the patient can void voluntarily. There are several types of urinary catheters.

Single-Use Straight Catheter

This catheter is used for only a short time to drain the bladder, and then it is removed. Some patients or caregivers are taught to insert the single-use straight catheter on their own.

Indwelling Foley Catheter

This catheter has a small inflatable balloon that encircles the catheter at the tip (**Figure P1-1**). When the balloon is inflated with sterile saline, it rests against the bladder outlet to anchor the catheter in place. The indwelling Foley catheter may have as many as three separate lumens within the body of the catheter.

Condom Catheter (Texas Catheter)

The condom catheter is used for male patients who are incontinent or comatose. These patients have complete and spontaneous bladder emptying.

Suprapubic Catheter

This catheter is surgically inserted into the bladder through the lower abdomen above the symphysis pubis (**Figure P1-2**). It is generally used for short periods of time for patients who have had gynecological or bladder surgery. It also may be used for patients who require a long-term alternative to catheterization due to incapacity to hold a Foley catheter in place. The suprapubic catheter is more comfortable than other catheters, as the patient may void naturally when the catheter is clamped.

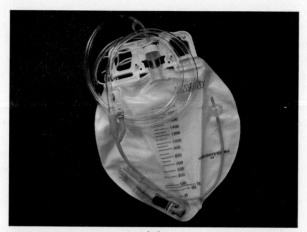

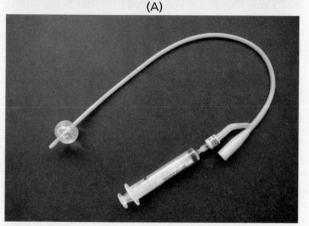

Figure P1-1 (A) Foley catheter and bag. (B) Foley catheter with the balloon inflated with sterile saline.
Courtesy of James Upchurch

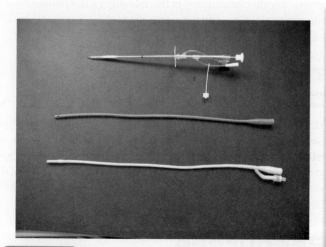

Figure P1-2 A suprapubic catheter shown at top, with Foley catheters beneath.
Courtesy of James Upchurch

Catheterization equipment includes personal protective equipment as well as a urinary catheter set, which contains the following:

- Sterile gloves
- Antiseptic solution
- Sterile cleansing sponges
- Sterile drapes or towels
- Syringe containing 5 ml of sterile water
- Connecting tubing and collection bag
- Water-soluble sterile lubricant
- Urinary catheter with 5-ml Foley balloon (usually 16F for males, 14F for females)

Preparation

Most patients will be apprehensive and frightened of bladder catheterization. The EMS provider should fully explain the procedure, reassure the patient, and make every effort to ensure privacy.

Procedure: Male Catheterization

1. Place the patient in a supine position and remove the patient's pants and undergarments.
2. Open the catheterization set using sterile technique.
3. Wash hands and don sterile gloves.
4. Place one sterile drape under the patient's penis and another above the penis to cover the abdomen.
5. Open a package of antiseptic solution and saturate sterile sponges or cotton balls.
6. Attach the syringe to the catheter and test the balloon to make sure it inflates.
7. Open a package of water-soluble lubricant and lubricate the first several inches of the catheter.
8. Grasp the patient's penis with one hand and retract the foreskin (if present).
9. With the other hand, cleanse the glans with a sterile sponge (maintaining hand sterility) and then discard the sponge. Repeat the procedure.
10. Raise the shaft of the penis upright to straighten the penile urethra and pass the tip of the catheter through the hole in the tip of the penis.
11. Continue passing the catheter with gentle, steady pressure, advancing the catheter 7 to 9 inches or until urine flows out the distal end of the catheter. Once urine appears, advance the catheter another 2 inches. If mild resistance is felt at the external sphincter, slightly increase traction on the penis and continue with steady, gentle pressure on the catheter. (If significant resistance is met, withdraw the catheter and consult with medical control).

12. Attach the syringe to the catheter and inflate the balloon with 3 to 5 ml of sterile water.
13. Gently pull back on the catheter until the balloon rests against the prostatic urethra. (Resistance will be encountered). Reposition the retracted foreskin of an uncircumcised patient. Attach the drainage bag to the catheter.
14. Run the catheter tubing along the patient's leg and tape the connecting tubing to the patient's thigh. Do not place any tension on the catheter.
15. Attach the collection bag to the bed or stretcher at a level below that of the patient to facilitate drainage by gravity.

Procedure: Female Catheterization

1. Place the patient in a supine position and remove the patient's pants and undergarments. Female patients should be positioned with knees bent, hips flexed, and feet resting about 24 inches apart. Note: This position may not always be possible for older female patients. Never force a patient's limbs, as this will cause ligament and muscle damage.
2. Open the catheterization set using sterile technique.
3. Wash hands and don sterile gloves.
4. Place one sterile drape under the patient's buttocks; position the drape with a central opening over the perineum, exposing the labia.
5. With one hand, separate the patient's labia to expose the opening of the urethra.
6. Cleanse the surrounding area with a sterile sponge or cotton ball (maintaining hand sterility) in downward strokes from anterior to posterior and then discard sponge. Repeat the procedure.
7. Introduce the tip of the well-lubricated catheter into the urethra using aseptic technique. Continue to advance the catheter 2 to 3 inches with gentle, steady pressure until urine flows out of the distal end of the catheter. Once urine appears, advance the catheter another 2 inches.
8. Attach a syringe to the catheter and inflate the balloon with 3 to 5 ml of sterile water.
9. Gently pull on the catheter until resistance is encountered.
10. Attach the collection tubing and bag to the catheter and secure the collection tubing to the patient's thigh as described above. Position the collection bag to facilitate drainage.

Possible Complications
Urinary Tract Infection

Urinary tract infection (UTI) is common and occurs in both sexes. The organisms most commonly associated with a UTI are gram-negative organisms normally found in the gastrointestinal tract, including *Escherichia coli*, *Klebsiella*, *Proteus*, *Enterobacter*, and *Pseudomonas*. These are frequently introduced from the hands of health personnel at the time of bladder catheterization. If allowed to progress, a UTI may lead to septic complications (urosepsis), which can be especially dangerous in the older patient. Steps to help prevent a UTI include:

- Never raise the bag above the level of the patient's bladder.
- The bag should be emptied every 8 hours via the drainage valve, using an alcohol wipe to clean the drainage tube before emptying.
- Hands should be washed and gloves worn before and after handling the catheter, bag, or tubing.
- Urine should not be allowed to collect in the tubing.
- Know and recognize the signs and symptoms of a UTI (refer to the *Other Medical Emergencies* chapter for a review of the signs and symptoms of a UTI).

Traumatic Removal of Indwelling Foley Catheter

When the catheter is pulled out with the balloon still inflated, the urethra can be traumatized. Cover the penis or vagina with a loose dressing and transport, replacing fluids as necessary. If the catheter is not totally dislodged, check with medical control to determine if the balloon should be deflated. After deflation, the catheter should not be pulled out.

Other Emergencies

Bladder distention from blockages can occur if the tubing becomes kinked or compressed externally, or disfigured internally from blood or sediment. The patient should be transported. Another emergency is the inability of the patient to self-catheterize. If this occurs, there is no field treatment other than to transport the patient.

Transport Considerations

When transporting a patient with a catheter in place, make sure that the tubing is secured to the leg of the patient, protect the patient's modesty, and do not pull on the tubing during transport. It is important to ensure that the bag is placed below the level of the patient's bladder, so that urine does not collect in the tubing.

Resources

National Association for Continence (www.nafc.org)

Ureterostomy

Introduction

A urinary diversion refers to the rerouting of the urinary tract when it is necessary to remove or bypass the bladder. The bladder may be removed due to cancer. A bypass procedure may be indicated for **neurogenic bladder**.

An **ileal conduit**, the most common type of urinary diversion in adults, is not a new bladder, but a tube or conduit constructed of small bowel that allows urine to drain to the outside of the body. Urine drains continuously through the stoma and requires an external pouch. When the ileal conduit cannot be constructed, a **ureterostomy** may be seen in adult patients. The ureter is brought to the abdominal wall to form a stoma. The ureterostomy has a higher rate of stenosis (narrowing), infection, and pouching difficulties.

Possible Complications

Emergencies related to this device are uncommon; however, the patient or family may have some questions or concerns. Additional considerations include:

- The stoma may be a source of bleeding. If the bleeding is visible, apply pressure and transport the patient to the emergency department.
- The stoma is not sensitive to touch, but the skin around the stoma can become sensitive if irritated by urine or the adhesive of the urostomy pouch.

Colostomy/ Ileostomy

Introduction

Certain illnesses or injuries prevent the normal passage of intestinal contents through the large and small bowels. A **colostomy** is a diversion involving the colon, in which a segment of diseased or injured colon is bypassed or removed and an end (or loop) of colon is brought through a small opening in the abdominal wall, forming a stoma. The removal of the entire colon and rectum results in the ileum being brought through the abdominal wall, forming an **ileostomy** stoma.

The bowel usually discharges liquid or solid feces into the bag (pouch) once or twice a day; the bag is then changed. Colostomy irrigation, ostomy care, and pouch changes are usually performed for home care patients by the patients themselves, family members, and home health practitioners. These procedures require special training and usually are not considered an acute intervention for EMS practice.

Possible Complications

Possible complications include:

- Bowel perforation
- Significant fluid/electrolyte imbalances from colostomy irrigation and diarrhea
- Stomal problems (i.e. bleeding, necrosis, retraction, stenosis, prolapse)
- Infection
- Obstruction

Tracheostomy

Introduction

A **tracheostomy** is a temporary or permanent surgical opening (stoma) through the third or fourth tracheal ring. Tracheostomies are performed when an endotracheal tube is contraindicated or cannot be passed, or when sustained ventilatory support is required. Patients who require a tracheostomy fall into one of two categories:

- Patients who have an obstruction at or above the level of the larynx, such as foreign body obstruction, carcinoma of the larynx, severe infection, or trauma to the tongue or mandible
- Patients who have no actual obstruction, but are unable to clear their own secretions and are in danger of hypoxia if secretions accumulate and are not removed from the chest

Patients in the latter group include those with paralysis of the chest muscles and diaphragm, patients who are unconscious or semiconscious with head injuries, and patients with fractured ribs or other chest injuries causing severe pain that inhibits them from coughing.

Tracheostomy tubes may be constructed of polyvinyl chloride (PVC) or silastic (silicone rubber) and may be single or double construction. The single tube has a built-in tracheal cuff and an obturator or stylet used for insertion. The cuff is inflated to prevent aspiration of upper airway secretions. The double tube has a similar attached cuff, as well as an inner cannula. The inner cannula is designed to be easily removed, cleaned, or replaced to maintain good air exchange. Some tracheostomy tubes have a small opening in the cannula that enables the patient to whisper or talk by moving air through the larynx. Once the tube is inserted in the neck, it is secured with sutures or soft cloth ties.

Rationale

The tracheostomy tube is inserted to allow passage of air and the removal of tracheobronchial secretions.

Emergencies and Complications

Emergencies

The three most common tracheostomy emergencies that the EMS provider may encounter are hemorrhage, tube dislodgement, and tube obstruction. Although a minimal amount of bleeding is expected after the tracheostomy is inserted or tubing is changed, continued bleeding at the site of the stoma or the vessels surrounding the incision may be cause for concern. If bleeding is more than minimal or does not stop on its own, the patient should be transported to the hospital.[1]

Another tracheostomy emergency is tube displacement that occurs during the early postoperative period when the stoma is not yet healed (healing takes approximately 1 week). Tube displacement may be complete or partial. Partial displacement occurs when the tip of the tube is dislodged and falls within a false passage anterior to the trachea. Tube displacement that occurs before the stoma has healed can result in stoma collapse and requires prompt action to manage the situation. Immediate treatment in complete tube displacement includes mask ventilation and replacement of the tracheostomy tube with an endotracheal tube. This is a risky procedure and should not be performed without specific training and medical direction. Alternatively, orotracheal intubation may be performed.

If tube displacement occurs in a stoma that is greater than 1 week old, the rate of closure depends on how long the tube has been dislodged. For these patients, the tube is replaced with the following steps:

1. Remove the inner cannula.
2. Insert the obturator into the outer cannula in order to cushion the tip of the tube and/or provide control of the tube upon reinsertion.
3. Insert the tube at a 90-degree angle.
4. Angle the tube downward 90 degrees more into position on the vertical plane and remove the obturator.[2]

Tube obstruction is the third serious tracheostomy emergency. If a tracheostomy patient is in respiratory distress, the inner cannula must be removed and inspected. A cannula that is clogged with secretions can be cleaned and/or replaced. If the patient remains in respiratory distress once the tube is reinserted, a suction catheter should be inserted. The catheter should easily pass and return tracheal secretions; resistance may indicate that the tube is clogged or lodged within a false passage. To manage this situation in a patient with an immature stoma, perform mask ventilation with a deflated cuff, and then insert an orotracheal tube. In a patient with a mature stoma, management involves replacing the entire tube. After the airway is secured, the tracheostomy can be reassessed under more controlled circumstances.[3]

Complications

Infection

The stoma itself may become infected, leading to redness, swelling, pus, and fever. Improper suctioning techniques may cause pulmonary infections and sepsis. The risk of infection can be reduced through the use of aseptic technique and good wound care.

Tracheal Stenosis

Stenosis occurs when the trachea narrows at the site of the cuff and may develop weeks or years after the tube has been inserted. Due to the reduced diameter of the trachea, the patient may develop dyspnea, stridor, decreased exercise tolerance, and recurring respiratory infections.

Tracheal Necrosis

Necrosis is associated with excessive cuff pressure and may occur as early as 3 to 5 days after insertion of the tube. In some patients, the necrosis may extend through the posterior wall of the trachea, causing an opening to develop between the trachea and esophagus. Necrosis may also cause erosion through the anterior wall of the trachea and into an artery, although this is rare. If this occurs, the tube may pulsate and/or show bright red blood.

Opening Between the Trachea and Esophagus

An opening or fistula between the trachea and esophagus allows air to escape into the stomach, which can cause oral and gastric secretions to be aspirated into the lungs. The patient may experience dyspnea, stridor, or evidence of aspiration pneumonia. If suction does not adequately keep the tube clear, consider inserting a slightly smaller endotracheal tube through the tracheostomy tube until the tip is just above the carina. If external bleeding is noted, use an absorbent dressing and apply slight pressure.

Subcutaneous/Mediastinal Emphysema

Subcutaneous/mediastinal emphysema appears immediately after initial tube insertion or reinsertion. Although rare, this condition can occur if the tube is displaced and air leaks into the surrounding tissues. The patient may experience mild to severe respiratory distress. The area beneath the skin may appear puffy and a crackling sensation (crepitus) may be palpated. Provide respiratory support and monitor the patient carefully. Refrain from using positive-pressure ventilation, as this may increase the extent of the air leak.

References

1. Morris LL Whitmer A, McIntosh E. Tracheostomy Care and Complications in the Intensive Care Unit. *Crit Care Nurs* 2013:33(5): 18–30, p. 24.
2. Ibid, pp. 25–26.
3. Ibid, p. 26.

Respirators/ Ventilators

Introduction

Historically, mechanical ventilators were only available in the intensive care units of hospitals. Portable units are now widely available for interfacility patient transport and home use. Mechanical ventilators are classified according to preset parameters that control the mechanism of the inspiratory phase (volume cycled, pressure cycled, and time cycled).

- *Volume ventilators* deliver a predetermined volume of gas with each cycle, after which inspiration is terminated. These types of ventilators deliver a constant tidal volume regardless of changes in airway resistance or compliance of the lungs and thorax. The volume stays the same unless high airway pressures are reached, in which case safety release valves stop the flow.
- *Pressure ventilators* are pressure-cycled devices that terminate inspiration when a preset pressure is reached. At this point, the gas flow ceases and the patient passively exhales. These types of ventilators are most often used for patients whose ventilator resistance is not likely to change.

- *Negative-pressure ventilators* use negative pressure to raise the rib cage and lower the diaphragm to then create negative pressure within the lungs so that air can flow in. These ventilators have settings for respiratory rate and pressure of the negative force exerted. They are used for patients with healthy lungs who have a muscular inability to exhale (spinal cord injury, neuromuscular disease).
- *Continuous positive airway pressure (CPAP) ventilatory support systems* are for patients who require continuous positive airway pressure and include mask systems and nasal systems. CPAP systems raise pressure in the patient's nose and pharynx, forcing air into the lungs during inspiration. After inspiration, pressure returns to a lower level.
- *Bilevel positive airway pressure (BiPAP) ventilator support systems* deliver two different levels of positive airway pressure. The system cycles spontaneously between a preset level of inspiratory positive airway pressure (IPAP) and expiratory positive airway pressure (EPAP). BiPAP systems, which are intended only to augment breathing, may be beneficial to patients with chronic obstructive pulmonary disease (COPD) or sleep apnea.

Rationale

Mechanical ventilators are used for home or transport patients who are unable to maintain spontaneous respirations for any length of time. Management goals include improving airway patency, ventilation, and oxygenation.

Emergency Care

When caring for a patient with a ventilator, evaluate the patient's work of breathing, tidal volume, peak flow, oxygen saturation, and quality of breath sounds. The following signs and symptoms of hypoxia should be recognized and treated:

- Restlessness
- Headache
- Confusion and mental status changes
- Hyperventilation
- Tachycardia
- Hypertension
- Dyspnea
- Cyanosis

Even if the patient's family is familiar with the ventilator, an onset of problems may initiate a call to EMS. Having a back-up ventilator is essential. You may encounter a wide variety of ventilators, but always remember to treat the patient and not the machine.

The initial step in managing a patient with a ventilator is to determine the patient's hemodynamic stability.[1] Hemodynamic instability in the ventilated patient can be caused by a worsening of the original pathology that necessitated intubation, or circumstances that are precipitated by the ventilator itself (such as tension pneumothorax and severe auto-positive end-expiratory pressure [auto-PEEP]).[2] (Auto-PEEP is gas trapped in alveoli at end expiration, due to inadequate time for expiration, bronchoconstriction, or mucus plugging. With this condition, work of breathing is increased, as the gas is not in equilibrium with the atmosphere and, therefore, exerts a positive pressure).

For patients who are in cardiac arrest or near arrest, the following steps should be implemented:

1. Disconnect the patient from the ventilator. A quick rush or a prolonged expiration of air from the endotracheal (ET) tube can be a sign of ventilator-induced auto-PEEP. Patients receiving CPR should not be connected to a ventilator.
2. Ventilate the patient with 100% oxygen utilizing a bag-valve mask (BVM) at 8 to 10 breaths per minute. Determine if there is equal rise and fall of the chest. Unequal chest rise can be a sign of a main-stem intubation, pneumothorax, or mucus plug.

3. Auscultate breath sounds. Decreased breath sounds could indicate main-stem intubation, pneumothorax, or atelectatic lung. Feel for subcutaneous crepitus, which may indicate pneumothorax, and assess for difficulty in hand ventilating, which may indicate low dynamic or static respiratory system compliance.
4. Determine that the ET is properly placed and functioning. Adjust the ET or re-intubate the patient if necessary. Some patients may bite the tube. If this occurs, insert a bite block.
5. If, after these procedures, the patient is still in cardiac arrest or near arrest, needle decompression (of both sides of the chest) should be considered. Medical control should be consulted prior to decompression.[3]

Special Circumstances: The Tracheostomy Patient
Unintentional Extubation

- Determine if the patient had a laryngectomy.
  - Oral intubation is an option if the patient did not have a laryngectomy.
- Determine the reason for the tracheostomy.
  - Anatomic reason, difficult or failed airway: oral intubation may not be an option.
  - Traumatic brain injury, chronic respiratory failure: oral intubation may be an option.
- Determine the age of the tracheostomy.
  - If the tracheostomy was performed less than 1 week prior, the site may not be mature enough for manipulation; in this case, there is a high risk of creating a false tract.
- Gently place a 6.0 ET tube in the stoma.
  - If available, fiberoptic visualization may be used to confirm placement.
  - Stop if there is any resistance.

Obstruction

- Remove inner cannula and replace with same-sized cannula.

References

1. Santanilla, Jairo I. "The Crashing Ventilated Patient," in *Emergency Department Resuscitation of the Critically Ill.* 2011, American College of Emergency Physicians, p. 15.
2. Ibid, p. 18.
3. Ibid, p. 19.

Patient-Controlled Analgesic Pumps

Introduction

Patient-controlled analgesia (PCA) provides safe, effective, and consistent pain relief to manage postoperative and chronic pain. The patient is allowed to have control over medication administration, with predetermined safety limits. A PCA pump is an electronically controlled infusion pump that will administer a preset amount of pain medication by continuous infusion or by self-administration of a preset bolus dose (**Figure P6-1**). A timing device sets the interval between patient-administered doses. The timer can be set to a specific interval that prevents additional doses from being administered until the time interval expires, regardless of how many times the button is pushed. Most pumps have a locked safety system to prevent tampering. At no time should anyone but the patient push the medication button. This prevents overmedication and is why it is called "patient-controlled analgesia."

The patient and caregivers can be valuable information resources concerning the PCA pump and medication. There should be written physician's orders in the home or on the medication cartridge stating the type of analgesic, loading dosage, concentration of analgesic mixture, and "lock-out interval" (minimum time allowed between doses). Overdose is uncommon, but should be considered in the patient who presents with an altered mental status that is not his or her baseline status.

The pump can administer medication via intravenous (IV) lines, subcutaneous needle, or epidural catheter.

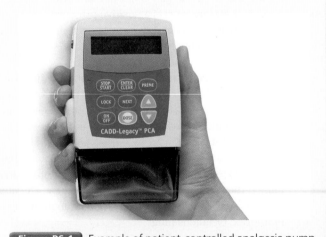

Figure P6-1 Example of patient-controlled analgesia pump.

© Smiths Medical

Rationale

Patient-controlled analgesia provides safe, effective, and consistent pain relief and allows the patient to control delivery of pain medication in a safe, effective, and reliable manner.

Equipment

Equipment that may be found in the patient's home includes the following:

- PCA infusion pump
- PCA administration set (pump tubing)
- IV tubing and fluid as applicable
- PCA infuser key
- PCA flow sheet
- Ordered narcotic analgesic vial, syringe, or cassette (mixed by pharmacy)
- Patient information booklet
- IV start kit (unless venous access is already available)

Possible Complications

Severe complications from pain medication administration include respiratory depression, respiratory arrest, and allergic reaction. Less-severe complications include nausea, vomiting, constipation, and increased somnolence. The combination of respiratory depression and neurological depression can make a patient at risk for atelectasis, pulmonary edema, and acute respiratory distress syndrome (ARDS). The administration of naloxone (Narcan) may be required. The patient's airway and breathing should be monitored closely.

Infiltration of the intravenous administration site can occur when IV fluids enter the subcutaneous space around the venipuncture site. Look for swelling and pallor (blanching) around the site, or note if the patient complains of a painful, burning sensation. Discontinue the infusion by shutting off the pump, and raise the extremity to promote venous drainage. Contact medical control for assistance.

Phlebitis is inflammation of the vein, and may be caused by the type of catheter, chemical irritation by medications, or the anatomical position of the catheter. The patient may complain of pain and tenderness at the vein site. The skin over the vein may be warm and red. Discontinue the infusion and apply warm, moist compresses over the site to provide relief.

Other risks include incorrect drug concentrations, incorrect rates, and calculation errors that lead to inaccurate drug delivery.

Enteral Feeding

Introduction

Enteral feedings are administered through a tube placed in the stomach or small intestine via the esophagus or directly through the abdominal wall. Common conditions that warrant enteral nutritional support include:

- Dysphagia
- Stroke
- Cancer
- Gastrointestinal disease
- Coma
- Cardiac or respiratory failure
- Depression

A gastric tube, or feeding tube, is a small polyurethane or silicone tube that is inserted through the nose to the stomach (nasogastric) or through the mouth to the stomach (orogastric) to provide liquid nutrition. Long-term effectiveness of these tubes is limited due to patient discomfort and irritation; therefore, they are used if the patient requires tube feeding for less than 6 weeks.

A gastrostomy, or G-tube, is used when prolonged or permanent (longer than 6 weeks) enteral feedings are needed. While the patient is under general or local anesthesia, a physician makes a small opening in the abdominal wall and inserts a special gastrostomy catheter through the wall and into the stomach. The tube usually extends 12 to 15 inches from the skin and is sutured into place. This provides a skin-level gastrostomy and eliminates the cumbersome external catheter. The button allows the attachment of a safety cap after removing the feeding tube.

A jejunostomy, or J-tube, is an intestinal tube that passes through the stomach and into a portion of the small intestine called the jejunum. This type of tube is used if the patient is at risk for aspiration or has severe esophageal reflux, obstruction, stricture (abnormal narrowing of duct), fistulae (abnormal passages of the GI tract), or ileus of the upper GI tract.

Rationale

Enteral feedings can be used to provide liquid nutrition for patients who have a healthy GI system, but are unable to swallow due to injury, paralysis, or unresponsiveness.

Indications

- Malnutrition risk or presence
- Inadequate intestinal digestion and absorption
- Absence of bowel obstruction

Possible Complications

Nausea, vomiting, and diarrhea can all be side effects from tube feeding. Diarrhea is the most common reported complication of tube feeding. The concentration of the formula, the rate of flow, and the amount of water provided can affect people differently.

Aspiration (the unintentional inhalation of food or fluids into the lungs) is one of the most serious complications in patients receiving enteral feeding and, due to resultant pneumonia, is among the leading causes of death in tube-fed patients. Although tube feeders may not be consuming food orally, they are still at risk for aspirating the enteral formula. These patients should avoid lying flat while receiving a tube feed or receiving an excessive amount of formula in a short period of time. To minimize the risk of aspiration, patients should be fed sitting up or at a 30- to 45-degree semirecumbent position. They should remain in the position at least one hour after feeding is completed.

Infection is a complication of a gastrostomy tube. The tube site is a wound that must be kept clean. Even with the best care, infection is still possible. An older person's recovery from infection can be further compromised if nutritional status is impaired, which is common in this age group. Excessive bleeding at the site may also occur until fully healed.

Metabolic and electrolyte imbalances are common complications associated with enteral feedings. Imbalances are often related to high or low serum levels of sodium, potassium, phosphorus, magnesium, zinc, copper, vitamins, trace elements, and water. Patients must be carefully monitored for fluid management in order to avoid electrolyte imbalances and fluid balance alteration.[1]

There are also many mechanical complications that can occur with feeding tubes. Obstructed or clogged feeding tubes are one of the most common mechanical problems encountered; tubes should be flushed with at least 30 ml to 60 ml of water after every feeding or medication administration. Leakage is another common complication associated with gastrostomy tubes. Tube leakage can cause severe skin excoriation and major hygiene problems. Approximately 25% of nasogastric tubes fall out or are pulled out inadvertently.[2]

References

1. Gavi S, Hensley J, Cervo F, Nicastri C, Fields S. Management of Feeding Tube Complications in the Long-Term Care Resident. *Annals of Long-Term Care* 2008:16(4):28–32.
2. Ibid.

Vascular Access Devices

Introduction

Many patients with cancer and other chronic illnesses require prolonged and frequent access to venous circulation. In the past, it was necessary for the patient to remain hospitalized or suffer repeated needle sticks to obtain blood or receive antibiotics at home. Today, medications, parenteral nutrition, and blood transfusions can be administered through a variety of vascular access devices.

These tubes are inserted into the central circulation where they remain for weeks or months, allowing reliable access to circulation. This allows more patients to be managed at home, and as a result, EMS providers encounter increasing numbers of patients with vascular access devices. The use of vascular access devices in the prehospital setting was initially strongly discouraged, but in critical situations, vascular access devices provide immediate and life-saving venous access.

Rationale

For the patient who requires immediate vascular access and offers no peripheral route, a vascular access device can provide a safe, rapid solution. However, only those who have received specialized training and whose protocols allow it should attempt to access a vascular access device.

Although many types of vascular access devices are in use, they may be classified into three general categories:

- Central venous catheters (CVC)
- Implanted ports
- Peripheral inserted central catheters (PICC)

Each category includes several types of catheters with a variety of uses and functions. Although the specifics are complex, a working knowledge of the general types and functions of vascular access devices is valuable for the EMS provider.

Features

Catheters implanted for long-term use have many common features. Most are constructed of radiopaque silicone or, less often, polyurethane. Silicone is strong, flexible, and less likely to cause clot formation than other materials. The location of the catheter will vary based on patient characteristics, patient preference, type and duration of therapy, and self- and home-care capabilities.

The venous catheter is inserted with the tip in the superior vena cava, just above the right atrium, thus the descriptive name of central venous catheter. The insertion site is usually one of the major veins of the chest or upper neck, or, in the case of peripheral access, one of the large veins of the arm or leg.

Vascular access devices are used for both bolus injections and continuous IV infusions. Examples include IV solutions, medications, total parenteral nutrition (TPN), blood, and blood products. Blood samples for laboratory studies are obtainable through most vascular access devices. The catheter may have one, two, or three lumens.

Central Venous Catheters

CVCs may also be referred to by the manufacturer's name (e.g., Broviac, Hickman, Groshong, Corcath). A CVC may be a single-lumen or multilumen catheter (**Figure P8-1**). The multi-lumen catheter is used for patients requiring complex therapy. Lumen sizes vary from 21- to 14-gauge. A small cap (referred to as an intermittent injection cap, buffalo cap, or heparin lock) covers each lumen and is filled with a heparin or saline solution to keep blood clots from blocking the catheter.

CVCs are inserted through the skin and then tunneled through the subcutaneous tissue to the site in which the catheter enters the vein (**Figure P8-2**). A cuff located in the subcutaneous portion of the catheter helps the catheter to imbed itself in tissue. Fibrous tissue then grows around the cuff, stabilizing the catheter and creating a barrier against infection.

Implanted Ports

Unlike a CVC, there is no external infusion site with an implanted, or subcutaneous, port. This port is like a tiny drum; it has a solid bottom and sides and is covered on top by a flexible material called the septum. The port is located at the distal end of the catheter and is implanted approximately 0.5 inch under the skin. The port is palpated through the skin, and a needle is inserted into the self-sealing septum.

Although not required, a dressing is often placed over the access site to add further protection. In routine circumstances, a special "Huber" needle is used to extend the life of the septum (**Figure P8-3**).

Peripheral Inserted Central Catheter

PICCs are small (23- to 16-gauge) single- or double-lumen catheters (**Figure P8-4**). Because of their smaller size, they are often used for neonates, very young children, or patients who require only short-term therapy.

PICC lines are less expensive than CVCs and have fewer major complications such as hemothorax, pneumothorax, and air emboli. They are also called nontunneled catheters, because they enter the skin near the point at which they enter the vein. PICC lines are often inserted at the antecubital space into the basilic or cephalic vein. Once inserted, the catheter may be sutured in place for stability.

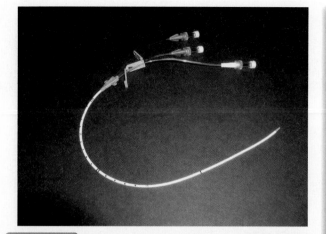

Figure P8-1 A CVC may be a single-lumen or a multilumen catheter. Here, a three-lumen catheter is shown.
Courtesy of James Upchurch

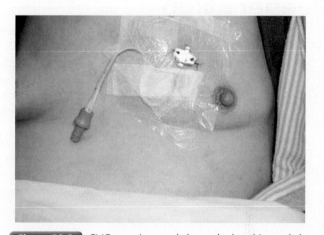

Figure P8-2 CVCs are inserted through the skin and then tunneled through the subcutaneous tissue to the site in which the catheter enters the vein.
Courtesy of James Upchurch

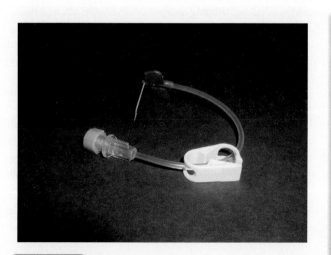

Figure P8-3 A Huber needle.
Courtesy of James Upchurch

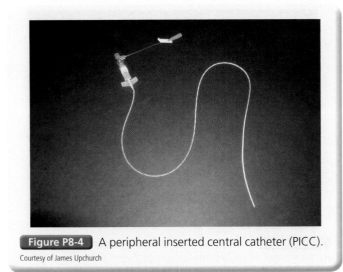

Figure P8-4 A peripheral inserted central catheter (PICC).

Courtesy of James Upchurch

Preparation

1. Rapid venous access is important in many medical and traumatic emergencies.
2. Standard methods of venous access, such as peripheral and external jugular access, and the intraosseous route, should always be attempted before using a vascular access device. Providers should follow their local protocols regarding methods of access.
3. The patient, family members, and other caregivers can often provide valuable information about the patient's medical condition and the use of the vascular access device, despite their limited knowledge of emergency situations.

Procedure

For the patient who requires immediate vascular access and offers no peripheral (or intraosseous) route, a vascular access device can provide a safe, rapid solution. However, only those who have received specialized training and protocols should attempt this.

1. Because of the extremely high risk of infection and sepsis, careful aseptic technique, including sterile gloves, must be used at all times.
2. The EMS provider should identify the location of the catheter or palpate the site of the implanted port.
3. The catheter can be clamped by folding it over, and smooth hemostats (no teeth) can be used to prevent infusion of air.
4. When clamping, use care to prevent tearing the catheter. If an infusion is in progress or a pump is attached,

the provider should ask for help from those familiar with the pump; the pump should be turned off, or the line coming from it disconnected.

5. If the vascular access device has multiple lumens, the pump may be left on and a "free" lumen can be used.
6. The EMS provider should remove the small injection cap covering the hub of the lumen and attach the syringe or IV tubing directly to the catheter.
7. The cap can also be left in place, and after cleaning the cap with alcohol or povidone-iodine, a needle (20 gauge or smaller) can be inserted through.
8. The EMS provider should then remove the clamp or unpinch the catheter.
9. Using a syringe, aspirate 3 to 5 ml of blood slowly, to avoid collapsing the catheter. This confirms placement and clears the line of heparin.
10. If called for in local protocols, blood samples can be obtained using a syringe or vacutainer (a vacutainer should not be used for PICC lines).
11. Be sure to pinch or clamp the lumen when attaching and removing syringes to avoid taking air into the catheter.
12. Using at least 10 ml of normal saline, the catheter should be flushed of blood.
13. The IV tubing should then be connected and carefully taped, using a loop of tubing to prevent inadvertent disconnection.
14. The infusion site should be monitored and the patient reassessed.

An implanted port may be used in much the same way as a central line or PICC. The port is usually implanted in the rib area or antecubital space.

1. Using a sterile-gloved hand, the provider should apply pressure around the edges of the port to slightly "stretch" the skin over the injection site.
2. If a Huber needle is not available, as small a needle as possible (preferably a 21 gauge or smaller) should be used to avoid port damage and leakage at the injection site.
3. The needle and syringe or IV tubing should be flushed first.
4. The needle must be inserted until it touches the back of the port; this may require a great deal of pressure to puncture the skin, scar tissue, and septum (**Skill Drill P8-1**).
5. The blood should then be aspirated; if it does not return freely, the device should not be used.
6. The port should again be flushed and infusion of medications or fluids begun.

SKILL DRILL P8-1

Huber Needle Insertion into a Subcutaneous Port

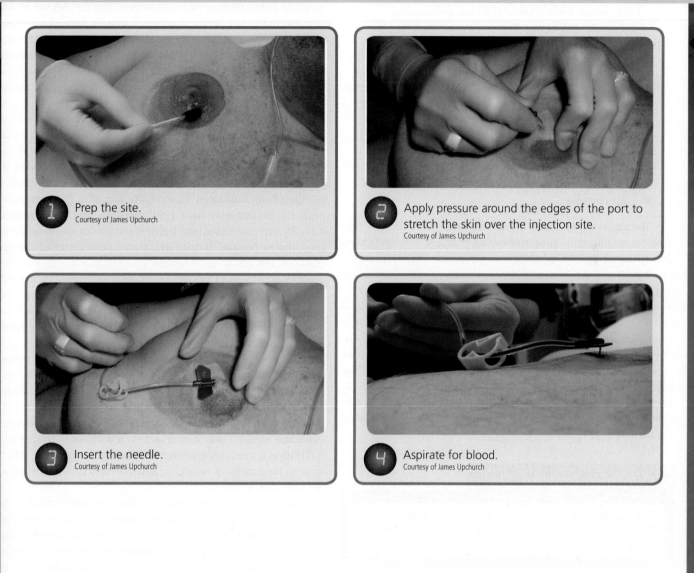

1 Prep the site.
Courtesy of James Upchurch

2 Apply pressure around the edges of the port to stretch the skin over the injection site.
Courtesy of James Upchurch

3 Insert the needle.
Courtesy of James Upchurch

4 Aspirate for blood.
Courtesy of James Upchurch

Possible Complications and Emergency Care

Patients with vascular access devices may call EMS for a variety of reasons, including complications of cancer, AIDS, or sickle cell disease; injuries; or problems with unassociated illnesses. Several difficulties related directly to the presence of a vascular access device may occur. The more common complications include:

- Infection of the exit site, tunnel, or port
- Systemic infection that develops from bacteria ascending through the catheter and entering the patient's circulation
- Catheter clot
- Venous thrombosis
- Catheter displacement
- Catheter leak
- Air embolus

Management of local infections may begin in the prehospital setting with simple dressing changes and caution to avoid further spread of infection. Systemic sepsis or septic shock will require standard management of circulation, airway, and breathing. The vascular access device itself may be used because IV access for fluid resuscitation of the critical patient may be difficult or impossible, and aseptic technique is essential (i.e. sterile gloves, alcohol, povidone-iodine). Intraosseous infusion should be attempted in the critical patient prior to accessing the vascular access device. It is important for the EMS provider to remember that the vascular access device itself may be the site of infection; if this is suggested by any clinical signs, the vascular access device should not be used for access.

Communication Tip

The patient, family members, and other caregivers can often provide valuable information about the patient's medical condition and use of the vascular access device.

Vascular access devices are usually flushed with a heparin or saline solution to prevent clotting. Despite proper care, clots may form in the catheter, disrupting the flow of solutions and medications. Sluggish flow or inability to infuse solutions requires rapid intervention. Never attempt to force or dislodge the clot. The catheter may require declotting with thrombolytics or may have to be replaced.

Thrombosis can develop in the vessel in which the catheter is inserted. The patient may complain of local tenderness or swelling in the arm, neck, or shoulder near the device. In addition, the patient or family may notice that the flow of solution or medication through the catheter is sluggish. Prehospital management of a thrombosis is similar to that of a deep vein thrombosis: the area should not be massaged; instead, the area or extremity must be immobilized, low-flow oxygen administered, and the patient transported to definitive care.

It is rare for the catheter or port to migrate or become displaced because vascular access devices are secured, usually with sutures. However, physical exercise or accidental "tugging" on the external apparatus can displace the catheter. The patient may complain of bleeding, burning upon infusion, or swelling from infiltrated fluid. Upon palpation of an implanted port, the patient may have pain, swelling, and bruising in the area. In extreme cases, the tip of the catheter can migrate and puncture or become lodged in a major vessel wall of the myocardium, leading to more severe symptoms. Patients who complain of shortness of breath, chest pain, dizziness, tachycardia, or hypotension should be treated by standard emergency protocols, with an awareness that the symptoms can result either from complications related to a special device or from an unrelated and potentially life-threatening event.

Occasionally a catheter develops a leak or tear, perhaps related to improper use. When this occurs, fluids or medications infiltrate into the surrounding tissues; the area will appear swollen and tender and the patient may complain of burning. The infusion should be stopped immediately, as certain medications can cause significant irritation and even necrosis of tissues when infiltration occurs. An appropriate dressing can be applied to the area to help prevent infection, and necessary measures should be used to stop bleeding.

Either improper occlusion of the catheter port or a tear in the catheter can lead to an air embolus. Because exact prehospital diagnosis is impossible, management is based on standard protocol and a complete patient assessment. The patient should be transported in a left lateral position with the legs slightly elevated and head lowered, to prevent an air embolus from migrating to the brain and causing a stroke. Oxygen, cardiac monitor, venous access, and rapid transport are indicated in these patients.

Dialysis

Introduction

The kidneys remove toxic materials from the body and maintain fluid, electrolyte, and acid–base balance. Dialysis uses the principles of osmosis, diffusion, and ultra-infusion to eliminate toxic materials from the body for patients with acute or chronic renal failure. Despite advances in therapies and transplants, nearly every patient with end-stage renal disease requires some form of dialysis. The two techniques are peritoneal dialysis and hemodialysis.

Peritoneal dialysis requires an implanted catheter, constructed of nylon or silicone rubber, which is fed into the abdominal cavity. Sterile dialyzing fluid (dialysate) bathes the peritoneal membranes that cover the abdominal organs and supporting capillary beds. Blood toxins travel from the abdominal capillaries into the dialysate fluid, which is then drained back through the catheter (**Figure P9-1**). This process lasts approximately 1 hour and is often repeated many times daily or throughout the night while the patient sleeps.

Hemodialysis involves shunting the patient's blood through a dialysis machine to facilitate removal of waste and toxins (**Figure P9-2**). Once the blood has been "detoxified," it is returned to the patient's circulation.

There are three common methods of vascular access for hemodialysis:

- *Arteriovenous (AV) fistula.* AV fistulas are created by establishing a surgical connection between an artery and an adjacent vein (anastomosed). The high pressures associated with arterial flow create a "bulge" or swelling of the vein known as a pseudoaneurysm (**Figure P9-3A**). Outflow of blood is accomplished by inserting a large bore needle into this "bulge."
- *Arteriovenous (AV) graft.* AV grafts are the most frequently used access points for chronic renal dialysis. Synthetic materials such as Gore-Tex or biological materials such as human umbilical veins are surgically implanted in the limb to create a U-shaped tunnel. The graft is connected to the vein and artery, and then secured just under the surface of the skin, which creates a raised area that looks like a large vessel (**Figure P9-3B**).
- *External arteriovenous (AV) shunt.* External AV shunts are seldom used today because of the advent of vascular access devices such as femoral and subclavian catheters. Similar to the AV graft,

the external AV shunt joins the vein and artery together. The tubing extends from each vessel tip outside the body and may be connected with a heparinized "T" device.

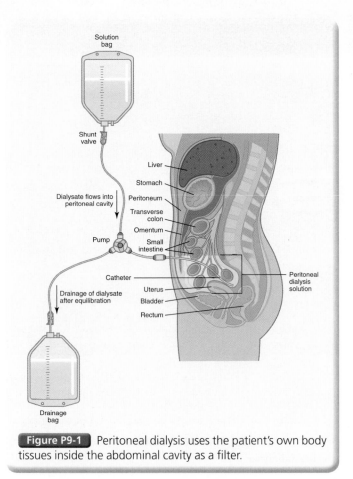

Figure P9-1 Peritoneal dialysis uses the patient's own body tissues inside the abdominal cavity as a filter.

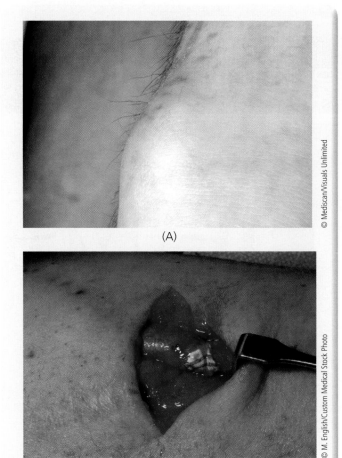

Figure P9-3 (A) With an AV fistula, a bulge is created by arterial pressure. (B) An arteriovenous graft creates a raised area that looks like a large vessel.

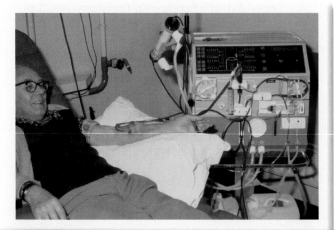

Figure P9-2 Hemodialysis is a method of mechanically cleansing the blood outside of the body, in order to remove various substances that would normally be cleared by the kidneys.

© Chris Priest/Science Source

Rationale

To maintain patency of access for dialysis and to detect complications of a hemodialysis access site related to infection, thrombosis, occlusion, bleeding, or cannula separation.

Assessment

Assessment should focus on the following:

- Status of the fistula, graft, or cannula site and dressing
- Location of shunt, fistula, or graft
- Vital signs
    - *Blood pressure assessments in the shunted extremity should be avoided because this procedure will obstruct blood flow.*
- Pulses distal to shunt, fistula, or graft
- Color, temperature, and presence of pain or numbness in the extremity in which the access is located

Possible Complications

- Infection, thrombosis, occlusion, bleeding, or separation from the cannula
- Too much water removal (hypovolemia, hypotension)
- Too little water removal (pulmonary edema, congestive heart failure)
- Electrolyte imbalances

Complications Specific to Peritoneal Dialysis

- Peritonitis (infection of the peritoneal cavity)
- Dialysate failing to drain from the peritoneal cavity due to catheter occlusion or the catheter tip lodging against the abdominal wall (Turning the patient from side to side or gently pressing on the abdomen may alleviate the fluid accumulation; however, it may be necessary for the physician to irrigate or replace the catheter.)
- Mild pain or discomfort with the procedure (Severe pain is not normal; consider the possibility of GI bleeding, myocardial infarction [MI], or aortic dissection.)
- Respiratory distress due to increase in pressure on diaphragm as dialysate is infused (Respiratory distress can be further compounded in the patient who is overhydrated; consider other causes of respiratory distress.)

Tips

Peritonitis, which is most often associated with organisms that have been introduced through the catheter itself, can cause severe sepsis and shock in a relatively short period of time. The patient experiences generalized abdominal tenderness and exhibits guarding upon exam.

Management of the septic patient includes ensuring adequate circulation, airway, and breathing; intravenous fluid administration (normal saline is the crystalloid of choice; lactated Ringer's should be avoided because of the higher concentration of potassium); cardiac monitoring; and rapid transport.

Emergency Care

If the patient develops bleeding at the site of an AV fistula or graft, the following steps should be taken:

- Apply direct pressure to the site. Most bleeding sites on AV fistulas or grafts are from needle insertions and are usually small holes. Since the graft makes a communication between the artery and the vein, the bleeding will be under pressure. Direct fingertip pressure with a single 4x4 over the hole will control the bleeding and not compromise the patency of the graft.

- Do not use a blood pressure cuff on the affected extremity to control the bleeding, as this will most likely clot off the graft.
- Do not use a bulky dressing between fingertip and graft because this will spread the pressure across the entire graft and not place it specifically on the bleeding point.

Prehospital Use of Dialysis Vascular Access Devices

IV access in the dialysis patient can be challenging. Always attempt to establish peripheral access (or intraosseous access) in a limb without a fistula or graft. If absolutely necessary and permissible by your local protocols, use the limb with an access site. A high infection and complication rate makes it important to avoid accessing fistulas and grafts. It should not be done without on-line medical direction.

Preparation

1. The decision to use a dialysis access device in the prehospital setting must be made based on training and local protocols.
2. Family or home caregivers may be able to provide useful information regarding the type and placement of the device.
3. The area should be gently palpated to locate the fistula or graft. A "thrill" or vibration should be felt over the fistula.
4. Any area that is red, tender, swollen, or draining, or shows other evidence of infection, should not be used.

Indications

Dialysis vascular access devices are to be utilized in the critical patient only after an attempt to obtain peripheral venous access (including the external jugular vein) or intraosseous access has failed. AV grafts, fistulas, and shunts can provide rapid and safe vascular access in the critical patient when routine access is impossible or not available.

Contraindications

A peritoneal dialysis catheter cannot be used for vascular access.

Equipment

- Povidone-iodine prep (alcohol should never be used, as it will damage synthetic materials)
- 14- or 16-gauge needle (standard steel or Teflon IV catheters may be used)
- 5-ml syringe for discard
- Syringe or vacutainer for blood samples
- 0.9% normal saline IV solution
- IV tubing (primed)
- Tape
- Constricting band (optional)

Procedure

1. The vein usually is sufficiently distended, but a constricting band can be placed proximal to the insertion site if needed.
2. Prep the site with povidone-iodine.
3. Stabilize the site before inserting the IV needle.
4. Insert the needle in the direction of venous flow (toward the head) at a slight angle (15 to 20 degrees), to prevent penetrating the posterior lumen of the vessel (**Skill Drill P9-1**).
5. The needle should be directed and the Teflon catheter advanced in the same manner as with standard IVs (watch for a "flashback" in the hub).
6. Next, 3 to 5 ml of blood should be aspirated and then discarded to confirm correct placement, as well as clear the shunt of heparin (grafts and fistulas are not heparinized).
7. Obtain the necessary blood samples per local protocols.
8. Remove the constricting band.
9. Attach the IV tubing and begin the infusion of normal saline or medications.
10. Use caution when administering fluids to avoid inadvertently overhydrating the patient.
11. Tape the IV tubing carefully and reassess the infusion site and the patient.

SKILL DRILL P9-1

Accessing a Dialysis Shunt

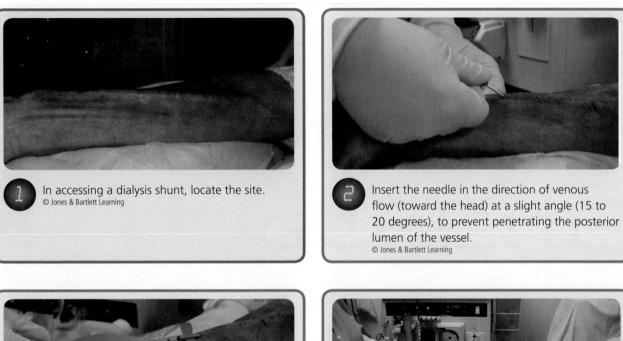

1 In accessing a dialysis shunt, locate the site.
© Jones & Bartlett Learning

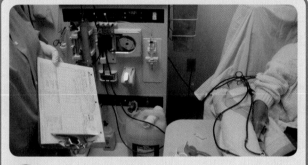

2 Insert the needle in the direction of venous flow (toward the head) at a slight angle (15 to 20 degrees), to prevent penetrating the posterior lumen of the vessel.
© Jones & Bartlett Learning

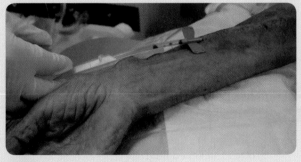

3 Aspirate 3 to 5 ml of blood to confirm correct placement and clear the shunt.
© Jones & Bartlett Learning

4 Continue to reassess the infusion site and the patient.
© Jones & Bartlett Learning

Ventricular Shunts

Introduction

A ventricular shunt is an implanted drainage system used to remove excess cerebrospinal fluid (CSF) in the brain. In patients with hydrocephalus, excess fluid in the brain can lead to increased intracranial pressure (ICP). A ventricular shunt consists of a primary catheter, a reservoir, a one-way valve, and the terminal drainage catheter (**Figure P10-1**). The primary catheter is surgically implanted into the lateral ventricle of the brain. The reservoir collects the fluid and the one-way valve prevents CSF from flowing back into the brain. Once implanted, the reservoir can be easily palpated through the skin, usually over the mastoid or parietal bone just behind the ear. The terminal (drainage) end of the catheter empties into the jugular vein (ventricular-atrial shunt) or in the peritoneal cavity (ventriculoperitoneal shunt).

Rationale

Increased intracranial pressure is a true medical emergency and requires rapid recognition and intervention to prevent brain stem herniation.

Possible Complications

- Plugging of the catheter with clotted blood or other thickened fluid
- Displacement of the primary or terminal end
- Dislodgement or damage to one or more components
- Infection

    - Initially, a ventriculoperitoneal shunt infection may not present with obvious neurological symptoms; however, symptoms can develop when the infection causes shunt obstruction and the resultant increase in intracranial pressure. The incidence of ventriculoperitoneal shunt infections in adults is between 1.6% and 16.7%. Shunt infection is most likely to occur shortly after shunt placement or revision (i.e. within 1 month).[1]

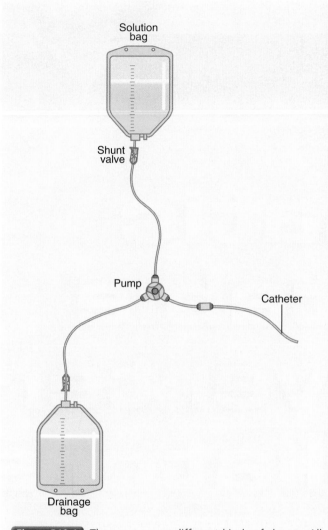

Figure P10-1 There are many different kinds of shunts. All have three basic parts: a ventricular catheter, a shunt valve, and a distal catheter.

Table P10-1	Signs of Increasing Intracranial Pressure
Early Signs	**Late Signs (Cushing's Triad)**
Headaches	Rising systolic blood pressure
Visual disturbances	Abnormal respirations
Irritability	Bradycardia
Vomiting	
Nausea	

Emergency Care

1. Recognize signs of increased intracranial pressure (**Table P10-1**).
2. Manage the airway with high-flow oxygen.
3. Intubate as needed per medical protocol.
4. Obtain venous access, but limit flow rate.
5. A plugged shunt may be pumped (per local protocol and medical direction).
   A. Locate the reservoir with palpation.
   B. Using one or two fingers, gently compress and release the reservoir several times.
   C. Pumping the reservoir may provide temporary relief.
   D. Do not delay airway management or rapid transport.

References

1. Wells DL, Allen JM. Ventriculoperitoneal Shunt Infections in Adult Patients. *AACN Adv Crit Care* 2013:24(1):13–14, p. 7.

PROCEDURE 11

Automatic Implantable Cardioverter Defibrillators

Introduction

More than 350,000 people die each year from sudden cardiac death. Of those resuscitated, over 50% will experience a second arrest within 2 years. The automatic implantable cardioverter defibrillator (AICD) was developed for high-risk patients with recurrent ventricular tachycardia or ventricular fibrillation.

The AICD consists of a pulse generator and leads. The unit is capable of sensing and terminating ventricular tachycardia, ventricular fibrillation, and bradyarrhythmias. The device, which is smaller than a deck of cards, is inserted under the skin in the upper chest area, and then wires are tunneled and inserted into the atria and ventricles. Once implanted, the generator can be palpated under the surface of the skin. The device is programmed to sense tachycardia and the width of QRS complexes. It will discharge when the ventricular rate exceeds set parameters (usually 170 beats/min) for 10 to 30 seconds. Most devices are capable of not only defibrillation and cadioversion, but also of pacing.

Rationale

AICDs are used in patients who experience lethal arrhythmias despite medical management to control ventricular tachycardia and ventricular fibrillation.

Possible Complications

- Most of the complications with the AICD occur in the inpatient setting and are related to a collection of blood at the site of insertion (hematoma) or dislodgement of the wires.
- The AICD may fail to fire if it has lost stored energy or battery power; if the sensing electrodes are damaged, disconnected, or displaced; or if the maximum rate is not set correctly despite evidenced ventricular tachycardia or ventricular fibrillation.

- The AICD may fire when no discharge is indicated. The patient's ECG must be monitored. EMS providers are able to deactivate the device when improper firing occurs. The patient should meet the following criteria:

  - Three or more distinct shocks, and
  - Obvious device malfunction with an EMS provider-witnessed inappropriate shock (i.e., alert patient in atrial fibrillation with rapid rate or supraventricular tachycardia)

Place an EMS donut (magnet) directly over the device to deactivate the device and ensure that shocks will no longer be delivered. After the defibrillator is deactivated, tape the magnet firmly in place. Regardless of the decision to deactivate the AICD device, be prepared to manage the underlying rhythm.

If the patient has a combination AICD and pacemaker, deactivating the AICD may or may not deactivate the pacemaker. If the patient becomes unstable or in the event of a rhythm change in which a shock is desired, remove the magnet to reactivate the AICD. If reactivation does not occur, use a manual defibrillator. If AICD deactivation indications are questionable or deactivation is unsuccessful (or a donut magnet is not available) and undesired shocks continue, medications may be administered for patient comfort.

Emergency Care

1. The AICD will not interfere with basic life support and is not a contraindication for standard external defibrillation. Follow the same arrhythmia protocols as for the patient without an AICD.
2. If the patient has received one or more internal countershocks, initial external shocks should be delivered at the maximum output (follow local protocols).
3. Defibrillation pads should not be placed directly over the generator, as this may cause permanent damage to the device.
4. If the first and second external countershocks are unsuccessful, consider using anterior-posterior placement of defibrillation pads.

Controversy

Although the AICD may discharge while treating a patient, studies show that this is not a hazard, as only approximately 2 joules of energy reach the body's surface, causing only a minor shock with no significant danger or physical harm.

Communication Tip

Provide emotional support to the patient and caregiver on any AICD-related call.

Ventricular Assist Devices

Introduction

A ventricular assist device (VAD) is a mechanical pump that is used to support heart function and blood flow in people who have weakened hearts. The device takes blood from a ventricle and helps pump it to the body and vital organs, just as a healthy heart would.

The VAD consists of three parts: a small tube that carries blood out of the heart into a pump; another tube that carries blood from the pump to the blood vessels, which delivers blood to the body; and a power source (**Figure P12-1**). The power source, which consists of either batteries or AC power, is connected to a control unit that monitors the VAD's functions. The batteries are carried in a case that is usually located in the holster of a vest wrapped around the patient's shoulders. The control unit gives warnings, or alarms, if the power is low or if it seems that the device is not working properly.

VADs include left ventricular assist devices (LVADs); right ventricular assist devices (RVADs); and biventricular assist devices (BiVADs), which involve two independent pumps. LVADs are the most common type of VADs and, therefore, are the focus of this section.

Prior to patient discharge from the hospital, family members of those receiving a VAD are provided extensive training in device operation, maintenance, response to device alarms, and what to do in case of emergency. The hospital will also usually notify the local EMS agency that the patient will be residing in the community. Information will be given regarding the type and manufacturer of the patient's device, as well as prehospital emergency care procedures specific to the device and emergency contact numbers for prehospital providers to access.

Rationale

LVADs are used in a number of situations. For most patients, they are a bridge to transplantation; however, they may also be used for patients who are candidates for transplantation or are recovering from a reversible condition, such as myocarditis, cardiogenic shock, or postcardiotomy failure, or for patients who will use them for the rest of their lives.[1]

Complications

Complications associated with LVADs include those that are related to the patient and those that are related to the device (**Table P12-1**). The most common complications mortality among patients with LVADs. Patients are at increased risk of having a neurologic event if they have a postoperative infection following device implantation or if they have a history of a previous stroke. The most common types of hemorrhage in patients with LVADs are epistaxis, gastrointestinal bleeding, and hematoma formation; the most common types of arrhythmias are atrial fibrillation and ventricular arrhythmias.[2]

Infection is the most common complication found in patients with LVADs and is a significant cause of morbidity and mortality, second only to heart failure as a leading cause of death among patients with LVADs. Infection can involve the surgical site, driveline, pump pocket, or the pump itself. Complications related to the device itself may also involve the driveline or pump, as well as the system controller, power source, or battery pack. In some cases, complications related to the device will trigger either visual or auditory alarms.[3]

Emergency Care

There are several different LVAD devices currently in use. Most patients have a tag located on the device's controller around their waist that indicates what type of device is implanted, what institution implanted it, and what number to call in case of an emergency. Most importantly, the tag will be a specific color; this color corresponds with an EMS Field Guide found on the MyLVAD web site (www.mylvad.com/ems), allowing providers to quickly locate management considerations for the specific device being cared for. Note: It is beyond the scope of this text to address the management of each device; instead, general emergency care procedures will follow.

Assessment of the patient with an LVAD begins with determining what type of device it is and what type of pump it uses (pulsatile pump or continuous-flow pump [most common]). The patient or patient's caregiver may have written directions or a device manual containing important information regarding the device. Additionally, the patient or caregiver should be able to provide the EMS provider with the contact information of the patient's VAD coordinator. On-line medical consultation with a physician may also be helpful when caring for patients with LVADs.

If an LVAD is improperly functioning, the device will emit an auditory and/or visual alarm on the system controller. An alarm may indicate pump failure, low power, loss of power, or the need to change the device's batteries or controller. An alarm may also indicate low pump flow, which may mean that the patient requires intravenous fluids to be administered, or that the driveline or a power source cable is not properly connected, requiring all connections to be checked. These troubleshooting issues should not delay patient transport.[4]

Assessment of the patient's airway and breathing is similar to other patients; however, patients with continuous-flow pump devices may have unreliable pulse oximetry readings, as the pulse pressure generated by the pump will be too low to detect (unlike that of the pulsatile pump, which should not affect the detection of pulse and blood pressure). The EMS provider will need to assess the patient's circulatory status by other means. The use of the ECG (including 12 leads) can provide important information regarding

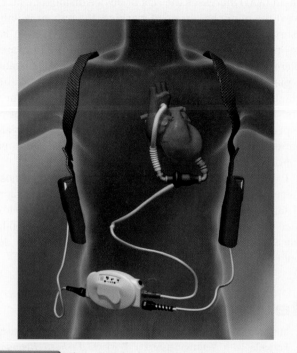

Figure P12-1 The ventricular assist device consists of three parts: a small tube that carries blood out of the heart into a pump, another tube that carries blood from the pump to the blood vessels, and a power source (AC or batteries). The batteries are carried in a case that is usually located in the holster of a vest wrapped around the patient's shoulders.

Reprinted with permission from Thoratec Corporation

Table P12-1 Complications Encountered in LVAD Patients

- Infection
- Bleeding
- Stroke/transient ischemic attack
- Hemolysis
- Arrhythmias
- Volume overload
- Dehydration
- Hypertension
- Hypotension
- Cardiac tamponade
- Recurrence of heart failure
- New right ventricular failure
- Aortic insufficiency

Data from: Mechem, C. Crawford. Prehospital Assessment and Management of Patients with Ventricular-Assist Devices. *Prehospital Emergency Care*, April/June, Volume 17, Number 2, p.226.

related to the patient include neurologic events, hemorrhage, and arrhythmias, with neurologic events (such as transient ischemic attack [TIA] or stroke) being a common cause of morbidity and

the patient's status. Assessment of the patient's neurologic status should include evaluation for stroke. Patients with stroke symptoms should be managed similar to other patients and transported to a stroke center, preferably one that is familiar with VADs.

The EMS provider should expose the patient, looking for signs of cable disconnect, but keep the driveline skin site covered unless visualization is absolutely necessary, as it is very important that this site remains sterile. Patient exposure and transport should be conducted with extreme caution in order to avoid inadvertently disconnecting, cutting, or dislodging cables.

Airway and respiratory interventions will be the same as for other patients. Large-bore intravenous access should be obtained in patients with hemodynamic compromise and intravenous fluids administered. Vasopressors, however, should be administered with caution, as an increase in afterload may worsen pump flow. Only symptomatic arrhythmias should be treated, with treatment based on standard protocols. There are no contraindications to either the administration of antiarrhythmics or to the performance of cardioversion or defibrillation. When performing defibrillation, however, the EMS provider should attempt to avoid placing the defibrillation pads directly over the device. Additionally, the system controller's cables may need to be disconnected before defibrillation in order to minimize damage to the electronic components of the device.[5]

After conducting a careful assessment of the patient's perfusion and the device's function, the EMS provider may need to decide whether or not to initiate chest compressions on the patient. Performing chest compressions on a patient with an LVAD increases the risk of device dislodgement. However, if the pump has stopped working, the patient is unlikely to survive without compressions! Additionally, there is the risk of thrombosis within the pump if compressions are not promptly initiated. Thrombosis will cause flow resistance if the pump is restarted and an increased risk of stroke if the patient survives. If the pump has stopped for a patient with a first-generation, pulsatile device, hand pumping—not chest compressions—should be started immediately; however, for a patient with a later-generation device, a hand pump is not an option.[6]

Patients with LVADs should be transported to a hospital familiar with the management of LVADs. All device equipment and family members or caregivers who are familiar with the device should also be transported with the patient. Non-LVAD medical and trauma emergencies in patients with the device should be managed according to local protocols.

References

1. Mechem CC. Prehospital Assessment and Management of Patients with Ventricular-Assist Devices. *Prehosp Emerg Care* 2013:17(2):223–229, pp. 223–224.
2. Ibid, p. 226.
3. Ibid.
4. Ibid, p. 227.
5. Ibid, p. 228.
6. Ibid.

abandonment   As it relates to elder abuse, a situation in which an older person is left at the emergency department by a family member or caregiver.

absorption   The process of a substance entering the blood circulation.

active adult community   A community that offers age restricted housing specifically for seniors who enjoy participating in physical and social activities. Also called active adult living and active retirement community.

active metabolites   Byproducts of a drug, created after it has been partially or fully degraded, that have drug effects on the body.

active neglect   The refusal or failure to fulfill a caregiving obligation; a conscious or intentional attempt to inflict physical or emotional stress. Examples include abandonment and denial of food or health-related services.

activities of daily living (ADLs)   Basic everyday activities needed to sustain life, such as feeding oneself, walking, dressing, getting up from a chair, and toileting.

acute myocardial infarction (AMI)   Heart attack; death of heart muscle following obstruction of blood flow to it. Acute in this context means "new" or happening right now.

acute pain   Pain with a rapid onset; the body's means of indicating the presence of a new injury.

acute pulmonary edema   Fluid accumulation in the lungs.

acute respiratory distress syndrome (ARDS)   A condition of severe lung injury after an acute event such as smoke inhalation, near drowning, aspiration, or severe bloodstream infection.

addiction   An overwhelming desire or need to continue using a substance at whatever cost, with a tendency to increase the amount or dose.

advanced healthcare directive (AHCD)   Written documentation that specifies medical treatment for a competent patient should the patient become unable to make decisions.

adverse drug withdrawal event (ADWE)   A set of clinical signs or symptoms caused by discontinuing a drug.

aerobic metabolism   The creation of energy through the combustion of carbohydrates and fats in the presence of oxygen.

ageism   Stereotyping of, and discrimination against, people who are old.

agonal   An abnormal pattern of breathing, characterized by gasping and labored breathing, and accompanied by strange vocalizations and myocionus (a brief, involuntary twitching of a muscle or a group of muscles).

alopecia   Hair loss, especially from the head, suggestive of normal aging (as opposed to traumatic alopecia, indicative of abuse).

Alzheimer's care facilities   Specialized facilities for those with signs of Alzheimer's disease or dementia.

andropause   A lessoning of testosterone and sexual activity in males later in life; also known as male menopause.

anemia   A deficiency in red blood cells or hemoglobin in the blood, resulting in a decrease in oxygen delivery to the tissues.

aneurysm   A swelling or enlargement of part of a blood vessel, resulting from weakening of the vessel wall.

angina   Chest pain or discomfort due to inadequate blood and oxygen supply to the heart tissue.

angina pectoris   Chest pain or discomfort due to inadequate blood and oxygen supply to the heart tissue.

angiodysplasia   A vascular legion in the gastrointestinal tract.

anhedonia   The sense that nothing is enjoyable anymore.

anthropometric   Relating to anthropometry (the study of human body measurement for use in anthropological classification and comparison).

antiarrhythmic medication   Medications used to treat abnormal heart rhythms.

apathetic thyrotoxicosis   Apathy and depression in the presence of hyperthyroidism.

aphasia   A language impairment that causes the inability to understand or produce speech; aphasia is caused by injury to the brain, most commonly stroke.

apraxia   An impairment in carrying out purposeful movements, which can also manifest as a speech impairment, with inability to produce speech with the correct rhythm and timing.

Area Agency on Aging (AAA)   A basic and universal resource that provides information services for older people; AAAs have senior information programs that track all resources in the community, and sponsor nutrition programs, senior centers, and transportation services.

arrhythmia   An abnormal or irregular heart rhythm resulting from an electrical disturbance in conduction; examples include atrial fibrillation, bradycardia, ventricular fibrillation, and ventricular tachycardia.

aspiration pneumonia   Pneumonia resulting from the inhalation of an object or secretions into the lungs.

assisted living   A residential facility that provides residents assistance with activities of daily living; also known as residential care, board and care, and boarding house.

asthma   Acute constriction of the air passages in the lungs.

atelectasis   Partial lung collapse.

atherosclerosis   A disorder in which cholesterol and calcium build up inside the walls of the blood vessels, forming plaque, which eventually leads to partial or complete blockage of blood flow. An atherosclerotic plaque can also become a site where blood clots can form, break off, and then embolize elsewhere in the circulation.

atrial fibrillation   Disorganized contraction of the atria, often described as chaotic twitching, that results in ineffective pumping of blood into the ventricles.

atrophy   Wasting or shrinkage of an organ.

autonomy   The right of an individual to make choices freely, in accordance with the individual's own goals and values.

bacteremia   Presence of bacteria in the blood.

baroreceptors   Sensory mechanisms in the aortic arch and carotid sinus that sense blood pressure changes and trigger a response to adjust the pressure.

Battle's sign   Bruising behind the ear over the mastoid process that may indicate skull fracture.

benign paroxysmal positional vertigo   One of the most common causes of vertigo; characterized by brief episodes of mild to intense dizziness. Symptoms are triggered by specific changes in head positioning, such as that caused by tipping the head up or down, and lying down, turning over, or sitting up in bed. Those with this condition may also feel out of balance when standing or walking.

bereavement   An extremely stressful time following a loss, during which grief and adaptation to that loss is experienced. Bereavement increases the risk of sleep disorders, suicide attempts, substance abuse (including alcohol, tobacco, and illicit drugs), and overall mortality.

beta-blockers   Medications that reduce blood pressure and lower heart rate; also known as beta-adrenergic blocking agents.

biliary colic   Sharp or crampy right upper quadrant pain that may radiate to the back and right shoulder; a classic symptom of gallbladder disease.

bradykinesia   Slowing down of movement.

brain death   The cessation of brain function.

brain herniation   The protrusion of the brain through the foramen magnum, or the opening at the base of the skull. Herniation is often fatal, as critical brain tissue is compressed.

bronchiectasis   Chronic dilatation of a bronchus or bronchi, with a secondary infection that usually involves the lower portion of the lung.

bruit   A whooshing sound heard upon auscultation with each heartbeat.

calcium channel blockers   Medications that can lower heart rate and treat a variety of conditions, such as high blood pressure; also known as calcium antagonists.

cardiac output   Amount of blood pumped out of the heart in 1 minute.

cardiogenic shock   Inadequate pumping action of the heart, often the result of acute myocardial infarction or congestive heart failure.

cervical spondylosis   Degenerative arthritis (osteoarthriris) of the cervical vertebrae and related tissues. If severe, it may cause pressure on nerve roots or the spinal cord with subsequent pain or numbness in the arms.

chemoreceptor   A sensory organ that responds to chemical stimuli.

cholangitis   Inflammation of the bile ducts.

cholecystitis   Infection of the gallbladder.

cholestasis   Any condition in which the flow of bile from the liver is slowed or blocked.

chronic bronchitis   Irritation of the major lung passageways, resulting from either infectious disease or irritants such as smoke.

chronic obstructive pulmonary disease (COPD)   A slow process of dilation and disruption of the airways and alveoli, caused by chronic bronchitis, emphysema, or asthma.

chronic pain   Pain experienced repeatedly or consistently over a long period of time and includes behavioral as well as physical factors.

cirrhosis   A chronic disease of the liver resulting in degenerative changes and death of functioning liver cells.

cognition   Refers to mental processes used for perceiving, remembering, and thinking.

cohort   persons who experience the same significant life event (i.e., birth, marriage) within a specified period of time

collagen   The substance that makes the skin and other connective tissues strong; both collagen and elastin decrease with age.

colostomy   A diversion involving the colon in which a segment of diseased or injured colon is bypassed or removed and an end or loop of colon is brought through a small opening in the abdominal wall and sutured, forming a stoma.

communication   The transmitting of information from a sender to a receiver and verification that the receiver received and understood the information.

crackles   High-pitched, popping breath sounds that occur during inspiration.

Crohn's disease   A chronic inflammatory condition of the gastrointestinal tract.

Cullen's sign   Bruising around the umbilicus; seen when there is blood in the free abdominal space (peritoneum).

cyanosis   Skin that appears bluish or gray in color, caused by decreased levels of oxygen in the blood.

deep vein thrombosis (DVT)   A blood clot in the leg or pelvis; the clot may result from prolonged immobility.

delirium tremens   A severe, potentially life-threatening withdrawal syndrome that can occur 24 hours to 1 week after an individual stops drinking.

dependency theory   A theory that attempts to explain the cause of elder abuse; maintains that frailty and medical illness set up the older person for abuse and neglect.

dependent lividity   A cutaneous dark spot on a dependent portion of a cadaver resulting from gravitational pooling of blood; also known as livor mortis.

depression Persistent mood of sadness, despair, or discouragement; depression may be a symptom of many different mental and physical disorders, or it may be a disorder on its own.

dermis The inner, living layer of the skin.

detrusor Muscle of the bladder wall.

diabetic neuropathy Nerve damage resulting from diabetes; causes pain and sometimes inflammatory lesions.

distribution The dispersion or dissemination of substances throughout the fluids and tissues of the body.

diverticulitis Infection of a diverticulum.

do not attempt resuscitation (DNAR) order Written documentation giving permission to medical personnel not to attempt resuscitation in the event of cardiac arrest; also known as a do not resuscitate (DNR) order.

do not resuscitate (DNR) order Written documentation giving permission to medical personnel not to attempt resuscitation in the event of cardiac arrest; also known as a do not attempt resuscitation (DNAR) order.

doctrine of informed consent The principle that allows a patient to decide against unwanted medical interventions.

dorsiflex To flex the foot upward.

duodenum The first section of the small intestine; begins after the stomach.

dysarthria A disorder of speech production, resulting from weakness, slowness, or incoordination of the speech mechanism due to damage to the nervous system; speech errors are highly consistent from one occasion to the next.

dyspepsia A gnawing, burning pain in the upper abdomen.

dysphagia Difficulty swallowing.

dyspnea Difficulty breathing; shortness of breath.

elastin The substance that makes the skin pliable.

elder abuse An all-inclusive term representing all types of mistreatment toward older adults; can be an act of commission (abuse) or omission (neglect), intentional or unintentional, and of one or more types: physical, psychological (or emotional), sexual, or financial, resulting in unnecessary suffering, injury, pain, loss or violation of human rights, and decreased quality of life.

elimination The process of removing compounds from the body.

emphysema A disease in which alveoli are destroyed with resulting loss of lung elasticity.

empyema A collection of pus in a body cavity, usually the pleural cavity.

enabling behavior Promoting the continued self-destructive behavior of an individual. Example: Spouse continues to make excuses for continued alcohol ingestion, stating, "He needs his beer daily to keep him happy."

encephalitis Infection or inflammation of the brain.

encephalopathy Any degenerative disease of the brain.

endocarditis Infection of the inner lining of the heart (endocardium).

enteral Within or by way of the stomach or intestine.

epidermis The outer, protective layer of the skin.

epigastric pain Pain in the upper middle region of the abdomen; can be an indication of a heart attack.

eschar A covering of black, dead tissue. This can form over a pressure ulcer, making it difficult to determine how deep the ulcer is.

esophageal reflux Regurgitation of food or acid from the stomach into the esophagus.

esophageal varices Enlarged venous channels in the esophagus that have the potential to rupture and cause uncontrolled, life-threatening bleeding.

ethnogeriatrics Health care for older persons from diverse ethnic populations.

euvolemia The presence of the proper amount of blood in the body.

excoriation Abrasion of the epidermis or of the coating of any organ by trauma, chemicals, burns, or other causes.

Federal Emergency Management Agency (FEMA) The United States Department of Homeland Security agency that coordinates the federal government's role in preparing for, mitigating the effects of, responding to, and recovering from domestic disasters.

financial/material exploitation Illegal or improper use of an older person's funds, property, or assets. Examples include cashing checks without permission, forging signatures, misusing money or possessions, forcing or deceiving into signing legal documents, and improper use of guardianship.

gait A person's manner of walking.

GEMS Diamond A concept developed to assist the prehospital professional when encountering the older patient. The GEMS Diamond has four components: G—geriatric patients; E—environmental assessment; M—medical assessment; S—social assessment.

geriatrics The branch of medicine concerned with the health of older people.

gerontology The study of aging.

gerophile A sexual predator targeting older people.

greater trochanter A bony prominence on the proximal lateral side of the thigh, just below the hip joint.

Grey Turner's sign Bruising of the abdominal flanks.

grief A multi-faceted response to loss.

Guillain-Barré syndrome A syndrome that typically occurs after a patient has had a viral respiratory illness; begins with weakness in the lower extremities that progresses toward the patient's head, and may lead to respiratory insufficiency or aspiration of stomach contents from the loss of the ability to cough.

half-life The time it takes for the amount of active medication in a person's system to decline by 50%.

hard site An area of soft tissue lying over a bony prominence; a high-risk spot for development of pressure ulcers.

hematemesis The vomiting of blood.

hematochezia Bright red blood in the stool.

hemodynamic Relating to circulation of the blood.

hemoptysis Coughing up of blood.

hemothorax A collection of blood in the pleural cavity.

hepatic metabolism   The liver's use of enzymes to break drugs down into more water-soluble compounds.

herpes zoster   A painful skin condition caused by reactivation of a virus.

home care   In-home services offered to patients with acute illness, long-term health conditions, permanent disability, or terminal illness. Services may include assistance with activities of daily living, administration of medication therapy, and IV therapy. Also known as home health care, personal care, or in-home care.

hospice   An interdisciplinary program of palliative care and supportive services that addresses the physical, spiritual, social, and economic needs of terminally ill patients and their families; this care may be provided in the home or at a hospice center.

hospice care   In-home or hospice care facility services provided to patients with a terminal illness. Services include supportive medical, social, and spiritual services to patients, and support for the patient's family.

Huntington chorea   Huntington's disease is an inherited disease that causes the progressive breakdown (degeneration) of nerve cells in the brain. Chorea is the most visible feature of Huntington's disease and often causes involuntary movements.

hypercarbia   Increased carbon dioxide in the blood.

hyperkalemia   An excessive amount of potassium in the blood.

hypertension   High blood pressure.

hyperthyroidism   Excessive amount of thyroid hormone produced by the thyroid gland.

hypertrophy   Enlargement of a muscle due to excessive strain put on that muscle.

hypnotic   A substance that induces sleep.

hypoglycemia   An abnormally low level of blood glucose.

hyponatremia   A decreased concentration of sodium in the blood.

hypothalamus   Organ at the base of the brain that controls many body functions through hormone systems.

hypothyroidism   Low levels of thyroid hormones, caused by changes in the thyroid gland.

hypoxemia   Decreased oxygen concentration in the blood.

hypoxia   A condition in which the body's cells and tissues do not have enough oxygen.

iatrogenic   Induced inadvertently by a physician or surgeon, or by medical treatment or diagnostic procedures.

idiopathic   Of unknown cause.

ileal conduit   A tube constructed of small bowel that allows for urine to drain to the outside of the body.

ileostomy   The removal of the entire colon and rectum, with the ileum being brought through the abdominal wall, forming a stoma.

immunosenescence   Refers to the gradual deterioration of the immune system brought on by natural age advancement.

incident command system (ICS)   A standardized, all-hazards incident management system that provides all users with a common organizational structure; the system supports five major functions: command, finance, logistics, operations, and planning.

infestation   The harboring of animal parasites. Common infestations in the setting of abuse and neglect are "bed bugs" (*Cimex lectularius*). The result of these infestations is hemorrhages in the skin, or wheals.

influenza   A contagious respiratory infection caused by a variety of flu viruses.

instrumental activities of daily living (IADLs)   Basic everyday activities that require a higher level of function, such as going shopping, making a meal, cleaning up, or using a telephone, which may become more difficult with age.

international normalized ratio (INR)   A system established by the World Health Organization (WHO) and the International Committee on Thrombosis and Hemostasis for reporting the results of blood coagulation (clotting) tests. Under the INR system, all results are standardized. For example, a person taking the anticoagulant warfarin would regularly have blood tested to measure the INR. The INR permits patients on anticoagulants to travel and obtain comparable test results wherever they are.

ischemia   A lack of oxygen that deprives tissues of necessary nutrients, resulting from partial or complete blockage of blood flow.

isolation theory   A theory that attempts to explain the cause of elder abuse; maintains that the older person's diminishing social network is a major risk factor in elder abuse.

kyphosis   A condition in which the back becomes hunched over due to an abnormal increased curvature of the spine.

kyphotic   Exaggerated curvature of the spine.

labyrinthitis   Inflammation of the inner ear structure (labyrinth).

life expectancy   The number of years that an average person of a given age may be expected to live.

listening   The act of receiving information. It includes observation of more than just words; it also includes observation of the volume, pitch, inflection, and tone of voice, as well as nonverbal aspects of communication.

livor mortis   A cutaneous dark spot on a dependent portion of a cadaver resulting from gravitational pooling of blood; also known as dependent lividity.

macroglossia   An abnormally large tongue.

macular degeneration   Deterioration of the central portion of the retina.

Medical Orders for Life Sustaining Treatment (MOLST)   A portable and enduring order form that makes a person's treatment wishes known to health care professionals through the identification of decisions regarding treatment preferences.

medication misuse   Unintentional or willful use of a medication in a way that differs from the prescribed dose or intent.

medication or substance abuse   Deliberate use of a drug for nonmedicinal reasons.

melanin   The pigment that provides color to the hair and skin.

melanocyte   Epidermal cell that produces melanin.

melena   Dark tarry stools that indicate bleeding somewhere within the gastrointestinal tract.

memorandum of understanding (MOU)   A document that outlines the terms of an agreement between two or more parties; generally recognized as binding.

Meniere's disease   A disease affecting the membranous inner ear; characterized by deafness, dizziness (vertigo), and ringing in the ear (tinnitus).

meningitis   An inflammation of the meningeal coverings of the brain; usually caused by a virus or a bacterium.

menopause   The process later in a woman's life during which menstruation ceases.

mesentery   The membrane(s) that connect organs to the abdominal wall.

metabolism   Describes how a drug is converted from its parent compound into its metabolites.

metastasis   The transfer of disease from one part of the body to another.

mitigation phase   The phase of emergency management that includes actions aimed at avoiding or lessening the impact of a disaster.

mobile integrated healthcare (MIH)   The provision of health care using patient-centered, mobile resources in the out-of-hospital environment that are integrated with the entire spectrum of health care and social service resources available in the local community.

myasthenia gravis   A condition from which patients complain of rapid muscle fatigue and loss of strength following the use of a muscle or group of muscles; occurs from the formation of immune system antibodies to the patient's own neurotransmitter (acetylcholine) receptors.

myocardial infarction   Death of heart muscle caused by hypoxia, as a result of obstruction of blood flow to the heart.

National Incident Management System (NIMS)   A standardized incident management system that enables all levels of government, nongovernmental organizations, and the private sector to work together during an emergency incident.

neglect   Refusal or failure on the part of the caregiver to provide life necessities, such as food, water, clothing, shelter, personal hygiene, medicine, comfort, and personal safety.

nephrons   The basic filtering units in the kidneys.

neurogenic bladder   A condition in which a person lacks bladder control due to a brain, spinal cord, or nerve problem, such as multiple sclerosis, Parkinson's disease, spina bifida, and stroke or spinal cord injury. Major pelvic surgery, diabetes, and other illnesses can also damage nerves that control the bladder.

neurons   Cells that make up nerve tissue and receive and transmit impulses.

nidus   A place in which bacteria may have multiplied or may multiply; a focus of infection.

nonadherence   Failure to comply with a medication regimen, whether by not taking medications or taking them only occasionally.

nonblanching erythema   Tissue redness that does not blanch (turn white) when pressed with a finger.

nonketotic diabetic acidosis   Metabolic acidosis in a person with type II diabetes; caused by hyperglycemia and dehydration, not by the formation of ketones. Patients with type II diabetes have insulin in their systems and, therefore, are not prone to the formation of ketones.

nonverbal communication   Communication consisting of eye contact, hand gestures, body position, facial expression, and touch.

nursing home   A facility where residents receive 24-hour nursing care. Also known as a skilled nursing facility, convalescent home, or long-term-care facility.

nystagmus   A lateral twitching of the eyes seen in a patient tracking the EMS provider's fingers from side to side across his or her visual field.

Occam's razor   A scientific and philosophic rule that entities should not be unnecessarily multiplied; interpreted as giving preference to the simplest of competing theories rather than the more complex, or that explanations of unknown phenomena be sought first in terms of known quantities.

old-age dependency ratio   The number of older people for every 100 adults between the ages of 18 and 64.

ombudsman   A resident advocate; responds to the needs of residents facing problems in long-term care facilities.

orthopnea   Difficulty breathing in the reclined position.

orthostatic hypotension   A decrease of 20 mm Hg in systolic blood pressure when moving from a sitting to a standing position; also called postural hypotension.

osteoarthritis   A progressive joint disease seen in older people, resulting in the destruction of cartilage, the formation of bone spurs in and around joints, and joint stiffness; thought to result from "wear and tear" and, in some instances, by repetitive trauma to the joints.

osteoblast   A cell that contributes to the body's continual process of remodeling bone by depositing newly formed bone.

osteoclast   A cell that contributes to the body's continual process of remodeling bone by absorbing bone.

osteomyelitis   Inflammation of the bone caused by infection; a frequent complication of pressure ulcers that can affect ulcer healing if the infection is not appropriately treated.

osteopenia   A decrease in the amount of bone tissue, regardless of the cause. Decreased bone density caused by failure of the rate of osteoid (resembling bone; the noncalcified matrix of young bone) tissue synthesis to keep up with the normal rate of bone lysis (dissolution or decomposition of; reduction or relief of).

osteophyte   A bony outgrowth, usually branched in shape. It is often a sign of osteoarthritis.

osteoporosis   A condition characterized by a decrease in bone mass, leading to a reduction in bone strength and a greater susceptibility to fracture, even after minimal trauma.

otosclerosis   A disease involving the middle ear capsule, specifically affecting the movement of the stapes (one of the three tiny bones in the middle ear).

ototoxic   Any drug with the potential to cause toxic reactions to structures of the inner ear.

palliative care   Care of patients whose disease is not responsive to curative treatment. Such care can include providing relief from pain and other distressing symptoms; neither hastening nor prolonging death.

palpitation   A subjective feeling of the heart "not beating right." This can manifest as skipped beats, rapid heart rate, or pounding in the chest.

pancreatitis Irritation or inflammation of the pancreas, usually caused by infection or chronic alcohol use.

paraplegia Paralysis of the lower half of the body, usually due to disease or injury of the spinal cord.

Parkinsonism Brain dysfunction that causes a loss of normal flexibility and fluidity of posture and movement, and the development of a hand tremor; due to a decrease in dopamine levels within the brain caused by either a primary disease such as Parkinson's disease, or as the result of trauma, medication use, or toxins.

Parkinson's disease A chronic nervous disease that is caused by degeneration of the dopamine-producing neurons within the brain, which leads to the development of Parkinsonism, and is characterized by a fine, slowly spreading tremor; muscle weakness and rigidity; and a peculiar gait.

passive neglect An unintentional refusal or failure to fulfill a caregiving obligation, which results in physical or emotional distress to the older person. Examples include abandonment and the non-provision of food and health services that are the result of the caregiver's lack of knowledge, laziness, infirmity, or addiction to drugs or alcohol.

pedal edema Swelling of the feet and ankles caused by a collection of fluid in the tissues; a possible sign of congestive heart failure (CHF).

penumbra Tissue surrounding the central area of a tissue involved in a stroke.

peptic ulcer disease Ulcerations or erosions occurring in the gastric mucosa and causing irritation or bleeding.

periorbital Surrounding the socket of the eye.

personality The essence of a person; the characteristics that make someone a unique, recognizable individual.

pharmacodynamics The pharmacologic or therapeutic effect of a medication or combination of medications.

pharmacokinetics Absorption, distribution, metabolism, and elimination of a drug.

physical abuse Force resulting in bodily injury, that is, from hitting, slapping, burning, unwarranted administration of drugs and physical restraints, force feeding, or physical punishment.

Physician Orders for Life Sustaining Treatment (POLST) An approach to end-of-life planning that ensures that seriously ill or frail patients can choose the treatments they want or do not want and that their wishes are documented and honored; see also Medical Orders for Life Sustaining Treatment (MOLST).

plantarflex To bend the foot downward.

pleural effusion Fluid in the thoracic cavity between the visceral and parietal pleura.

pleuritic chest pain Chest pain related to breathing; usually indicative of lung, chest wall, or other noncardiac chest problems.

pneumonia An inflammatory condition of the lung primarily affecting the alveoli.

pneumothorax A partial or complete accumulation of air in the pleural spaces.

portal hypertension Increased resistance to venous blood flow through the portal vein and liver, which displaces fluid in the abdomen, causing liver enlargement and increased size of venous channels in the esophagus.

postprandial hypotension A condition in which there is a systolic blood pressure drop of 20 mm Hg in a supine/sitting position within 120 minutes of eating a meal.

power of attorney (POA) A type of advance directive that names a future decision maker and anticipates a future situation in which decisions about CPR and other forms of life-sustaining treatment must be made, but the patient is unable at that time to make them; also known as a health care proxy or a health care agent.

preparedness phase The phase of emergency management that includes actions taken before an emergency occurs, in order to prepare for the emergency.

presbycusis Hearing loss associated with aging.

pressure ulcer A sore, initially of the skin, due to prolonged pressure, usually in a person who is lying down; it can form at any site, but are most common over bony prominences. The combination of pressure, shearing forces, friction, and moisture lead to the death of tissue due to lack of blood supply. Also referred to as decubitus ulcer, pressure sore, or bedsore.

prodromal An early symptom indicating the onset of a disease.

proprioception Perception of movement and the body's position, mediated by sensory nerve endings in muscles and tendons.

psychoactive A type of drug that affects the mind or behavior; there is a strong relationship between drugs of this type and the occurrence of falls.

psychological or emotional abuse Infliction of anguish, emotional pain, or distress. Includes verbal assaults, threats, intimidation, harassment, and forced social isolation.

psychopathology of the abuser theory A theory that attempts to explain the cause of elder abuse; maintains that the abuser's problems (such as personality disorders or substance abuse) can lead to the abuse or neglect.

psychotropic A type of drug that is capable of affecting the mental state; there is a strong relationship between drugs of this type and the occurrence of falls.

pulmonary edema A buildup of fluid in the lungs, usually as a result of congestive heart failure.

pulmonary embolism The lodging of a clot in the vessels of the lungs.

pulmonary embolus A blood clot that breaks from a large vein and travels to the blood vessels of the lung, causing obstruction of blood flow.

pulmonary fibrosis A disease in which tissue deep in the lungs becomes thick and stiff, or scarred, over time.

pulsus paradoxus A loss of more than 10 to 12 mm Hg of blood pressure during inspiration.

purulent sputum Sputum that contains pus; it is a physical finding in pneumonia.

quadriplegia Paralysis of all four limbs, usually due to disease or injury of the spinal cord.

quality of life The general well-being of an individual, which is affected by five interrelated factors: emotional health, physical health, social connections, economic security, and safety.

raccoon eyes Bruising around the eyes that indicates possible basal skull fracture.

recovery phase The phase of emergency management that includes actions taken after the disaster has subsided, in order to help the community return to a pre-disaster level of function.

reserve capacity The body's ability to respond to increased demands under stress, such as illness and exercise.

residual volume The amount of air left in the lungs after the maximum possible amount of air has been expired.

respite care Provides temporary relief for caregivers, ranging from hours to days.

response phase The phase of emergency management that includes actions to address the acute and short-term effects of an emergency or disaster that is in progress.

rhabdomyolysis Disintegration of muscle fibers that results in excretion of myoglobin (pigment of the muscle) in the urine; typically associated with death of muscle as occurs in compartment syndrome.

rheumatoid arthritis A systemic inflammatory disease that affects the body's joints; symptoms include inflammation in and around the joints in the hands, wrists, ankles, and feet, and less often in the knees and spine.

rhonchi Coarse, low-pitched breath sounds heard in patients with chronic mucous in the airways.

rigor mortis The stiffness that occurs in the deceased.

rotator cuff A tendon supporting the shoulder joint, composed of four muscles that attach to the humerus to allow motion and provide stability to the arm and shoulder; highly susceptible to injury in older people due to progressive degeneration.

rule of symmetry A principle that states that physical findings found on both sides of a patient's body are more likely to be normal than findings found on only one side of the body.

sedative A substance that decreases activity and excitement.

self-neglect Behaviors on the part of the older person that threaten his or her own health or safety. Generally manifests itself in refusal or failure to provide self with adequate food, shelter, or personal safety.

separation anxiety Anxiety that may be experienced by an older person when there is a threat of being taken away from family, friends, neighbors, or pets.

sepsis Disease state that results from the presence of microorganisms or their toxic products in the bloodstream.

sequelae A pathological condition resulting from a prior disease.

sexual abuse Nonconsensual sexual contact of any kind, including with a person incapable of giving consent. Includes but not limited to unwanted touching, sexual assault or battery such as rape, sodomy, coerced nudity, and sexually explicit photographing.

social learning theory A theory that attempts to explain the cause of elder abuse; maintains that violence is learned: if a person was abused as a child, that person will abuse his or her parents. Also called transgenerational theory.

status epilepticus The term used to describe a continuous seizure, or multiple seizures without a return to consciousness, that occurs for 30 minutes or more.

stenosis Abnormal narrowing of a blood vessel.

stressed caregiver theory A theory that attempts to explain the cause of elder abuse; maintains that when the caregiver reaches a certain stress level, abuse and neglect will occur.

stroke volume The amount of blood pumped out of the heart in one beat.

subarachnoid hemorrhage Bleeding between the arachnoid and pia matter in the brain.

subdural hematoma Bleeding into the area between the brain and the meningeal layer called the dura matter.

substance abuse A maladaptive pattern of behavior in regard to the use of chemically active agents that leads to clinically significant impairment or distress.

suicidal ideation Thoughts about or plans of committing suicide.

sundowners Also referred to as Sundowner's Syndrome or sundowning; defined as mood and behavior changes that occur a few hours before or during twilight.

synapse The junction between two neurons.

tamponade To close or block in order to stop bleeding.

thermoreceptors Temperature-sensing mechanisms throughout the body that send information to the hypothalamus.

thromboembolism The blocking of a blood vessel by a particle that has broken away from a blood clot at its site of formation.

thyroid storm A rare, life-threatening condition of hyperthyroidism, usually triggered by a stressful event or increased volume of thyroid hormones in the circulation.

thyrotoxicosis A morbid condition due to the overactivity of the thyroid gland.

tracheostomy A temporary or permanent surgical opening (stoma) through the third tracheal ring.

tramline A bruise appearing as a pale linear central area lined on either side by linear bruising.

transgenerational theory See social learning theory.

transient ischemic attack (TIA) A disorder of the brain in which brain cells temporarily stop working because of insufficient oxygen; causes stroke-like symptoms that resolve completely.

tuberculosis An airborne infectious disease caused by *Mycobacterium tuberculosis.*

ulcerogenic Tending to produce or develop into ulcers or ulceration.

ureterostomy A method of diverting urine in which the ureter is brought to the abdominal wall to form a stoma.

urethritis Inflammation of the urethra.

urine burn Reddening of the skin that occurs around the inner thighs and buttocks when the older person is allowed repeatedly to lie for prolonged periods of time in his or her own urine.

vasculitis Inflammation or infection in a blood vessel.

vasovagal syncope A common cause of syncope. When the vagus nerve is overstimulated, the body's blood vessels dilate and the heart slows down. This anti-adrenaline effect decreases the ability of the heart to pump blood upward to the brain against gravity.

ventilation   Movement of air in and out of the lungs produced by chest wall movement

verbal communication   Communication consisting of words and the volume, pitch, inflection, and tone of voice.

vertigo   A sensation in which a person feels that he or she is spinning, the surroundings are spinning, or both the person and the environment are spinning; often caused by a problem in the inner ear, but can also be caused by low blood pressure, dehydration, and anemia.

vesicles   Tiny blisters.

vital capacity   Volume of air moved during the deepest inspiration and expiration.

wheezes   High-pitched, whistling breath sounds caused by air traveling through narrowed air passages within the bronchioles, characteristically heard on inspiration in patients with asthma or chronic obstructive pulmonary disease (COPD).

Note: Page numbers followed by *f* or *t* indicate material in figures or tables respectively.

A

AAA. *See* area agency on aging
AARP. *See* American Association of Retired Persons
abandonment, 213
abdomen, 57
    assessment, 48
    pain in, 56–57
abdominal bruising, 223
abnormal neurological examination, 162
abrasions, 221, 221*f*
absence seizures, 162
absorption, 197–198
abuse
    evidence of, 226
    and neglect in long-term care facilities, characteristics of, 214*t*
    and restraints, rights regarding, 215*t*
    theories of, 218–219
    types of, 214*f*
abuser, profiles of, 218*t*
ACE inhibitors, 207
ACS. *See* acute coronary syndrome
active adult communities, 9–10
active metabolites, 199
active neglect, 212
activities of daily living (ADLs), 4, 16, 40, 42, 108, 113, 158, 223, 240
acute coronary syndrome (ACS), 134
acute myocardial infarction (AMI), 134, 135
acute pain, 106
acute pulmonary edema, 121
acute respiratory distress syndrome (ARDS), 127
addiction, 74
additional assessment pearls, 223
adequate nutrition, 234
ADLs. *See* activities of daily living
adult (active adult) communities, 9–10. *See also* care facilities
adult, older, 93, 94
Adult Protective Services (APS), 213
advanced health care directives (AHCD), 89
advanced life support (ALS), 154
adverse drug events (ADEs), 200, 206–207
    in older people, 207
adverse events, common categories of, 206–207

adverse medication-related events in older patients, ways to preventing, 208
aerobic metabolism, 120
Affordable Care Act, 231
ageism, 4–6
aggressive behavior, 167
aging. *See* geriatric patient(s)
aging skin, infection in, 178
agonal, 86
AHCD. *See* advanced health care directives
AICD. *See* automatic implantable cardioverter defibrillator
airway, assessment, 43–44
alcohol abuse, 219
alert, verbal, painful stimuli, unresponsive (AVPU) scale, 150
"all-hazards" approach, 241
alopecia, 221
ALS. *See* advanced life support
altered mental status (AMS), 41, 156–157, 157*t*
Alzheimer's care facilities, 10
Alzheimer's disease, 159–160
    medications used to treat, 161*t*
American Association of Retired Persons (AARP), 246
AMI. *See* acute myocardial infarction
amitriptyline, 203
AMS. *See* altered mental status
andropause, 6
anemia, 126
aneurysm, 21, 56
angina, 54
angina pectoris, 78, 134–135
angiodysplasia, 179
anhedonia, 68
animal abuse, 227
animal cruelty, 226–227
anomic aphasia, 32
antacids, 200
anthropometric measurements, 184
antiarrhythmic medications, 43
anticholinergic effects, 206
anticholinergic medications, 206
anticholinergics, 77*t*
antidepressants, for depression, 70
antipsychotics, 160
anxiety, fear of separation and, 34
aortic arch chemoreceptors, 20
    decreased sensitivity with aging, 20
aortic valve disorders
    regurgitation, 138–139
    stenosis, 138

apathetic thyrotoxicosis, 174
aphasia, 32, 33, 155
apraxia, 34
APS. *See* Adult Protective Services
ARDS. *See* acute respiratory distress syndrome
area agency on aging (AAA), 235–237
aricept, 160, 161*t*
arm movement, 153
arrhythmias, 20, 43, 140, 142
arteriovenous (AV) fistula, 274, 274*f*
arteriovenous (AV) graft, 274, 274*f*
aspiration pneumonia, 44
assessment
    of geriatric patient
        airway in, 43–44
        breathing, 44
        circulatory status in, 42–43
        common complaints encountered in, 52–62
        detailed physical exam, 51, 52
        "diamond" concept of, 3–4, 3*t*
        environmental/scene size-up, 40–41, 41*f*
        Five I's of Geriatrics, 40
        initial, 41–45
        medication use in, 44–45
        mental status in, 41–42
        Occam's razor approach, 39
        ongoing, 51
        physical examination, 48–49, 51, 52
        principles of, 40
        priority identifications, 50
        scene size-up/environmental, 40–41, 41*f*
        SPLATT for, 104, 104*t*
        trauma, 45–49, 45*f*
    of nutritional status, 184–185, 185*t*
assisted living facilities, 10, 243. *See also* care facilities
assisted living, responsibilities of, 244–245
assistive devices, use of, 113
asthma, 123–124, 124*f*
atelectasis, 99
atherosclerosis, 20, 21, 133, 134
atrial fibrillation, 20, 140, 142–143, 143*t*
atrophy, 148
    of brain, 17, 18
atrovent, 206
attitude, and EMS–providers, 4–6
audiologist, 31
automatic implantable cardioverter defibrillator (AICD), 143, 279
    complications, 280–281
    emergency care, 281

autonomy and consent, 89
AV fistula. *See* arteriovenous (AV) fistula
AV graft. *See* arteriovenous (AV) graft
AVPU scale. *See* alert, verbal, painful stimuli, unresponsive (AVPU) scale
AV shunt. *See* external arteriovenous (AV) shunt
azilect, 161

B

backboard(s), padding needed with, 47
bacteremia, 177. *See also* sepsis
balance training, 108–113
baroreceptors, 21
basic life support (BLS) providers, 154
Battle's sign, 164
Beers Criteria, 203
behavior, enabling, 81
behavioral emergencies, 166–167
    threatening to caregiver, 167
    threatening to patient, 166–167
    uncooperative patients and refusal of transport, 167
benign paroxysmal positional vertigo, 58
benzodiazepines, 81, 160, 162, 201, 207
bereavement, 93–94
beta-blockers, 43, 78*t*
"better safe than sorry" approach, 235
bilateral bruising, 222
biliary colic, 182, 182*f*
biliary pain. *See* biliary colic
bladder catheterization, 254
blanket roll, 107
bleeding, gastrointestinal tract
    intracranial, 17
    subcutaneous, 21, 22
blindness, communication in presence of, 28
blood pressure. *See also* hypertension
    low, postural changes and, 21
    measurement of, baseline determination, 43
blood sugar, 162
blood-thinning medications, 221
BLS providers. *See* basic life support (BLS) providers
blunt trauma, 223
bones, loss of, 100
bradykinesia, 161
brain, atrophy, 17, 18
    hematoma between dura mater and, 17
brain cancer, 166
brain death, 87
brain herniation, 163, 164
brain tissue, 152
breath, shortness of, 52
breathing capacity/vital capacity, age-related changes, 20, 52, 53
breathing, shortness of, 120
Broca's aphasia, 32
bronchiectasis, 121
bronchitis, chronic, 123
bruises, 221–223, 221*f*
bruising, 49
burns, 189–190, 222
    management, 190
    prevention, 190, 191*t*

C

CAD. *See* coronary artery disease
calcium channel blockers, 43, 77*t*
cancer, 191–193
    in nervous system, 166
cane, 113
cardiac and central nervous system (CNS) drugs, 200
cardiac arrest, 145
cardiac arrest resuscitation (CPR), 91
cardiac output, age-related changes, 20
cardiac pacemakers, 86
cardiovascular assessment
    AMI, 134
    angina pectoris, 134–135
    aortic valve disorders, 138–139
    atherosclerosis, 133, 134
    cardiac arrest, 145
    electrical disturbances, 142–143
    hypertensive assessment, 143
    mitral valve disorders, 139–140
    syncope, 144
    thromboembolism, 134
cardiovascular disorders, 165
cardiovascular drugs, 108
cardiovascular system
    age-related changes in, 20–21
    problems, 206
    substance abuse and, 78
cardioverter defibrillator, implantable, 55, 56
care facilities
    active adult communities, 9–10
    Alzheimer's disease management in, 10
    apartments, senior, 10
    assisted living, 10
    caregiver stress, 159
    congregate housing, 10
    hospice care, 11
    nursing homes, 10–11
    respite care, 11–12
cataracts, 149
catechol-O-methyltransferase (COMT) inhibitors, 161
catheterization, 254
    bladder, 254
    female, 256
    male, 255–256
catheters, types of, 268
cells, types of, 100
central cord syndrome, 102
central nervous system (CNS)
    infection, 157
    problems, 206
central venous catheters (CVCs), 269
cerebral vascular disease, 152–154
cerebrospinal fluid (CSF), 278
cervical extension/distraction injury, 102
cervical injuries, 101–102
cervical spondylosis, 102
chaffing, 221
chemoreceptor, 20
chemotherapies, 166, 193
chest pain, 54–56
CHF. *See* congestive heart failure

chief complaints, of geriatric patients, 52–62
child abusers, 227
cholangitis, 182
cholecystitis, 182
cholestasis, 171
cholinergics, 77*t*
cholinesterase inhibitors, 160
chronic alcohol use, 166, 166*f*
chronic bronchitis, 123
chronic condition, 170
chronic obstructive pulmonary disease (COPD), 232
    vs. congestive heart failure, 55
    respiratory assessment
        asthma, 123–124, 124*f*
        emphysema and chronic bronchitis, 123
chronic pain, 106
cigarette burns, 222
Cincinnati Prehospital Stroke Scale, 153, 153*t*
circulatory assessment, 42–43
cirrhosis, 78
CISD. *See* Critical Incident Stress Debriefing
CISM. *See* Critical Incident Stress Management
clinical assessment, 220–223
clinical death, 86
Clostridium difficile (C. diff), 172
cognition, 66
collagen, 21
colorectal cancer, 182
colostomy, 258
communication with aged patient
    in cases of hearing loss. *See* hearing loss, aging and
    in cases of speech impairment, 31, 32
    in presence of visual impairment, 28–29
    in stress situations, 35, 36
    techniques for, 35
    with families, 91–93
community-based resources, 236
community-dwelling *vs.* nursing home residents, 170
community health needs assessment, 232
community paramedicine, 231
community strategies for emergency preparedness, 242–244
compulsive/obsessive "hoarding" syndrome, 236
COMT inhibitors. *See* catechol-O-methyltransferase (COMT) inhibitors
condom catheter, 254
confusion, 206
congestive heart failure (CHF), 128, 140, 141
    vs. chronic obstructive pulmonary disease, 55
    program, 233
consciousness. *See* mental status
Consensus formula, 190
consent
    autonomy and, 89
    implied, 90
constipation, 182–183
continuous positive airway pressure (CPAP), 262
COPD. *See* chronic obstructive pulmonary disease
coronary artery disease (CAD), 133

CPAP. *See* continuous positive airway pressure
CPR. *See* cardiac arrest resuscitation
crackles, 122
cranial nerve function, 148–149
crime, influence in aging, 6
Critical Incident Stress Debriefing (CISD), 94
Critical Incident Stress
      Management (CISM), 94
Crohn's disease, 181
CSF. *See* cerebrospinal fluid
Cullen's sign, 223
Cushing's triad, 164
CVCs. *See* central venous catheters
cyanosis, 81

D

daily living, activities of, 4, 16, 17
deafness, aging and, 18
death
      brain, 87
      causes of, 16, 16*t*
      certification of, 87
      definition of, 86–87
      determination of, 86–87
      epidemiology of, 87
      good death, 88
      impending, 88
      notification of, 92*t*
      pronouncement of, 87
decision making, influence in aging, 6
decubitus ulcer. *See* pressure ulcers
deep vein thrombosis (DVT), 125
degeneration, macular, 28
dehydration, 183–186, 220
      assessment for, 184–185, 186*t*
      management, 185–186
      prevention, 186
delirium, 157–158
      vs. dementia, 159
delirium tremens (DTs), 81
dementia, 32, 158–159
      communication in presence of, 33
      delirium *vs.*, 159*t*
dementia-related complaints, 159
dentures/dental appliances, 19, 31
      handing to patients, 31, 32
Department of Homeland Security, 245
dependency theory, 219
dependent lividity, 86
depression, 166. *See also* suicide
      age-related psychological changes
            Geriatric Depression Scale, 69
            impact of, 68
            OPQRST, 67
            "red flags," 68
            symptoms of, 67
            treatment of, 69
            in United States, 67
dermal–epidermal junction, 174, 174*f*
dermis, 174, 175
detailed physical examination, 51, 52
detrusor instability, 40
deviated septum, signs of, 223
diabetes, 172–173
diabetic neuropathy, 60
dialysis, 273

assessment, 274
      complications, 275
      emergency care, 275
      rationale, 274
      shunt, 277–278
diarrhea, 61–62
diphenhydramine, 203, 207
disaster
      checklists, 241
      long-term care facilities during, 244–245
      planning, 240, 243
distal femur fractures, 103
distribution, 198
diuretics, 207
diverticulitis, 181, 181*f*
diverticulosis, 180
dizziness, 58–59
DNAR order. *See* do not attempt resuscitation
      (DNAR) order
DNR orders. *See* do not resuscitate (DNR)
      orders
do not attempt resuscitation (DNAR) order,
      89–91
do not resuscitate (DNR) orders, 7, 89–91
doctrine of informed consent, 89
documentation, 94, 226
domestic violence, 226–227
donepezil, 161*t*
dopamine agonists, 161
dorsiflex, 151
drug-induced mental impairment, 201
drug interactions, 199–203, 222
      drug–disease interactions, 201
      drug–drug interactions, 200
      drug–herb interactions, 202–203
      drug–nutrient interactions, 200–201
      and toxins, 166
drug metabolism, 200
drug-related adverse events, 222
drug–disease interactions, 201
drug–drug interactions, 200, 200*t*
drug–herb interactions, 202–203
drug–nutrient interactions, 200–201
duodenum, 179
dura mater, hematoma between brain
      and, 17
DVT. *See* deep vein thrombosis
dysarthria, 34
dyspepsia, 180
dysphagia, 121, 179
dyspnea, 81, 120

E

ear(s), age-related changes in appearance/
      function, 18, 52*t*. *See also* hearing aids
EBR. *See* evidence-based research
Echinacea, 202
economic security, 235
edema, pedal, 50
effective prehospital acute stroke
      care, 155
effusion, pleural, 122
elastin, 21
eldepryl, 161
elder abuse, 212, 226–227
      in long-term care facilities, 213–217

observing for clues to, 219–224
elder mistreatment in long-term care facilities,
      characteristics of, 214
elimination, 198–199
embolism, 54
      pulmonary, 20
emergency department, 9
emergency management model, 241
emergency management phases,
      241, 242
emergency medical services, 241
emergency planners, 242
Emergency Preparedness Packet for Home
      Health Agencies, 242
emergency services personnel, 245
emergency warning systems, 244
emotional abuse, 212
emotional health, 234
emotional suffering, 224
emphysema, 123
empyema, 125
EMS provider(s), 219, 225, 246, 283
      assessment of older patient. *See* assess-
            ment, of geriatric patient
      attitude toward older patients, 4–6
      bereavement and grief, 93–94
      communication with families, 91–93
      death. *See* death
      ethical and legal considerations, 89–91
      vs. MIH providers, 232
      palliative and hospice care, 87–88, 87*f*
      role of, 94
enabling behavior, 81
encephalitis, 166
encephalopathy, 148
end-of-life care, 6
endocarditis, 138
endocrine emergencies, 172–174
      diabetes, 172–173
      thyroid disorders, 173–174
            treatment, 174
endocrine system, age-related changes, 23
endotracheal (ET) tube, 263
enteral feedings, 266
      rationale, 266
environmental assessment, 4, 219–220, 235
environmental emergencies, 187–189
      prevention, 189
ephedra, 202
epidermis, 174
epigastric pain, 55
eschar, 177
esophageal cancer, 179
esophageal reflux, 121
esophageal varices, 78
esophagus, 260–261
ET tube. *See* endotracheal tube
ethnogeriatrics, 12–13
euvolemia, 61
evidence-based research (EBR), 203
excoriations, 221
exelon, 161*t*
exercise and strength training, 100*f*
explicit memory, 66
external arteriovenous (AV) shunt, 273
extremities, deformity of, 49

eye(s)
    age-related changes in, 52t
    jerky movements of, 58
    movements, 151

F

face, physical changes with aging, 52t
facial droop, 153, 153t
facility administration, participation in, 215t
fall(s), 97–98
    assessment following, 104–105
    fear of, 98
    head trauma from, 98
    hip fracture due to, 97
    and injuries in older people, 107–116
        exercise and balance training, 108–113
        reducing medications, 108
    intrinsic risk factors for, 105t
    psychological and social impacts of, 98
    SPLATT for, 104t
    trauma due to, 97
fall-risk increasing drugs (FRID), 201, 202t
false teeth, 19, 31
    handing to patients, 31, 32
fatal injuries, 201
fatigue, 151
FDA. See Food and Drug Administration
fecal incontinence, 182–183
Federal Emergency Management Agency (FEMA), 241
feeding tube, 266
FEMA. See Federal Emergency Management Agency
fever, 59–60
fibrillation, atrial, 20, 140, 142–143, 143t
fibrinolytic therapy checklist for ischemic stroke, 154, 154t
financial exploitation, 212, 223
fire, prevention, 190, 191t
Five I's of Geriatrics, 40
flail chest, 46, 48
    in older patients, 102
flame, 190
flovent inhaler, 204
fluid resuscitation, 190
flumazenil, 207
focal neurological function, sudden loss of, 155–156
Food and Drug Administration (FDA), 203
footwear, 115
fractures, 222f
    distal femur, 103
    hip, 100, 102–103, 107
        falling and, 102
    odontoid, 102
    rib, 102
fraud, 223
FRID. See fall-risk increasing drugs
Future of Health Care of Older People, The, 88

G

G-tube, 265
gait, 149–150

galantamine, 161t
gallbladder, 179
    disease, 182, 182f
gallstones, prevalence of, 182
gastric tube, 266
gastroesophageal reflux disease (GERD), 179
gastrointestinal bleeding, 179–182
gastrointestinal emergencies, 178–183
    age-related changes in, 178–179
gastrointestinal problems, 206
gastrointestinal (GI) system
    age-related changes in, 23–24
    substance abuse and, 78–79
gastrointestinal (GI) tract, 197
gastrostomy tube, 266
GEMS Diamond, 3–4, 3t
generalized pain, 60–61
generalized weakness, 156
GERD. See gastroesophageal reflux disease
Geriatric Depression Scale, 69, 69t
geriatric patient(s)
    activities of, 16, 17
    age-related changes in, 197–199
    aging process, history of, 2–3
    assessment of. See assessment, of geriatric patient
    cardiovascular assessment
        AMI, 134
        angina pectoris, 134–135
        aortic valve disorders, 138–139
        atherosclerosis, 133, 134
        cardiac arrest, 145
        electrical disturbances, 142–143
        hypertensive assessment, 143–144
        mitral valve disorders, 139–140
        syncope, 144
        thromboembolism, 134
    cohorts, 2
    communication, with aged patient
        in cases of hearing loss. See hearing loss, aging and
        in cases of speech impairment, 31, 32
        in presence of visual impairment, 28–29
        in stress situations, 35, 36
        techniques for, 35
    death of, 16t
    demographic profile of, 7–9
    EMS provider
        assessment by, 2
        attitude and, 4–6
    ethnic identity of, 12–13
    GEMS assessment, 3–4
    geriatrics, 2
    gerontology, 2
    health care system and. See care facilities
    medications, 197–199
    psychological changes in, 19
    psychosocial changes in. See psychosocial changes, age-related
    respiratory assessment
        ARDS, 127–128
        CHF/APE, 128–129
        cigarettes, controlling use of, 130
        COPD. See chronic obstructive pulmonary disease (COPD)

history of, 122
    influenza, 125
    lung cancer, 126–127
    physical examination, 122
    pneumonia, 120
    pulmonary embolism, 125–126
    pulmonary fibrosis, 128
    signs and symptoms, 120–122
    tuberculosis, 127
    vaccinations, 129, 130
sociology of aging and, 5–6
geriatric trauma
    assessment of, 104–105
    management of, 105–107
geriatrics, 2
gerontology, 2
gerophile, 224
GI. See gastrointestinal
ginkgo, 203
Glasgow Coma Scale, 48, 48t
glaucoma, 149
global aphasia, 32
glove injury, 222f
glucometer, 163
gradual hearing loss, 149
greater trochanter, 115
Grey Turner's sign, 223
grief, 93–94
Guillain-Barré syndrome, 156, 164

H

half-life, 198
haloperidol (haldol), 167
hard site, 176
head, physical changes with aging, 48
head trauma, 165
    falls and, 98
health and safety problems, signs of, 236
health care reform, 231
healthcare access, 244
hearing aids, 30–31
    first aid for, 30–31
    types of, 30
hearing loss
    aging and, 29–31. See also hearing aids
    patients with, 149
heart
    chest examination, 48
    output and stroke volume, 20
    pacemaker, 55
    reduced responsiveness to adrenal hormones, 21
heart rhythm
    disturbances in, 20
    pacemaker, 55, 142, 143
heat-related deaths in United States, 188
hematemesis, 179
hematochezia, 180
hematoma subcutaneous, 21, 22
hemodialysis, 273f, 274
    vascular access for, 274
hemodynamic stress, response of aging kidneys, 24
hemoptysis, 121

hemorrhagic stroke, 152
symptoms of, 153
hemothorax, 223
hepatic metabolism, effects of aging, 23
hepatic system, substance abuse and, 78
hepatitis, 171
hepatitis B virus infection, 171
hepatitis C virus infection, 171
herbal medications by older patients, use of, 202
herpes zoster, 178
hip fractures, 100, 107
falling and, 102
splinting, 111
hip protectors, 115
HIV, infection, 171
home care, 11
workers, 244
hospice care, 11, 87f, 87–88
House Select Committee on Aging, 212
"Huber" needle, 269f
insertion in subcutaneous port, 271
human bone, 100
Huntington chorea, 159
Hurricane Katrina, 240
Hurricane Sandy, 240
hydration, 234
hygiene, 220
hypercarbia, 20
hyperkalemia, 199, 207
hypertension, 78
hyperthermia, 188–189
management, 189
hyperthyroidism, 173
symptoms of, 174
treatment of, 174
hypertrophy, 134
hypnotic(s), 78, 202t
hypoglycemia, 79
older patients with, 173
hyponatremia, 199
hypotension, 157
orthostatic, 21
hypothalamus, 187, 187f
hypothermia, 187–188
management of, 187–188
signs and symptoms of, 187
hypothyroidism, 173
clinical presentation of, 173, 174, 174t
older patient for, treatment, 174
sign of, 173
hypoxemia, 127
hypoxia, 121
signs and symptoms of, 263

I

IADLs. See instrumental activities of daily
living
iatrogenic symptoms, 39
IBD. See inflammatory bowel disease
ICS. See Incident Command System
idiopathic, 149
idiopathic pulmonary fibrosis (IPF), 128
ileal conduit, 257
ileostomy, 258
immersion burns, 222

immobilization
of kyphotic patient, 47
of older trauma patient, 106
padding of board, 47
problems with, 47
immune function, age-related changes of,
170, 175
immune system
age-related changes in, 24
substance abuse and, 79
immunosenescence, 171
impaired sensory systems, 150
implantable defibrillator, 55, 56
implanted ports, 269
implicit memory, 66
implied consent, 90
inadequate care, 213
incidence, 213
Incident Command System (ICS), 245
incident management concept, 245
indwelling Foley catheter, 254
traumatic removal of, 256
infection, age-related risk factors, 170t
infectious disease, 170–171
infestations, 221
inflammatory bowel disease (IBD), 181
influenza, 125
information, rights to, 215t
initial assessment, 41–45
injuries. See also trauma
fatal, 99
intrinsic risk factors for, 105t
lower extremity, 103
in older patients, 98t
reduce risk of, 116
upper extremity, 103
inner cannula, 259f
innovative programs in MIH, 236
instrumental activities of daily living (IADLs),
16, 240
integumentary system, age-related changes in,
21, 22, 174–175
international normalized ratio
(INR), 43
intracranial bleeding, 17
intracranial pressure, 279
intravenous therapy, 106
IPF. See idiopathic pulmonary fibrosis
iptratropium bromide, 206
ischemia, 54, 78, 134
ischemic colitis, 181
ischemic stroke, 152
fibrinolytic therapy checklist for, 154t
vs. hemorrhagic stroke, symptoms of,
153t
isolation theory, 219

J

J-tube, 266
jaw thrust, in airway management, 44
jejunostomy tube, 266

K

kidney(s), 198–199
function, age-related changes, 24

knife wounds, 221f
kyphosis, 100, 100f
kyphotic patient, 22, 107f
immobilization of, 47
to long backboard, immobilizing, 109
respiratory problems in, 20

L

labyrinthitis, 58
lacerations, 221, 221f
left ventricular assist devices (LVADs), 55,
56, 282
complications encountered in, 283t
emergency care, 283–284
rationale, 283
life (daily), activities of, 16, 17
life expectancy, 2
listening, communication skill, 28
liver, 199
livor mortis, 86
local stakeholder group, 232
long-term care facilities, 243, 244
characteristics of
abuse and neglect in, 214t
elder mistreatment in, 214
during disaster, 244–245
elder abuse in, 213–217
long-term care ombudsman,
217, 237
lower extremity weakness, 108
lower gastrointestinal bleeding,
180f, 180–181
treatment, 181–182
lung cancer, 126–127
chronic obstructive disease
embolus, 20
residual volume, 20
COPD vs. CHF, 55
embolus in, 54
LVADs. See left ventricular assist devices

M

macroglossia, 173
macular degeneration, 28
malnutrition, 183–186, 220
assessment for, 184–185, 186t
management, 185–186
material exploitation, 212, 223
Matter of Balance, A, 236
MCI. See mild cognitive impairment
"Meals on Wheels" program, 234
mechanical ventilators, 262
emergency care, 263
rationale, 263
medical assessment. See assessment, of
geriatric patient
Medical Orders for Life Sustaining Treatment
(MOLST), 90f
medication abuse, 75
medication classes, 205
medication containers, 199f
medication misuse, 75
medication nonadherence
behavioral interventions for, 204

medication toxicity/adverse effects, assessing problems related to, 203–207
  adverse drug events, 206–207
  drug withdrawal problems, 207
  history, 204–205
  medication nonadherence, 205
medications
  geriatric patient, 197–199
  passage of, 197–199
  usage of, 201, 222–223
melanin, 21
melanocyte, 175*t*
melena, 179
memantine, 161*t*
memorandum of understanding (MOU), 243
memory, 66–67
Meniere's disease, 29, 58
meningitis, 166
menopause, 6
mental function, 148
mental status, 148
  assessment of, 41–42
mesenteries, age-related changes, 24
metabolic disturbances, 206–207
metabolic encephalopathies from systemic illness, 165
metabolism, 198–199
  hepatic, aging effect on, 23
metastasis, 151*t*
Michigan Alcoholism Screening Test, 79, 80
MIH. *See* mobile integrated healthcare
mild cognitive impairment (MCI), 160
Mini-Nutritional Assessment Short-Form (MNA-SF), 184, 185*t*
misuse, medication, 222–223
mitigation phase, 241, 242
mitral valve disorders
  regurgitation, 139–140
  stenosis, 139
mixed nonfluent aphasia, 32
MNA-SF. *See* Mini-Nutritional Assessment Short-Form
mobile integrated healthcare (MIH), 231
  program development, 232
  providers, EMS providers *vs.*, 232
  and quality of life, 234–236
  role of primary care physician in, 233–234
  types of, 233
MOLST. *See* Medical Orders for Life Sustaining Treatment
monoamine oxidase (MAO) inhibitors, 70, 70*t*
motor function, 149
motor vehicle collisions, 98–99
MOU. *See* memorandum of understanding
mouth, insertion of dentures, 31, 32
multi-lumen catheter, 269
musculoskeletal system, 22–23
  assessment of, 48
  substance abuse and, 79

myasthenia gravis, 156
  patients with, 156
myocardial infarction, 78

N

NAHC. *See* National Association for Home Care and Hospice
Namenda, 160, 161*t*
narcotic overdose, 164
National Association for Home Care and Hospice (NAHC), 242
National Center on Elder Abuse (NCEA), 212, 213, 214
National Elder Abuse Incidence Study, 213
national Eldercare Locator, 237
National Incident Management System (NIMS), 245
National Institute of Justice, 214
natural disasters, 243
nausea, 61–62
NCEA. *See* National Center on Elder Abuse
"near poor" geriatric patients, 8
necrosis, 260
negative-pressure ventilators, 262
neglect, 212
  evidence of, 226
  in long-term care facilities, characteristics of abuse and, 214*t*
  theories of, 218–219
nephrons, loss with aging, 24
nervous system
  age-related changes in, 17–18
  cancer in, 166
  complaints related to
    altered mental status, 156–157
    Alzheimer's disease, 159–160
    delirium, 157–158
    delirium *vs.* dementia, 159
    dementia, 158–159
    focal neurological function, sudden loss of, 155–156
    generalized weakness, 156
    head and spine trauma, 165
    loss of consciousness, 163–164
    lowered level of consciousness, 162–163
    paraplegia and quadriplegia, 164–165
    Parkinson's disease, 160–161
    secondary neurological disorders, 165–166
    seizure disorders, 161–162
    stroke and cerebral vascular disease, 152–154
    transient ischemic attack, 155
neurogenic bladder, 257
neurons, loss with aging, 17
neuropathy, diabetic, 60
neurotransmitter (acetylcholine) receptors, 156
nidus, 172
NIMS. *See* National Incident Management System
911 program, frequent users of, 233
non-accidental bruising, 222
nonadherence, with medical regimens, 45
nonblanching erythema, 176

nonketotic diabetic acidosis, 151*t*
nonsteroidal anti-inflammatory drugs (NSAIDs), 201
nonverbal communication, 27–28
normal age-related changes in nervous system
  cranial nerve function, 148–149
  mental function and status, 148
  motor function, 149
  posture and gait, 149–150
  sensation and reflexes, 149
normeperidine, 199
NSAIDs. *See* nonsteroidal anti-inflammatory drugs
nursing homes, 10–11
  evacuation of, 244*f*
  residents, rights of, 215*t*–216*t*
  top complaints of residents in, 217*t*
Nursing Home Reform Act, 215, 217, 223
nursing home residents, community-dwelling *vs.*, 170
nutrition, 234
nutritional supplements, 201
nystagmus, 58

O

observation admission avoidance program, 233
Occam's razor approach, 39
odontoid fractures, 102
old-age dependency ratio, 9
OLD CART mnemonic, 60
older adults, 93, 94
  diabetes in, 172
  viral hepatitis in, 171
Older Americans Act, 236
older patients
  assessment of, 153
  chronic conditions in, 102
  distal femur fractures in, 103
  exercise goal for, 113
  with hypoglycemia, 173
  injuries in, 98*t*, 101–104
  management of, who has fallen, 105
  medication history of, 204*t*
  neurological examination of, 150–151
  rib fractures, 102
older people
  preparedness strategies for
    agency, 242
    community, 242–244
    personal, 241
    resource for, 236–237
older person
  neurological examination in, 223
  in shelters, needs of, 246
older person's gait, evaluating and documenting, 149
older population
  burns, 99
  epidemiology of trauma in, 97–99
ombudsman, long-term care, 217
Omnibus Budget Reconciliation Act, 215
ongoing assessment, 51
Onset, Provocation, Quality, Radiation, Severity, Time (OPQRST), 60, 67–68
open book fractures, 102
ophthalmologic assessment, 223

opioids, 76t, 151
OPQRST. *See* Onset, Provocation, Quality, Radiation, Severity, Time
orthopnea, 55, 121
orthostatic hypotension, 21, 58, 108
osteoarthritis, 101, 101f
osteoblasts, 100
osteoclasts, 100
osteomyelitis, 177
osteopenia, 102
osteophyte, 102
osteoporosis, 22, 100–101
OTC. *See* over-the-counter
otosclerosis, 29
ototoxic medications, 29
over-the-counter (OTC)
    medications, 200
    remedies, 203

P

pacemakers, 142, 143
pain
    in abdomen, 56–57
    chest, 54–56, 121
    epigastric, 55
    generalized, 60–61
palliative care, 11, 87–88
palpitations, 135
paraplegia, 164–165
Parkinsonism, 160
Parkinson's disease, 34, 159–161
passive neglect, 212
patient-controlled analgesia (PCA) pump, 264f
    complications, 264
    rationale, 264
patients
    companions of deceased, 91–93
    interviewing, 224–225
PCA pump. *See* patient-controlled analgesia (PCA) pump
PCP. *See* primary care physician
PE. *See* pulmonary embolism
pedal edema, 50
pelvis, physical changes with aging, 52t
penumbra, 152
peripheral inserted central catheters (PICCs), 269–270, 270f
peripheral nerves, 150
peritoneal dialysis, 274f, 275
perpetrators of elder abuse, 227
personal emergency response system (PERS), 115–116, 116f
personal funds, protection of, 216t
personal rights, 215t
personality, 67
pharmacodynamics, 197
    interactions, 200
pharmacokinetics, 151, 197
phenytoin, 198
phlebitis, 265
physical abuse, 212
physical examination, 48–49, 51, 52t
physical health, 234
Physician Orders for Life Sustaining Treatment (POLST), 90
physiological changes

age-related
    endocrine system, 23
    hepatic function, 23
    immune system, 24
    integumentary system, 21
    musculoskeletal system, 22–23
    nervous system, 17–18
    renal function, 24
    in respiratory system, 44
    sensory function, 18–19
    with aging, 99–101
    pulmonary system, 99
PICCs. *See* peripheral inserted central catheters
pink puffer, 55t
plantarflex, 151
plasma-protein binding, 198f
pleuritic chest pain, 121
pneumonia, 120, 125
    aspiration, 44
pneumothorax, 223
POA. *See* power of attorney
POLST. *See* Physician Orders for Life Sustaining Treatment
"poor/near poor" geriatric patients, 8
portal hypertension, 78
post-disaster phase SWiFT level tool in, 248t
postherpetic neuralgia, 178
postprandial hypotension, 43
postural hypotension, 21
posture, 149–150
potential stroke patient, 156
poverty, among geriatric patients, 8
power of attorney (POA), 89
prehospital care professionals, 219
prehospital care providers, 240, 241
prehospital management
    of patient, 181
prehospital providers, 154
prehospital stroke scales, use of, 154
preparedness phase, 241, 242, 243
presbycusis, 29, 149
pressure, backboard (prevention), 47
pressure ulcers, 176f, 176–178, 177f, 220
    complications, 177
    disease, 179
    prevention and care, 177–178
    stages, 176–177, 176f
    treatment, 178, 178t
pressure ventilators, 262
primary care physician (PCP), 233
    in MIH, role of, 233–234
primary care replacement model, 232
priority patients, identification of, 50
prodromal, 178
proprioception, 149
prosthetic joint replacements, injuries with, 103–104, 103f
proton pump inhibitors, 179, 179t
providers, 243
proximal fractures, 103
psychoactive, 108
psychological abuse, 212, 224
psychological changes, age-related, 19
psychopathology of the abuser theory, 219

psychosocial changes, age-related
    assessment, goals of, 79
    chemical dependency and substance abuse. *See* substance abuse
    cognition, 66
    depression. *See also* suicide
        Geriatric Depression Scale, 69
        impact of, 68
        OPQRST, 67
        "red flags," 68
        symptoms, 67
        treatment of, 69
        in United States, 67
    enabling behavior, 81
    environmental observation, 80
    history questions, 80
    management considerations in, 82
    medical examination, 81
    memory, 66–67
    personality, 67
psychotropic medication, 108, 201, 222
pulmonary disease, chronic obstructive *vs.* CHF, 55
pulmonary edema, 120, 128–129
pulmonary embolism (PE), 20, 125–126
pulmonary fibrosis, 128
pulmonary system, changes in, 99
pulse(s), in geriatric patients, 43
pulsus paradoxus, 55, 124
pupil(s)
    aging and, 18
    assessing, 162

Q

quadriplegia, 164–165
quality of life, MIH and, 234–236

R

raccoon eyes, 165
racial identity, influence in aging, 6
range of motion (ROM), 48
razadyne, 161t
recovery phase, 241, 242
rectal bleeding, 223
Red Cross, 246
reflexes, 149
reflux, esophageal, 121
regurgitation
    aortic valve, 138
    mitral valve, 139
reserve capacity, 120
residual volume, age-related changes in, 20
resources for older people, 236–237
respiratory assessment, geriatric patient(s)
    ARDS, 127–128
    CHF/APE, 128–129
    cigarettes, controlling use of, 130
    COPD. *See* chronic obstructive pulmonary disease (COPD)
    history of, 122
    influenza, 125
    lung cancer, 126–127
    physical examination, 122
    pneumonia, 120
    pulmonary embolism, 125–126

pulmonary fibrosis, 128
  signs and symptoms, 120–122
  tuberculosis, 127
  vaccinations, 129, 130
respiratory muscle weakness causes of, 156
respiratory problems, kyphosis and, 20, 22
respiratory system
  age-related changes in, 19, 20, 44
  substance abuse and, 78
respite care, 11–12
response phase, 241, 242
restraints, 223
rhabdomyolysis, 98
rheumatoid arthritis, 101
rhonchi, 122
rib fractures, 102
rigor mortis, 86
rivastigmine, 161*t*
ROM. *See* range of motion
rotator cuff, 103
rule of symmetry, 49

S

safety, 235–236
scene size-up, 40–41, 41*f*
schizophrenia, 161
secondary neurological disorders, 165–166
sedative(s), 78
sedative-hypnotics, 76*t*
seizure disorders, 161–162
selective serotonin reuptake inhibitors (SSRIs), 70, 70*t*, 76*t*, 77, 203
self-determination, rights to, 215*t*
self-neglect, 212
"senile" tremor, 149
senior information programs, 237
Seniors Without Families Triage (SWiFT) assessment instrument, 246
sensation, 149
sensory function, age-related changes in, 18–19
sensory impairments, 149
separation anxiety, 34
sepsis, 171–172
septicemia. *See* sepsis
septum, 269
sequelae, 178
serotonin and norepinephrine reuptake inhibitors (SNRIs), 70, 70*t*
serotonin syndrome, 203
services and activities, provision of, 215*t*
severe respiratory compromise, evidence of, 156
sexual abuse, 212
sexual assault in elderly, 224
shelters, 245–246
short-duration disasters, 244
shortness of breath (dyspnea), 52–54, 120
sinemet, 161
single-use straight catheter, 254
skin, 174, 174*f*, 220–221
  age-related changes, 21, 22
smoke alarms, 190
smoking, 100
social assessment, of older person, 223–224.
    See also assessment, of geriatric patient
social learning theory, 219
speech impairment, 31, 32

speech test, 153, 153*t*
spinal injuries, 101–102
spine trauma, 165
SPLATT, for assessment of patient, 104
SSRIs. *See* selective serotonin-reuptake inhibitors
St. John's Wort, 203
stakeholders
  engaging, 232
  importance of collaboration with, 232
State Long-Term Care Ombudsman Programs, 217
status epilepticus, 162
stenosis, 260
  mitral valve, 139
stocking, 222*f*
stomach cancer, 179
stomach lining, 179
stressed caregiver theory, 219
stroke, 152–154
stroke assessment tool, 155
stroke volume, age-related changes in, 20
subcutaneous hematoma, 21, 22
subcutaneous fat layer, 175
subcutaneous/mediastinal emphysema, 261
subdural hematoma, 17, 81
substance abuse, 66, 74, 219
  early and late onset drinkers, 74, 75
  older adults, pathophysiology
    cardiovascular system, 78
    gastrointestinal system, 78–79
    hepatic system, 78
    immune system, 79
    musculoskeletal system, 79
    respiratory system, 78
  risk factors for, 75–76, 76*t*
  screening for, 79
suicidal ideation, 72
suicide
  DOs and DON'Ts, 73
  IS PATH WARM, 72, 73
  long-term care facilities, 72
  older people and, 68, 71
  risk factors
    alcoholism, 72
    hopelessness, 71
    life roles, changes in, 72
    loneliness, 72
    loved one, death of, 71
    physical illnesses, 71
  in United States, 70, 71
sundowners, 160
suprapubic catheter, 254, 255*f*
surrogate decision makers, 89
suspected abusers, interviewing, 225–226
Symmetrel, 161
symmetrical bruising, 49
sympathomimetics, 76*t*
synapses, loss with aging, 17
syncope, 144
systemic illness
  metabolic encephalopathies from, 165

T

tachycardia, 180
tamponade, 21

TBI. *See* traumatic brain injury
teeth, false, 19, 31
  handing to patients, 31, 32
temperature regulation,
    age-related changes in, 187
Texas catheter, 254
thermoreceptors, 187, 187*f*
thromboembolism, 134
thrombosis, 272
thyroid disorders, 173–174
thyroid gland, 173, 173*f*
thyroid hormones, 173
thyroid storm, 59
thyrotoxicosis, 174
tooth (teeth), false, 19, 31
  handing to patients, 31, 32
torso trauma, 102
toxins, drug interactions and, 166
trachea, 260–261
tracheal necrosis, 260
tracheal stenosis, 260
tracheostomy, 259
  complications, 260
  emergency, 260
  patient, 263
tramline bruising, 222
transgenerational theory, 219
transient ischemic attack, 155
transport considerations, 255
transportation, 243
trauma. *See also* trauma scene
  assessment, 45–49
  chest, 48
  disorders related to, 166
  epidemiology of, 97–99
  falls and, 97
  getting up safely, 116
  Glasgow Coma Scale, 48
  in older population, 97–99
  physiological changes associated with, 99–101
  torso, 102
trauma scene assessment, mechanism of injury, 45
traumatic aortic injury, 102
traumatic brain injury (TBI), 97
tricyclic antidepressants, 70, 70*t*
tube feedings, 201
tuberculosis, 127

U

ulcerative colitis, 181
ulcerative proctitis, 181
ulcerogenic, 179
unequal pupils, 164, 164*f*
upper extremity injuries, 103
upper gastrointestinal bleeding, 179–180, 180*f*, 181
urban model, 232
ureterostomy, 257
urethritis, atrophic, 40
urinary catheters, 253

complications, 256
rationale, 254
resources, 256
urinary tract infection (UTI), 172, 256
management, 172
signs and symptoms of, 172
urine burns, 221
urine retention, 172
UTI. *See* urinary tract infection

V

VAD. *See* ventricular assist device
vaginal bleeding, 223
valvular heart diseases
aortic valve disorders, 138
mitral valve disorders, 139–140
vascular access devices, 268
complications, 272
emergency care, 272
preparation, 270
procedure, 270–271

rationale, 268–270
use of dialysis, 275–278
vasculitis, 151*t*
vasovagal syncope, 144
venous catheter, 269
ventilation, 20
ventilators, mechanical, 262
ventricular assist device (VAD), 282
ventricular shunt, 278
complications, 279
emergency care, 279
verbal communication, 27–28
vertigo, 58–59
vesicles, 178
virus infection, 171
vision, impaired, 28–29
aging and, 17, 18
communication in presence of, 28
visual impairment, 149
vital capacity/breathing capacity,
age-related changes, 20, 52, 53

vitamin C, 151, 151*t*
vitamin D, 151, 151*t*
vitamin K, 201
volume ventilators, 262
vomiting, 61–62

W

walker, 113
warfarin, 198, 201
warning systems, 244
We Can Do Better Conference,
246, 248*t*
weight gain, 173
Wernicke's aphasia, 32
wheezes, 122
working memory, 67

Y

youth, changes in physiology from, to old
age. *See* physiological changes,
age-related